Flow Controlled Ventilation Mode Through a Straw Size Tube

Nabil A. Shallik
Editor

Flow Controlled Ventilation Mode Through a Straw Size Tube

Springer

Editor
Nabil A. Shallik
Clinical Anaesthesiology Department
Weill Cornell Medical College in Qatar
Doha, Qatar

ISBN 978-3-031-77476-8 ISBN 978-3-031-77477-5 (eBook)
https://doi.org/10.1007/978-3-031-77477-5

This Springer imprint is published by the registered company Springer Nature Switzerland AG
The registered company address is: Gewerbestrasse 11, 6330 Cham, Switzerland

Preface

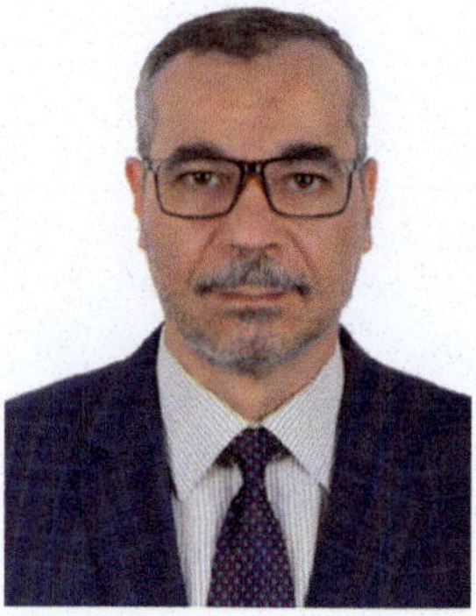

Breathing is the first act of life and the last. Our very life depends on it. (Joseph Pilates)

In the realm of medicine, artificial respiration and mechanical ventilation stand as monumental achievements. Among these innovations, the flow-controlled ventilation mode represents one of the most sophisticated developments in airway management. Since its inception, there has been a palpable need for a concise yet thorough clinical review book on flow-controlled ventilation and its clinical use; a comprehensive reference that is easy to read and can provide practical advice for both trainees and experienced practitioners alike.

With great enthusiasm, we present to you the realization of that vision in the form of this book, *Flow Controlled Ventilation Mode Through a Straw Size Tube*. It is designed to be more than a mere manual; it is a practical companion intended for use in the clinical environment. Emphasizing the clinical aspects of flow-controlled ventilation and the utilization of ultra-thin endotracheal tubes, it serves as an invaluable resource for anesthesia trainees, consultants, intensive care physicians, emergency physicians, ORL-HNS surgeons, maxillofacial surgeons, chest surgeons, anesthesia nurses, anesthesia technical staff, and pulmonologists alike.

While every effort has been made to ensure accuracy and reliability, readers are encouraged to notify us of any errors or discrepancies. It is important to note that this handbook is a supplement to, not a substitute for, professional judgment and consultation.

Doha, Qatar Nabil A. Shallik

Acknowledgments

We would like to extend our gratitude to our authors for their participation in writing this important book once again. Their clinical wisdom and commitment have been invaluable at every step of the journey.

A special thanks is extended to Mr. Abil Luez, who artistically captured all images and video clips of the book.

I am profoundly grateful to my sons and my daughter for their unwavering support throughout the creation of this book.

I would also like to thank Dr. Hanan Mawlana for her patience and constant support during the editing of this book.

We are immensely grateful to the Anesthesia Chairman (Dr. Mohammad Hilani), Deputy Chairman (Dr. Mashael Al Khelaifi), anesthesiologists, anesthesia technicians, and anesthesia technologists at Hamad Medical Corporation, Doha, Qatar, for their assistance and support.

We hope you find this work enjoyable and useful in your daily practice. Please read the disclaimer in the next chapter (Introduction).

Contents

Abbreviations

$\{(A\text{-}a)\ O_2\}$	Alveolar–arterial oxygen
3D	Three-dimensional
ΔEELV	Relative end-expiratory lung volume
ΔP	Alveolar driving pressure
ABG	Arterial blood gas
AC	Assist control
AC–PCV	Assist control–pressure control ventilation
AC–VC	Assist control–volume-controlled ventilation
AEC(s)	Airway exchange catheter(s)
AP	Anterior–posterior
APAP	Auto-titrating (adjustable) positive airway pressure
APRV	Airway pressure release ventilation
ASA	American Society of Anesthesiologists
ASV	Adaptive support ventilation
ATC	Automatic tube compensation
atm	Atmospheric pressure
BCV	Biphasic cuirass ventilation
BiLevel	Bilevel positive pressure
BiLevel PCV	Bilevel positive airway pressure
BMI	Body mass index
C	Compliance
C5	Cervical vertebra 5
CE marking	The CE marking (an acronym for the French "Conformite Europeenne") certifies that a product has met EU health, safety, and environmental requirements
CFI	Cross-field intubation
CICI	Cannot intubate, cannot intubate
CICO	Cannot intubate, cannot oxygenate
CICV	Cannot intubate, cannot ventilate
CINMA	Critical illness neuromuscular abnormalities
CmH_20	Centimeter water
CO_2	Carbon dioxide
COPD	Coronary obstructive pulmonary disease
CORE index	Compromise, oxygenation, respiration, effort index

CORP index	Compliance, oxygenation, rate, pressure index
COVID-19	Coronavirus disease 2019
CPAP	Continuous positive airway pressure
CSA	Central sleep apnea
CSV	Continuous spontaneous ventilation
CT	Computed tomography
CTA	Conventional tube adapter
CTM	The cricothyroid membrane
DAS Guidelines	Difficult Airway Society Guidelines
DLT	Double-lumen tube
DP	Driving pressure
E	Elastance
eFONA	Emergency front of neck access
EADi	Electrical activity of the diaphragm
ECLS	Extracorporeal life support
ECMO	Extracorporeal membrane oxygenation
EELV	End-expiratory lung volume
EEP	End-expiratory pressure
EIT	Electrical impedance tomography
El_{Th}	Global thoracic electrical impedance
ENT	Ear, nose, and throat
EPAP	Expiratory positive airway pressure
$ETCO_2$	End-tidal CO_2
ETT	Endotracheal tube
EVA	Expiratory ventilation assistance
EVLP	Ex vivo lung perfusion
F	Rate/frequency
FCaV	Flow-controlled automatic ventilator
FCmV	Flow-controlled manual ventilator
FCV	Flow-controlled ventilation/ventilator
FEES	Fiber-optic endoscopic evaluation of the swallowing
FIC	Frova intubating catheter
FIO_2	Inspired oxygen fraction
FLEX	FLow-controlled EXpiration
FONA	Front of neck access/front of neck airway
FRC	Functional residual capacity
GCS	Glasgow Coma Scale
GFRE	Gas flow reversing element
HFJV	High-frequency jet ventilation
HFNC	High-flow nasal cannula
HFNO	High-flow nasal oxygen
HLI	Heart lung index
HME	Heat and moisture exchanger filter
I	Current /flow
I:E	Inspiratory to expiratory ratio

IAP	Intra-abdominal pressure
ICs	Intubating catheters
ICU	Intensive care unit
ID	Internal diameter
IEQ	Inspiratory effect quotient
IMV	Intermittent mandatory ventilation
IPAP	Inspiratory positive airway pressure
IT	Intra-tracheal
I-time	Inspiratory time
LASER	Light amplification by stimulated emission of radiation
LED	Light-emitting diode
LFJV	Low-frequency jet ventilation
LMA	Laryngeal mask airway
MAD	Mucosal atomization device
MICU	Medical intensive care units
MLS	Micro-laryngoscopy surgery
MLT	Micro-laryngoscopy tube
mmHg	Millimeter mercury
MP	Mechanical power
MRI	Magnetic resonance imaging
MV	Mechanical ventilation
MV	Minute volume
NAVA	Neurally adjusted ventilatory assist
NEEP	Negative end-expiratory pressure
NPO	Nil per oral
OD	Outer diameter
OLV	One-lung-ventilation
PACU	Post-anesthesia care unit
Pair	Atmospheric pressure = pressure at the mouth
Palv	Pressure in the alveoli
PAV	Proportional assist ventilation
PC	Pressure control
PC-IMV	Intermittent mandatory ventilation
PC-PSV	Pressure control with pressure support
PC-SIMV	Synchronized intermittent mandatory ventilation
PC-VG	Pressure-controlled volume-guaranteed
PCO_2	Partial pressure of CO_2
PCV	Pressure-controlled ventilation
PCV-VG	Pressure-controlled ventilation volume-guaranteed mode
PEEP	Positive end-expiratory pressure
Pinsp	Inspiratory pressure
PIP	Peak inspiratory pressure
PITS	Post-iatrogenic post-intubation
P_{mean}	Mean pressure
Pmus	Expiratory muscle systems

PO_2	Partial pressure of O_2
POCUS	Point-of-care ultrasound
PP	Pause Pressure
Ppaw	Proximal airway pressure
Ppeak	Peak pressure
P_{plat}	Plateau pressure
PRVC	Pressure-regulated volume control
PS	Pressure support
PSV	Pressure support ventilation
PTTS	Post-tracheostomy tracheal stenosis
PV Loop	Pressure–volume Loop
PVR	Pulmonary vascular resistance
Q	The flow
R	Resistance of the air passages
RAAS	Richmond agitation sedation scale
RCT	Randomized clinical trial
RER	Respiratory exchange ratio
RS	Respiratory system
rs	Respiratory system
RSBI	Rapid shallow breathing index
SAD	Supraglottic airway device
SARS-CoV-2	Severe acute respiratory syndrome coronavirus 2
SAT	Spontaneous awakening trial
SAT	Spontaneous awakening test
SBT	Spontaneous breathing trial
SGAD	Supraglottic airway device
SGS	Subglottic stenosis
SICU	Surgical intensive care unit
SIMV	Synchronized intermittent mandatory ventilation
STRIVE-Hi	SponTaneous Respiration using Intra-VEnous Anesthesia and High-flow nasal oxygen
TCI	Target-controlled infusion
TIVA	Total intravenous anesthesia
TLM	Transoral LASER microsurgery
USG	Use of ultrasonography
V	Voltage; potential difference
VALI	Ventilator-associated lung injury
VAPS	Volume assured/guaranteed pressure support
VATS	Video-assisted thoracoscopic surgery
VC	Volume control
VC-PS	Volume control with pressure support
VC-SIMV	Synchronized intermittent mandatory ventilation
VCV	Volume-controlled ventilation
VE	Virtual endoscopy
VILI	Ventilator-induced lung injury

V-Q mismatch	Ventilation-perfusion mismatch
VS	Volume support
vs	Versus
VSV	Variable pressure support or volume support ventilation
ZEEP	Zero (or equal to atmospheric pressure) end-expiratory pressure

Introduction

Sahar Abida Mahadik and Nabil A. Shallik

1 Book Overview

Breathing is the first act of life and the last. Our very life depends on it (Joseph Pilates)

In the evolving landscape of respiratory care, the search for optimal ventilation strategies has been marked by important moments of innovation driven by challenging clinical circumstances. Our management is refined with the improved understanding of respiratory physiology, the development of highly intelligent devices and a drive for advancement. The advent of flow-controlled ventilation (FCV) represents one such paradigm shifts in respiratory therapy. As we embark on a comprehensive exploration of FCV in this textbook, we invite readers to delve into the intricate interplay between respiratory physics, mechanical ventilation strategies, and the clinical applications of FCV across diverse clinical scenarios.

As opposed to conventional ventilators which rely on active inspiration to deliver tidal volume and a passive expiration, flow-controlled ventilators employ active processes for both inspiration and expiration. This flow can be set to be low and constant, allowing gradual inspiration and expiration with more homogeneous distribution of air. It also mitigates the high pressure generated through airway

S. A. Mahadik
Anaesthesia, ICU and Perioperative Medicine Department, Hamad Medical Corporation, Doha, Qatar

N. A. Shallik (✉)
Anaesthesia, ICU and Perioperative Medicine Department, Hamad Medical Corporation, Doha, Qatar

Clinical Anaesthesiology Department, Weill Cornell Medical College in Qatar, Doha, Qatar

Clinical Anaesthesiology Department, College of Medicine Qatar University, Doha, Qatar

Anaesthesia and SICU Department, Tanta University, Tanta, Egypt
e-mail: nshallik@outlook.com

N. A. Shallik (ed.), *Flow Controlled Ventilation Mode Through a Straw Size Tube*, https://doi.org/10.1007/978-3-031-77477-5_1

stenosis or smaller diameter endotracheal tubes with conventional modes when achieving adequate tidal volumes. This evolution in ventilation provides the precise regulation of airflow to optimize patient outcomes and enabling practitioners to tailor ventilation strategies to the unique needs of each patient.

2 How to Navigate This Book?

Although you may explore this text as a journey from start to finish, we intend each chapter to also stand alone as a reference for review of the topic on its own. For example, if you wish to learn about the ultrathin tube or straw size tube, it would not be required to read any other chapter to understand the topic in totality. The textbook commences with a foundational understanding of respiratory physics, airflow dynamics, and physiology during FCV. Through a review of pressure-volume relationships, fluid mechanics and the theoretical basis for gas exchange, readers will gain insight into the fundamental principles that govern FCV and its impact on pulmonary function. Following this overview, the basics of ventilation and the traditional modes of ventilation are reviewed to build upon our existing understanding of the commonly used ventilation modes.

After building this foundation, we turn our attention to the specifications of non-traditional modes of ventilation, which provide a framework for us to understand FCV ventilators. You may find a particular focus on the only commercially available FCV ventilator, the "Evone®" ventilator, due to the lack of other examples and not as an endorsement of the product. By reviewing the design of the apparatus including the components, their functions and the array of features, readers will develop a comprehensive understanding of the framework behind this modern technology. Although exposure to the use of this ventilator in workshops and at the bedside is essential, the text can sow the seeds of understanding this novel device.

A key innovation in FCV technology that comes hand-in-hand with the ventilator is the ultrathin tube or straw size endotracheal tube, exemplified by the Tritube®. In subsequent chapters, we explore the utility of Tritube® in various clinical contexts, including its use in oral surgery and segmental tracheal resection. Through case-based discussions and procedural explanations, readers will gain practical insights into the integration of Tritube® and FCV techniques into their clinical practice.

Any experienced practitioner understands the significance a manual, hand-held method of ventilation provides in emergency situations when even the most high-tech devices are deemed faulty. Here, we introduce the flow-controlled manual ventilator (FCmV), exemplified frequently by the Ventrain®, merely because there is no alternative of its kind on the market. This ventilator represents another advancement in FCV technology, based off of the fundamentals of fluid mechanics, the Bernoulli's principle. By examining the uses of Ventrain® in diverse clinical scenarios, readers will appreciate its versatility and potential to optimize patient outcomes in critical care settings.

As we venture further into the realm of clinical practice, we explore the utility of FCV in laparoscopic abdominal surgeries, ICU settings, and pediatric care. This book aims to provide a comprehensive review of evidence-based research and clinical best practices through which readers can gain a deeper understanding of the role of FCV in enhancing surgical precision, optimizing respiratory support, and improving patient safety and clinical outcomes.

A vital step in any patient's journey to recovery is the liberation from mechanical ventilation. The assessment of readiness, weaning (in a stepwise fashion), and the independence of a patient's own respiratory function constitute a set of unique challenges in critical care. In this chapter, we examine the science and art of ventilation liberation, exploring strategies for optimizing weaning protocols, minimizing complications, and promoting successful extubation in patients undergoing FCV and other modes of mechanical ventilations.

Finally, we reflect on the past, present, and future of FCV, tracing its evolution from its inception to its current state, envisioning its potential to shape the future of respiratory care. Through a synthesis of historical perspective, technological innovation, and clinical insight, readers will gain a holistic understanding of the transformative impact of FCV on the practice of respiratory medicine.

In each chapter of this textbook, we aim to provide readers with a comprehensive resource that integrates theoretical knowledge with practical application. Hence, we strongly advise readers to analyze the images, diagrams, photos, and videos to accompany the descriptions. After all, "a picture is worth a thousand words," and a complex idea can be conveyed with a single image. It is our hope that this textbook will serve as a guide for clinicians, researchers, and educators alike as we navigate the complexities of FCV and strive toward excellence in respiratory care.

This book serves as a useful resource rather than merely being pursued and forgotten on a bookshelf. The team behind this creation have diligently aligned the techniques and procedures outlined in this text with the latest recommendations and practices at the time of its publication. Nevertheless, given the dynamic evolution of respiratory care, continual updates are inevitable. *We conclude* our work by emphasizing that sharing knowledge stands as one of humanity's greatest acts; as Lao Tzu once said 'give a man a fish and you feed him for a day. Teach him how to fish and you feed him for a lifetime'.

Disclaimer *This book aims to summarize the published materials and some clinical pearls. Although care has been taken to ensure information is correct, this is not guaranteed, and no responsibility is accepted for clinical decisions based on material within this book. Clinicians are advised to check the primary literature and their clinical sense. The opinions stated within this book do not constitute clinical advice. They are opinions, not facts, and others may take a different view of our interpretations of these trials. Please refer to the appropriate clinical guideline issued by the relevant society or scientific body for the management of any specific condition.*

Here we introduce the flow-controlled manual ventilator (FCmV), exemplified frequently by the Ventrain®, merely because there is no alternative of its kind on the market and also you may find a particular focus on the only commercially available FCV ventilator, the "Evone®" ventilator, moreover using of (Tritube®) instead of ultrathin or straw sized ETT nomenclature due to the lack of other examples and not as commercial endorsement of the products.

Conventional Mechanical Ventilation—I
History, Mechanics, and Indications

Muhammad Shakeel Riaz, Mohammed Shafee Shaikh,
Wael Khalaf, Abdul Gafoor Tharayil, Arshad Chanda,
and Siddhartha Banerjee

Breathing is the first act of life and the last. Our very life depends on it. (Joseph Pilates)

1 Introduction

Artificial breathing or mechanical ventilation is one of the most sophisticated developments in modern medicine. Mechanical ventilation is not merely filling the lungs with air but an intricate interplay of pressure, volume, flow and time to achieve an optimum gas exchange to maintain homeostasis and thus, sustain life.

2 Brief History of Mechanical Ventilation

History is the link of the future. If you know the history, you will know the future. (Asep Kambali)

Mechanical ventilation started in 1700s with the discovery of oxygen followed by an understanding of importance of respiration in the delivery of oxygen. However, traces of ventilatory assistance can be found in ancient times. The father of modern medicine, Hippocrates (460–370 BCE), had described tracheal intubation as a method to artificially ventilate the lungs. Claudius Galen (129–199 CE), the Greek physician and surgeon, has described in one of his experiments, in his landmark text "On the parts of the human body" inflating the lungs of various dead animals with

M. S. Riaz (✉) · M. S. Shaikh · W. Khalaf · A. G. Tharayil · A. Chanda · S. Banerjee
Surgical ICU, Department of Anesthesia, ICU and Perioperative Medicine, Hamad Medical Corporation, Doha, Qatar
e-mail: MRiaz2@hamad.qa; MShaikh10@hamad.qa; WKhalaf1@hamad.qa; atharayil@hamad.qa; achanda@hamad.qa; SBanerjee1@hamad.qa

N. A. Shallik (ed.), *Flow Controlled Ventilation Mode Through a Straw Size Tube*, https://doi.org/10.1007/978-3-031-77477-5_2

bellows. He described the trachea as "a rough artery", a conduit for the passage of air, to and from the lungs.

However, it took a long time for a description of the positive pressure ventilation to appear in the medical texts when in 1543 a medical researcher, Andreas Vesalius, published in his anatomy text, the first reference to the positive pressure ventilation; "But that life may be restored to the animal, an opening must be attempted in the trunk of the trachea, into which a tube of reed or cane should be put; you will then blow into this, so that the lung may rise again and take air". Paracelsus, in 1493 and later in 1541, experimented with resuscitating patients by placing a tube in the mouth and blowing air to the lungs with bellows. In 1667, Robert Hooke, used positive pressure for continuous supply of oxygen to keep a dog alive. The first case of mouth-to-mouth breathing was reported by William Tossach in 1774. The first non-invasive ventilator, a bag-and-mask manual ventilator, was described by Chassier. The now common term 'barotrauma" was first demonstrated by Leroy, in 1827, when he showed that positive pressure ventilation could be hazardous and overinflation of lungs could lead to lung damage.

"The tank ventilator" was the first negative pressure full body ventilator. Described by the Scottish physician John Dalziel in 1838 in which the patient was required to maintain a sitting position in an airtight box while the air was manually pumped in and out of the box.

Later, the first "iron lung" was introduced by the Frenchman, Dr. Woillez, in 1876, who called it a Spirophore. In 1910, a non-invasive mechanical ventilator was developed, named "rhythmic inflation apparatus" by Green and Janeway. It could easily be referenced to present CPAP helmets as in "rhythmic inflation apparatus", patient's head was placed into the apparatus with a secure seal around the neck and positive pressure applied to patient's head.

Dräger, designed a positive pressure ventilator in 1911, known as "Pulmotor". It used a naso-buccal mask to deliver a mixture of compressed air or oxygen with ambient air to the patient. The cylinder of oxygen or compressed air was used as a source of energy for the pulmotor functioning. In 1928, Dr. Phillip Drinker (1894–1972) and Dr. Louis Shaw (1886–1940) at Harvard University developed the first widely used negative pressure respiration apparatus. This generated a pressure down to 60 cm of H_2O at a rate between 10 and 40 breaths per minute. The "iron lung" was later improved and patented by Dr. Emerson in 1931. The iron lungs were used for polio patients with respiratory insufficiency during the first half of the twentieth century.

In July 1952, a Polio outbreak occurred in Copenhagen after a super spreader event a year earlier (an international conference on Polio which was attended by physicians and patients). Bjørn Ibsen, an anaesthetist, used the combination of performing a tracheostomy and manual ventilation as respiratory support for polio patients. This decreased the mortality from more than 80% down to 30%. This also demonstrated that positive pressure ventilation was safe and effective when used even longer periods of time.

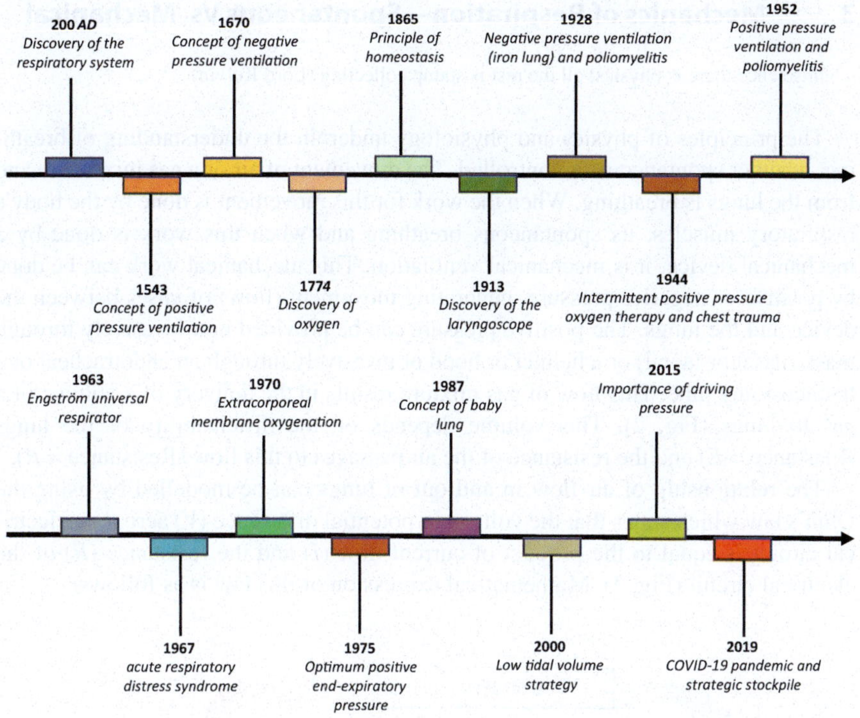

Fig. 1 The scientific discoveries and inventions leading to the modern practices of mechanical ventilation

The development of blood gas measurements using the CO_2 (Severinghaus) and O_2 (Clarks) electrodes helped in the refinement of mechanical ventilation goals. Positive pressure ventilation became a widely practised mechanical ventilation approach while the negative pressure approach diminished due to various reasons.

Initial positive pressure ventilation devices were only volume controlled with no alarms, monitors, or trigger sensitivities for spontaneous breathing by patients. With the engineering advancements, in second generation positive pressure ventilators, triggering by the patient was possible and in addition pressure control and pressure support modes were introduced to clinical practice. The next generation of ventilators had microprocessors which made the flow triggering possible as well as the monitoring of gas delivery and other ventilator parameters. The modern ventilators come with a plethora of advanced modes and a wide array of monitoring parameters to individualise the mechanical ventilation for each patient according to their disease and demographics. This scientific culmination of complexity and safety makes the practice of mechanical ventilation, for present day physicians, a clinical art (Fig. 1).

3 Mechanics of Respiration—Spontaneous Vs. Mechanical

In science there is physics; all the rest is stamp collecting (Lord Kelvin)

The principles of physics and physiology underpin the understanding of breathing, whether spontaneous or controlled. The movement of air or a gas mixture to and from the lungs is breathing. When the work for this movement is done by the body's respiratory muscles, its spontaneous breathing and when this work is done by a mechanical device, it is mechanical ventilation. This mechanical work can be done by positive or negative pressure, generating movement (flow) of gases between the device and the lungs. The positive pressure can be provided non-invasively through mask (nasal or facial) or a helmet or hood or invasively through an endotracheal or a tracheostomy tube. This flow of gas mixture results in the delivery of a volume of a gas to lungs (Fig. 2). This volume depends on the distensibility of the lungs (Elastance = E) and the resistance of the air passages to this flow (Resistance = R).

The relationship of air flow in and out of lungs can be modelled by using the Ohm's law which states that the voltage or potential difference (V) across an electrical circuit is equal to the product of current flow (I) and the resistance (R) of the electrical circuit (Fig. 3). Mathematical expression of this law is as follows:

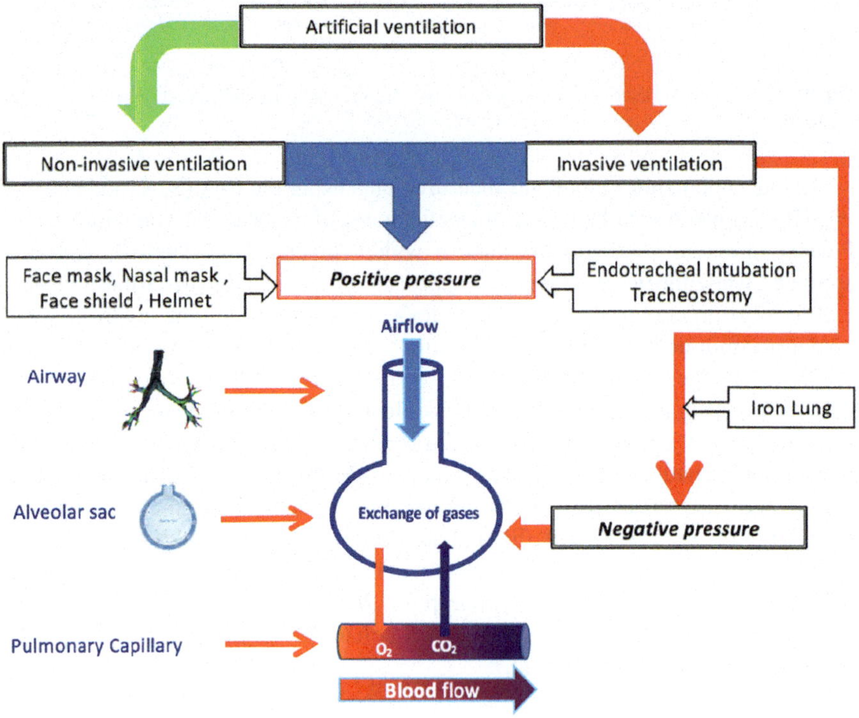

Fig. 2 Mechanical ventilation

Fig. 3 Ohm's law

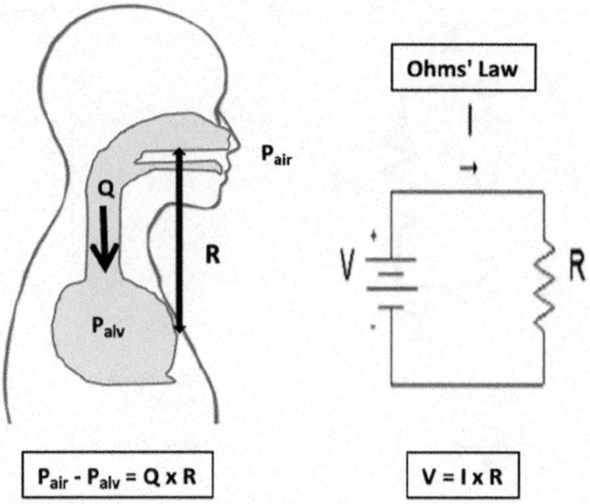

$$V = I \times R \text{ or } I = V / R \text{ or } R = V / I$$

In the context of respiratory mechanics, the equivalent of voltage or potential difference is the pressure difference between the proximal and the distal end of the respiratory circuit. The flow (Q) of air is equivalent to the current flow (I), while the resistance of the air passages (R) is equivalent to the resistance of the electrical circuit (R) (Fig. 4a).

In the case of spontaneous breathing (Fig. 4b), the proximal pressure is at the mouth and equal to the atmospheric pressure (Pair) while the distal pressure is the pressure in the alveoli (Palv). During spontaneous natural ventilation, the lung volume increases due to the work of respiratory muscles, i.e., contraction of diaphragm and other respiratory muscles during inspiration. This increases the lung volume which leads to the drop of pressure in the alveoli (Palv) below the proximal pressure at the mouth (Pair). This pressure difference (Pair—Palv) leads to the flow of air into the lungs as flow becomes a positive value. Using Ohm's principle, the equation for flow would be as following:

$$Q = \frac{\text{Pair} - \text{Palv}}{R}$$

During positive pressure ventilation (Fig. 4c), i.e., invasive mechanical ventilation using endotracheal tube (ETT) or tracheostomy tube (TT), the proximal pressure is at the proximal end of the ETT or TT (the end of the tube closer to airway is the proximal end and the end farther away from the airway and closer to the ventilator is the distal end of the tube). This proximal airway pressure is commonly labelled as peak airway pressure (Paw) or peak inspiratory pressure (PIP). The distal pressure is the pressure in the alveoli (Palv) and this could be zero, if no positive end expiratory pressure (PEEP) is used or positive and equal to the PEEP. This pressure difference (Paw—PEEP) leads to the flow of gas into the lungs as flow is a positive value. However, the work to generate this flow is done by the mechanical ventilator

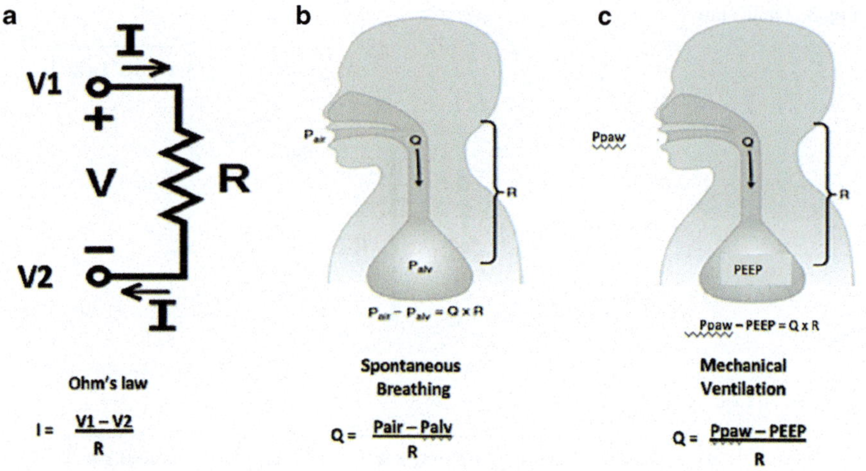

Fig. 4 Application of Ohm's law for modelling respiratory mechanics. $I = Q$; $V = P$; $R = R$; Pair = Pressure at mouth; Palv = Pressure at alveoli; Ppaw = Proximal airway pressure; PEEP = Positive end expiratory pressure

and is independent of the respiratory muscles activity which may be inactive due to sedation or paralysis during controlled mechanical ventilation. The Ohm's equation for flow may be written as following:

$$Q = \frac{\text{Paw} - \text{PEEP}}{R}$$

In case of non-invasive positive pressure ventilation, the proximal pressure is at the mouth through the mask or helmet or supraglottic airway device and is higher (positive) than the atmospheric pressure. This is set as CPAP (continuous positive airway pressure) or IPAP (Inspiratory positive airway pressure) in case of BiPAP. The distal pressure, i.e., alveolar pressure is always positive and work for the movement of air into the lungs is mainly done by the patient's respiratory muscles activity.

The movement of gas out of the lungs, i.e., expiratory flow or expiration, is mostly passive both in spontaneous as well as mechanical ventilation. However, some advanced modes of mechanical ventilation may provide some active expiration like flow controlled ventilation (FCV).

Conventionally, the inspiratory flow or inspiration is considered as positive, and the expiratory flow or expiration is considered a negative. This is demonstrated in the flow-time scalars of the ventilators with waveform displays.

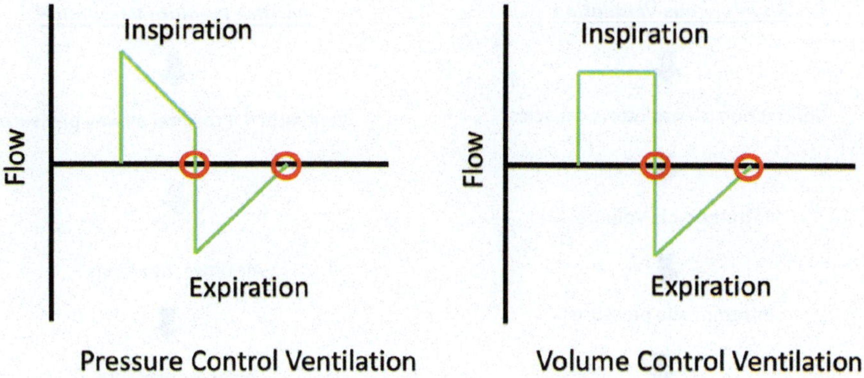

Fig. 5 Flow-time waveforms with inspiratory and expiratory pauses

It is also important to note from the flow-time waveform that when proximal airway pressure (Pair or Ppaw) and the distal alveolar pressure (Palv or PEEP) become equal, the flow becomes zero, i.e., there is no flow of gas in either direction. This occurs normally at the end of both inspiration and expiration, i.e., twice in each breath cycle. These points are shown as red circles in the (Fig. 5) and are known as inspiratory and expiratory pauses, respectively. Modern ventilators have these pauses as functional capabilities to measure certain ventilatory parameters when the flow is paused for few seconds at the end of inspiration or at the end of expiration. The inspiratory pause function is used to measure plateau pressure (Pplat) which is the pressure inside the lungs when there is no flow. The plateau pressure provides valuable information about the lung compliance as well as airway resistance. The expiratory pause function is used to measure the intrinsic PEEP or auto-PEEP also known as dynamic hyperinflation. It can also be used to evaluate the expiratory flow limitations in obstructive airway disease patients.

The sequence of events leading to flow of gases into the lungs is also different during spontaneous and mechanical ventilation and is summarised in Fig. 6.

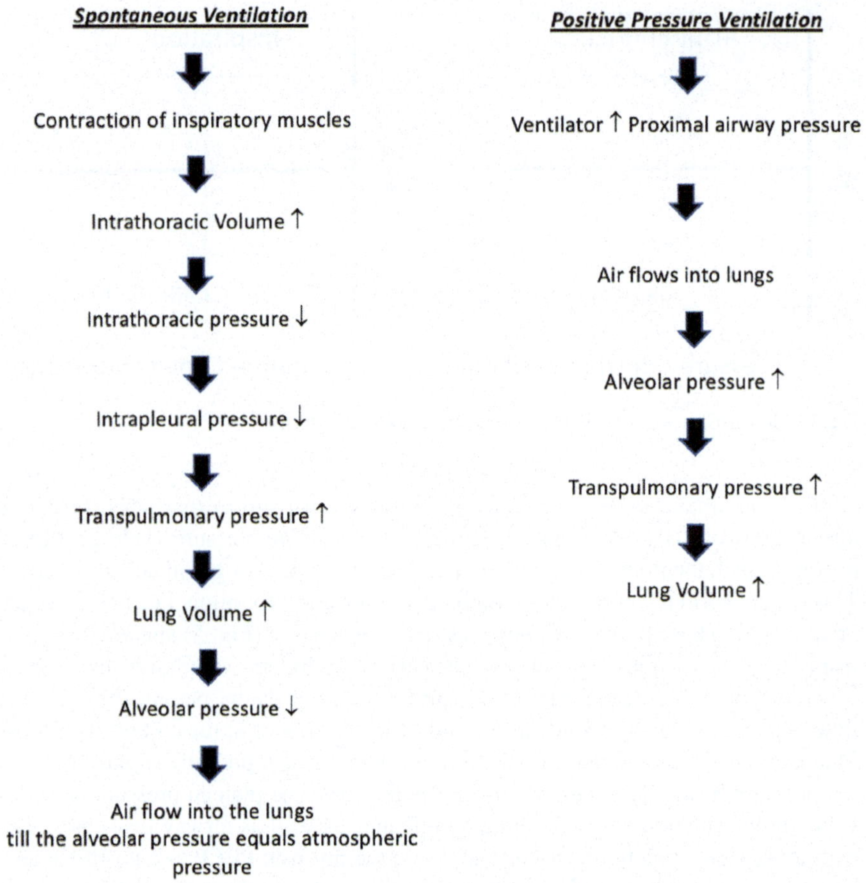

Fig. 6 Sequence of events during spontaneous vs. mechanical ventilation

4 Indications of Mechanical Ventilation

> Do not be afraid to take a big step if one is indicated. You cannot cross a chasm in two small jumps. (David Llyod George)

Invasive mechanical ventilation is a lifesaving and life sustaining intervention and remains an absolute indication for admission to critical care units. It is a big clinical step in the treatment course of any patient. Timing of initiation of mechanical ventilation and the choice of an appropriate ventilation mode is a crucial clinical decision. However, there is little evidence to help clinicians with this decision since patients are critically ill when this decision must be made which transfers the onus of this decision to their clinical judgement. An understanding of the pathophysiology of the processes leading to the need for mechanical ventilation may improve clinical judgement on when and how to initiate the mechanical ventilation.

Mechanical ventilation is usually indicated when patient is unable to ventilate the lungs to such an extent that the gas exchange across the alveolo-capillary membrane is deranged and cellular function is compromised. There are few fundamental processes that may lead to this pathological state, e.g., inability of patient to maintain or protect the airway, demand–capacity imbalance of respiratory muscles, compromised alveolar patency or abnormal alveolor-capillary membrane interface, and failure of ventilatory control.

The main purpose of invasive mechanical ventilation is to maintain normal gas exchange, i.e., to maintain normal O_2 and CO_2 tensions in the blood and to offload the respiratory muscles by taking over the work of breathing, either partially or completely. This is achieved through an artificial airway as a bridge between patient and ventilator which provides oxygen rich positive pressure breaths to maintain minute ventilation appropriate to the patient's requirements. So, the mechanical ventilation may be indicated.

- When there is a need for an artificial airway to maintain or protect the airway, i.e., airway patency and/or protection.
- When there is a need to offload tiring or impaired respiratory muscles which are not able to maintain the minute ventilation, i.e., demand–capacity imbalance.
- When there is a need to maintain the alveolar patency due to an inflamed alveolo-capillary membrane or alveolar units are flooded with mucous, fluid or blood leading to compromised gas exchange, i.e., abnormal alveolo-capillary interface.
- When there is a need to maintain an adequate minute ventilation (number and volume of breaths) in patients who have lost the ability to self-regulate this, i.e., control failure.

These physiological processes are interlinked and interdependent. If an abnormality in one is not treated by timely initiation of mechanical ventilation, it may lead to compromise in the other processes, e.g., a compromised airway may lead to respiratory muscle fatigue due to increased work of breathing to maintain the minute ventilation. The muscle fatigue can result in abnormal CO_2 and O_2 tensions in the blood which in turn can cause obtundation of the respiratory control centre. This chain of events can occur in the reverse order as well and due to this interdependence of these physiological processes the categorisation of any indications for mechanical ventilation is merely arbitrary.

Leading on from the above description, the main indications for invasive mechanical ventilation can be grouped as follows:

4.1 Airway Patency/Protection

- Proximal airway obstruction, e.g., angioedema, facial injury, facial burns, smoke inhalation, and stridor.
- Distal airway obstruction, e.g., acute severe asthma, acute exacerbation of COPD.

- Airway protection may be indicated when conscious level is decreased due to drugs, toxins, CNS pathology, e.g., cerebrovascular accidents.
- Airway protection may be indicated in case of dynamic airway, e.g., from trauma or due to oropharyngeal infections.

Clinically, a compromised airway can manifest as high work of breathing, inadequate ventilation, stridor, poor or weak cough needing frequent suctioning, aspiration, etc. In these instances, low inspiratory pressure ventilation is an appropriate strategy if the indication for mechanical ventilation is airway compromise.

4.2 Demand–Capacity Imbalance

The demand on respiratory muscles is due to the need to maintain adequate minute ventilation to meet the metabolic demands (O_2 consumption and CO_2 production) which drive the minute ventilation. The elastance and compliance as well as the resistance properties of the lung also contribute to the demand load on respiratory muscles. The capacity of the respiratory system is the strength and endurance of the respiratory muscles which in turn depends on patient's general state of health and physiological reserves. It may be affected by inflammation, nutrition, electrolyte imbalance etc. This imbalance is usually seen in conditions like sepsis and septic shock, but it can happen in all types of shocks, i.e., hypovolemic, hypoxic, cardiogenic. The increased metabolic demand is manifested as severe metabolic acidosis in these conditions. This demand–capacity balance is particularly delicate in chronic lung disease patients as the chronically high demand leads to poor functional capacity of respiratory muscles. Minimal increase in demand or decrease in capacity in these patients due to any trigger will lead to exacerbation of their lung condition and a requirement for mechanical ventilation (Fig. 7).

Clinically, excessive demand or loading of respiratory muscles is associated with sympathetic overdrive resulting in the use of accessory muscles of respiration, sweating, abdominal breathing, inability to speak full sentences, etc. Mechanical ventilation is focussed on offloading the respiratory muscles by taking over the work of breathing through positive pressure ventilation. However, an assist control mode, rather than a full control mode, with patient triggering as per patient comfort could be a better strategy to avoid atrophy of respiratory muscles.

4.3 Impaired Alveolo-Capillary Membrane

Impaired gas exchange at the level alveolo-capillary membrane leads to ventilation-perfusion VQ mismatch. This could be on due to defects on the alveolar side of the interface like pneumonia, pulmonary oedema, acute respiratory distress syndrome etc. or on the vascular side leading to ventilation-perfusion (VQ) mismatch, e.g., due to massive pulmonary embolism, air, or fat embolism. The defect could also be

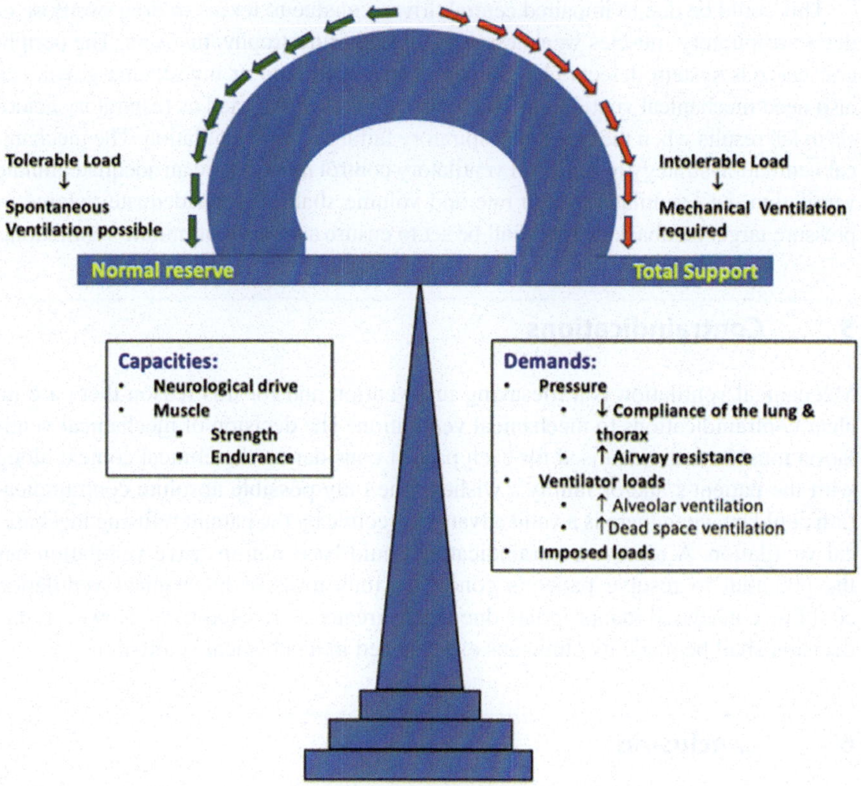

Fig. 7 Demand–capacity balance

in the membrane itself, e.g., due to pulmonary fibrosis. These defects are usually manifested as hypoxemic (Type I) respiratory failure.

Clinical signs of inadequate oxygen delivery could be altered mental status, arrythmias, other organ dysfunctions like acute kidney injury or liver injury, etc. Judicious use of PEEP is an important consideration when initiating mechanical ventilation due to impaired alveolo-capillary membrane.

4.4 Respiratory Control Impairment

The respiratory system control centre is in the medulla oblongata in the brain stem. This centre receives input from mechanoreceptors in lungs and chest wall and central and peripheral chemoreceptors which sense pH, pCO_2, and pO_2. The cortical signals to this centre regulate the respiratory centre response to voluntary activities. Although, some central nervous system conditions may lead to hyperventilation, the respiratory control impairment usually leads to hypoventilation and hypercapnic (type II) respiratory failure.

This could be due to impaired central drive, e.g., due to toxins or drug overdose or due to respiratory muscles weakness, e.g., muscular dystrophy, myositis. The peripheral nervous system defects like Guillain-Barré syndrome or myasthenia gravis can also need mechanical ventilation. The hypercapnia is manifested as respiratory acidosis in lab results when the cause of respiratory failure is hypoventilation. The mechanical ventilation strategy in impaired ventilatory control must ensure an adequate minute ventilation, i.e., ventilator breath rate and volume shall be set. Adequate volume or pressure target feedback alarms shall be set to ensure adequacy of minute ventilation.

5 Contraindications

Mechanical ventilation is a lifesaving intervention and for this reason there are no clear contraindications to mechanical ventilation. The decision of mechanical ventilation must be individualised for each patient considering the clinical context along with the patient's and/or family's wishes. The only possible absolute contraindication could be when there is a valid advance directive by the patient refusing mechanical ventilation. A relative contraindication could be if non-invasive ventilation has the potential to resolve patient's condition, thus invasive mechanical ventilation could be considered inappropriate due to the greater associated risks. However, this decision shall be made by clinicians experienced in mechanical ventilation.

6 Conclusion

In conclusion, this chapter offers an outline of major milestones in the history of mechanical ventilation from ancient times to modern microprocessors-based mechanical ventilators. This historical outline is followed by a simple application of Ohm's law to understand the basic mechanics of respiration. The three variables of Ohm's law (V, I, and R) can easily be translated into the fundamental variables of respiratory mechanics i.e., pressure, flow, volume, and resistance. This understanding of mechanics lays the ground for understanding the pathophysiological perspective of indications of mechanical ventilation in the next section. The indications for mechanical ventilation are broadly divided into airway management, demand–capacity imbalance, gas exchange membrane integrity, and nervous system control impairment.

Bibliography

1. Hidalgo J, et al., editors. Personalized mechanical ventilation. Cham: Springer; 2022. https://doi.org/10.1007/978-3-031-14138-6_2.
2. Brochard LJ. Mechanical ventilation: negative to positive and back again. Crit Care Clin. 2023;39:437–49. https://doi.org/10.1016/j.ccc.2022.12.002.
3. Bellani G, editor. Mechanical ventilation from pathophysiology to clinical evidence; 2022. https://doi.org/10.1007/978-3-030-93401-9_2.

4. H. Poor, Basics of mechanical ventilation, 2018. https://doi.org/10.1007/978-3-319-89981-7_1.
5. MacIntyre NR. Indications for mechanical ventilation. In: Webb A, editor. Oxford textbook of critical care, Oxford textbook. 2nd ed. Oxford: Oxford Academic; 2016; online edn. https://doi.org/10.1093/med/9780199600830.003.0091.
6. Hickey SM, Giwa AO. Mechanical ventilation. [Updated 2023 Jan 26]. In: StatPearls [Internet]. Treasure Island: StatPearls Publishing; 2024. Available from: https://www.ncbi.nlm.nih.gov/books/NBK539742/
7. Mora Carpio AL, Mora JI. Ventilator management. [Updated 2023 Mar 27]. In: StatPearls [Internet]. Treasure Island: StatPearls Publishing; 2024. Available from: https://www.ncbi.nlm.nih.gov/books/NBK448186/
8. Chatburn RL, El-Khatib M, Mireles-Cabodevila E. A taxonomy for mechanical ventilation: 10 fundamental maxims. Respirat Care. 2014;59(11):1747–63. https://doi.org/10.4187/respcare.03057.
9. Poor H. Phase variables. In: Basics of mechanical ventilation. Cham: Springer; 2018. p. 11–27. https://doi.org/10.1007/978-3-319-89981-7_2.
10. Hasan A. Understanding mechanical ventilation: a practical handbook. London: Springer; 2010.
11. Hasan A. Understanding mechanical ventilation. London: Springer; 2010. https://doi.org/10.1007/978-1-84882-869-8_4.
12. Bellani G, editor. Mechanical ventilation from pathophysiology to clinical evidence. Cham: Springer; 2022. https://doi.org/10.1007/978-3-030-93401-9_4.
13. Poor H. Basics of mechanical ventilation. Cham: Springer. https://doi.org/10.1007/978-3-319-89981-7_2.
14. Ward J, Noel C. Basic modes of mechanical ventilation. Emerg Med Clin N Am. 2022;40:473–88. https://doi.org/10.1016/j.emc.2022.05.003.

Conventional Mechanical Ventilation—II
Nomenclature and Basic Modes

Muhammad Shakeel Riaz, Mohammed Shafee Shaikh, Wael Khalaf, Abdul Gafoor Tharayil, Arshad Chanda, and Siddhartha Banerjee

What's in a name? That which we call a rose by any other name would smell just as sweet. (William Shakespeare)

1 Introduction

The terminology used in the field of mechanical ventilation is extensive and often perplexing. The knowledge of basic nomenclature of mechanical ventilation is fundamental in developing a sound understanding of various modes of mechanical ventilation. The basis of any mode of mechanical ventilation remains the interplay of key fundamental variable of respiratory mechanics, i.e., pressure, volume, and flow.

2 Nomenclature of Mechanical Ventilation Modes

What Americans call cross-ventilation, the English call draughts. (Hermione Gingold)

2.1 A Breath

A breath can be described as a single iteration of both inhalation (positive flow) and exhalation (negative flow), as outlined by the flow-time curve.

M. S. Riaz (✉) · M. S. Shaikh · W. Khalaf · A. G. Tharayil · A. Chanda · S. Banerjee
Surgical ICU, Department of Anesthesia, ICU and Perioperative Medicine, Hamad Medical Corporation, Doha, Qatar
e-mail: MRiaz2@hamad.qa; MShaikh10@hamad.qa; WKhalaf1@hamad.qa; atharayil@hamad.qa; achanda@hamad.qa; SBanerjee1@hamad.qa

N. A. Shallik (ed.), *Flow Controlled Ventilation Mode Through a Straw Size Tube*, https://doi.org/10.1007/978-3-031-77477-5_3

2.2 Anatomy of a Mechanical Breath

Every mechanical ventilation breath is an event with four phase variables which defines and determines the nature and structure of this breath. These variables are related to following processes:

1. How the inspiration is initiated—*Trigger*.
2. How the flow is delivered during inspiration—*Target*.
3. How the inspiration is ended—*Cycling*.
4. How the proximal airway pressure behaves during expiration—*Baseline*.

Figure 1 shows a schematic representation of these phase variables.

1. *How the inspiration is initiated —Trigger*

   Inspiration can be initiated (triggered) either by the ventilator or by the patient.

   Ventilator triggering is also called *time triggering* as the ventilator initiates a breath after a set amount of time has elapsed from the beginning of the previous breath. This "time" is most commonly a factor of the set rate on the ventilator, e.g., if the ventilator rate is set to 15 breaths per minute, then each breath cycle would be of 4 seconds duration and ventilator will trigger a breath at the start of every fifth second. A time-triggered breath is a control breath as it is triggered by the ventilator.

   Patient triggering occurs when the ventilator delivers a breath due to a pressure drop or a baseline flow change in the ventilatory circuit due to patient's effort. With patient's inspiratory effort, the pressure in the circuit drops as described in the mechanics of respiration. This drop in pressure is sensed by the ventilator and a breath is delivered to the patient if the drop is more than the set pressure on the ventilator for triggering a breath. This is called *pressure triggering*. The other type of patient triggering is due to change in bias flow. The bias flow is the continuous baseline flow of gas that is delivered to the patient circuit during both inspiration and expiration. This flow maintains a baseline pressure within the circuit. With patient's inspiratory effort, some of this flow from the inspiratory limb will enter the patient. This will decrease the flow in the expira-

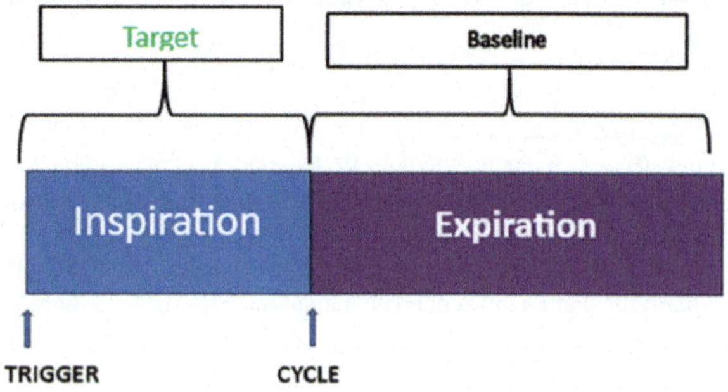

Fig. 1 Phase variables in a mechanical breath

tory limb of the ventilatory circuit below baseline flow. The ventilator will deliver a breath if this change in flow is more than the set flow on the ventilator for triggering a breath. This is called *flow triggering.* These pressure or flow triggered breaths are *assisted breaths* as ventilator assists patient's efforts of initiating a breath.

Both patient trigger and ventilator trigger can be combined in a hybrid manner and the breaths delivered like this are called *Assist-Control* breaths. In this modality, if the ventilator's time trigger goes by without the patient initiating a breath, the ventilator will start a "control" breath. However, if the patient triggers the ventilator by means of the pressure or flow trigger before the time trigger duration elapses, the ventilator will initiate an "assist" breath, as per the preset parameters and the time trigger timer will be reset. There is no difference between the control and assist breaths in terms of the volume, flow or pressure generated. Figure 2 depicts the characteristics of assisted vs. controlled breath.

2. *How the flow is delivered during inspiration —Target (limit)*

The target variable is the one which determines how the flow is delivered during the inspiration. This is also called "control" or "limit" which is a source of confusion when used interchangeably. The target variable could be either pressure or flow. Although volume or tidal volume may be mistaken as a target variable but technically volume could not be target variable as it is derived variable of flow. Volume delivered in per unit time is defined as the flow and merely setting a volume does not describe how the inspiration would be delivered, i.e., at a high flow rate (fast) or a low flow rate (slow). Hence, flow, not the volume, is a target variable.

The flow and pressure are interrelated and work in tandem in the context of target variables of mechanical breath. The set target variable is the independent variable and the other becomes the dependent variable and their relationship is defined by the Ohm's law as described earlier in mechanics of respiration and explained below.

When target variable is set as flow, the ventilator delivers this flow independent of any other variables. However, the pressure (proximal airway pressure) is a dependent variable and depends on the resistance and the distal airway pressure. The pattern of flow may also be selected as constant flow in which the

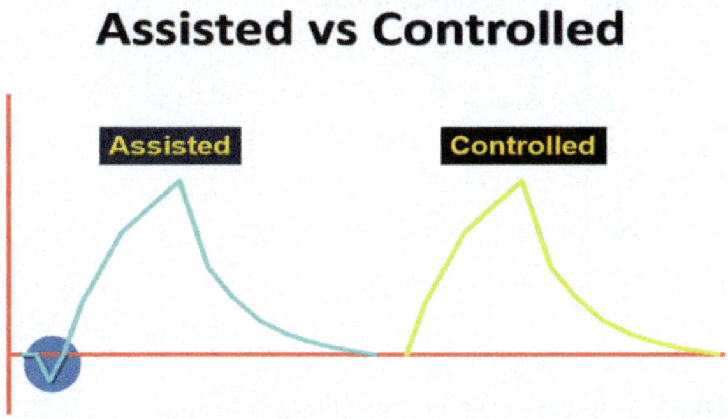

Fig. 2 Assisted vs. controlled breaths in assist-control

inspiratory flow rises quickly to the set rate and is maintained throughout the inspiration. This is also called square wave or rectangle wave flow. The other pattern of flow is decelerating flow in which the flow is highest at the beginning of inspiration and decreases to baseline flow by the end of inspiration. This is also called ramp flow (Fig. 3).

When target variable is set as pressure, the proximal airway pressure becomes the independent variable. The flow now is a dependent variable and changes with the resistance and the distal pressure. The flow waveform in pressure target is always a ramp waveform as the flow quickly increases at the beginning of respiration to achieve the set target pressure. The flow decreases as the difference between the proximal and distal pressure decrease with rise of alveolar pressure as the inspiratory phase proceeds. This results in a ramp waveform (Fig. 3).

The target variables (flow or pressure) are the fundamental variables in defining the basic modes of ventilation as volume or pressure modes.

3. *How the inspiration is ended—Cycling*

The "cycling" in the mechanical ventilation terminology refers to the termination of Inspiration. The mostly used three cycling variables are volume, time, and flow, i.e., a breath can be volume-cycled, time-cycled, or flow-cycled. In volume-cycled breaths, inspiration ends when a set volume is delivered, in time-cycled breaths, inspiration ends when a set inspiratory time has elapsed and in flow-cycled breaths, inspiration ends when the flow has decreased to a set percentage of the flow. In pressure-targeted modes (PCV) inspiration ends when inspiratory time elapses which is determined by the respiratory rate and I:E ratio. In volume-controlled ventilation (*VCV*), cycling occurs when the set tidal volume is delivered. In pressure support mode (*PSV*), cycling occurs when a preset proportion of flow rate is reached from the initial flow rate. Pressure cycling is not common but employed as a safety mechanism in VCV if the pressure exceeds the safety limit.

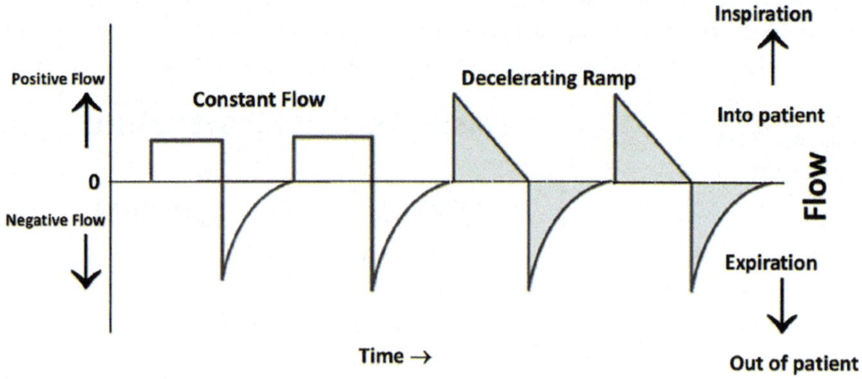

Fig. 3 Constant and decelerating flow waveforms

Table 1 Variables defining common ventilator modes

Mode	Trigger	Control	Cycling
Volume control	Time or patient initiated (pressure or flow)	Flow	Volume
Pressure control	Time or patient initiated	Pressure	Time
Pressure support	Patient initiated	Pressure	Flow

4. *How the proximal airway pressure behaves during expiration—Baseline.*
   The baseline variable refers to the proximal airway pressure during the expiratory phase of breath cycle. This could be zero, i.e., equal to atmospheric pressure and called as ZEEP.
   The baseline pressure can also be set above the atmospheric pressure, i.e., a positive value above zero and is called as positive end expiratory pressure (PEEP). PEEP is the most common baseline variable in the modern mechanical ventilatory practices.
   The phase variables of a mechanical breath can be used to define a basic mode of mechanical ventilation. The trigger variable would define if a mode were control mode (time-triggered) or an assist mode (pressure or flow triggered) or an assist-control mode (hybrid triggering). The target (control or limit) variable would define if a mode were volume control (flow) mode or a pressure-control mode. The cycling variable would define if a mode were volume-cycled (volume control mode) or a time-cycled (pressure control mode) or a flow-cycled mode (pressure support mode). This is summarized in Table 1.

2.3 Anatomy of a Mode of Mechanical Ventilation

A mode of mechanical ventilation can be characterized as a pre-established pattern governing the interaction between the patient and the ventilator. This pattern is established through the combination of three fundamental variable components (Fig. 4):

1. The variable that controls the ventilator breath (Breath Control).
2. The sequence of breaths (Breath Sequence).
3. The strategy for achieving specific targets (Targeting Scheme).

2.4 Breath Control Variable

The ventilator can control or assist a breath either by pressure or volume as a control variable. Volume, here, is an integration of flow. The equation of motion for respiratory system can be used to understand the theoretical basis of these control variables. The equation, describes the relationship of pressure (P or Paw), volume (V), and flow (Q) as functions of time, as following:

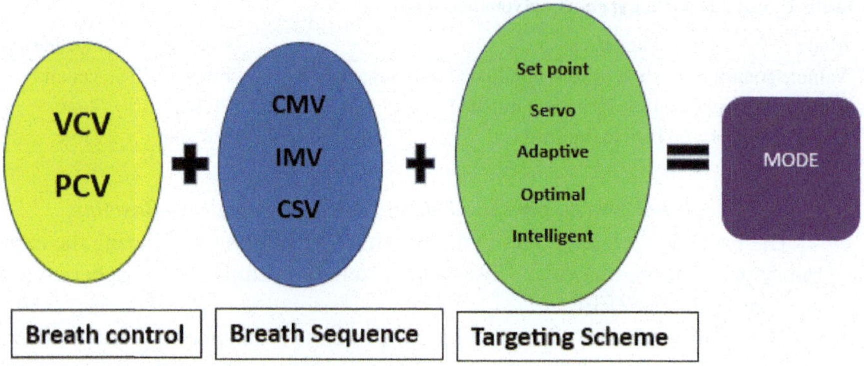

Fig. 4 Patient-ventilator interaction framework. *VCV* volume control ventilation, *PCV* pressure control ventilation, *CMV* control mechanical ventilation, *IMV* intermittent mechanical ventilation, *CSV* continuous spontaneous ventilation

$$P(t) = EV(t) + RQ(t)$$

Or

$$\text{Paw}(t) = V(t) / \text{Crs} + \text{Rrs} \times Q(t) + \text{PEEP} - \text{Pmus}(t)$$

According to the equation of motion, if any of the functions, i.e., pressure, volume or flow is known, the other two can be determined. It also shows that there can only be one control variable, i.e., flow (Q) or pressure (Paw) at any given time because all the other elements of the equation are either respiratory system (rs)'s constants like elastance (E), compliance (C), and resistance (R) or a derived variable like volume or determined by the independent control system which is inspiratory and expiratory muscle systems (Pmus). During fully controlled mechanical ventilation with no respiratory effort by the patient, the Pmus is zero.

The control variable means the one which is controlled or predetermined and pre-set prior to the inspiration.

In case of *volume as a control variable* this would mean that both volume and flow are pre-set prior to inspiration. This would be volume *control ventilation (VCV)* when both volume and flow are pre-set as setting only volume or only flow would not be sufficient to call it a VCV mode. Some pressure control modes allow to set the tidal volume and allow the ventilator to determine the flow. Similarly, some pressure control modes allow to pre-set the inspiratory flow while tidal volume will depend on the inspiratory pressure.

In case of *pressure as a control variable*, the inspiratory pressure as a function of time is pre-set prior to inspiration, in which the inspiratory pressure as a function of time is predetermined. This would be labeled as *pressure control ventilation (PCV).*

3 Breath Sequence Variable

A breath sequence is a particular pattern of spontaneous and/or mandatory breaths. A mandatory breath is the one in which patient has no control over its timing or frequency and its start and end are independently controlled by the ventilator according to the set parameters. A ventilator can deliver three basic breath sequences, i.e., a controlled mandatory (CMV), intermittent mandatory (IMV), and continuous spontaneous (CSV).

1. *Controlled Mandatory Ventilation (CMV)*
   The breath sequence in CMV prevents any occurrence of spontaneous breaths between mandatory breaths, as every patient-triggered signal within the trigger window results in a ventilator-initiated inhalation, meaning a mandatory breath takes place. Mandatory breaths are breaths delivered by the mechanical ventilator according to preset parameters. This is also called assist-control mode. The set frequency in this mode is minimum breath rate and the mandatory breath rate can be higher than this but never below the set rate.
2. *Intermittent Mandatory Ventilation (IMV)*
   During IMV, the set frequency of mandatory breaths is the maximum frequency (in contrast to CMV where mandatory frequency is the minimum frequency) since every patient signal between the mandatory breaths initiates a spontaneous breath. Spontaneous breathing is allowed, and mandatory breaths are delivered in three ways, either at set frequency or only when spontaneous frequency falls below set frequency or when measured minute volume falls below a preset value. The ventilator delivers a set number of mandatory breaths (or controlled breaths) at a fixed rate or frequency. These controlled breaths are delivered to ensure a minimum level of ventilation and oxygenation, especially when the patient is not breathing adequately on their own. In addition to the mandatory breaths, IMV allows the patient to take spontaneous breaths when they want to. These spontaneous breaths are triggered and cycled by the patient's own respiratory effort. This feature is important as it permits some degree of patient control and effort in the breathing process.

Synchronized Intermittent Mandatory Ventilation (SIMV): It works like the IMV, but ventilator detects the patient's respiratory efforts and delivers mandatory breaths in coordination with those efforts. This synchronization helps the patient to take control of their own breathing while receiving support when needed. The support rate and the level are decided by the preset parameters which can be pressure targeted as in P-SIMV or volume controlled as in V-SIMV.

3. *Continuous Spontaneous Ventilation (CSV)*
   Only spontaneous breathing is allowed. Spontaneous breath can be an unsupported breath or supported by the ventilator in which the patient decides the respiratory rate and initiates the breath, but the flow is delivered by the ventilator to quickly achieve and maintain the set proximal airway pressure, e.g., pressure support ventilation (*PSV*).

Based on the two breath control variables and three breath sequences, ventilators can have five basic patterns of operations. *A ventilatory pattern* is a combination of breath control variable, i.e., volume (VC) or pressure (PC) and breath sequence, i.e., CMV, IMV or CSV. Thus, there are five basic ventilatory patterns, namely VC-CMV, VC-IMV, PC-CMV, PC-IMV, and PC-CSV. The VC-CSV combination is not possible because volume control implies ventilator cycling, and ventilator cycling makes every breath mandatory, not spontaneous.

3.1 Targeting Schemes

Targeting schemes are further sophistication of the breath. A targeting scheme can be described as a model that outlines how operator inputs and ventilator outputs are interconnected to attain a particular ventilation pattern, typically configured as a feedback control system. Within every ventilation pattern, various categories can be identified based on the strategies they employ for achieving their objectives (set-point, dual, biovariable, servo, adaptive, optimal, and intelligent). These targeting schemes help to understand the advanced and more sophisticated modes of mechanical ventilation.

The Nomenclature of mechanical ventilation is summarized in Fig. 5.

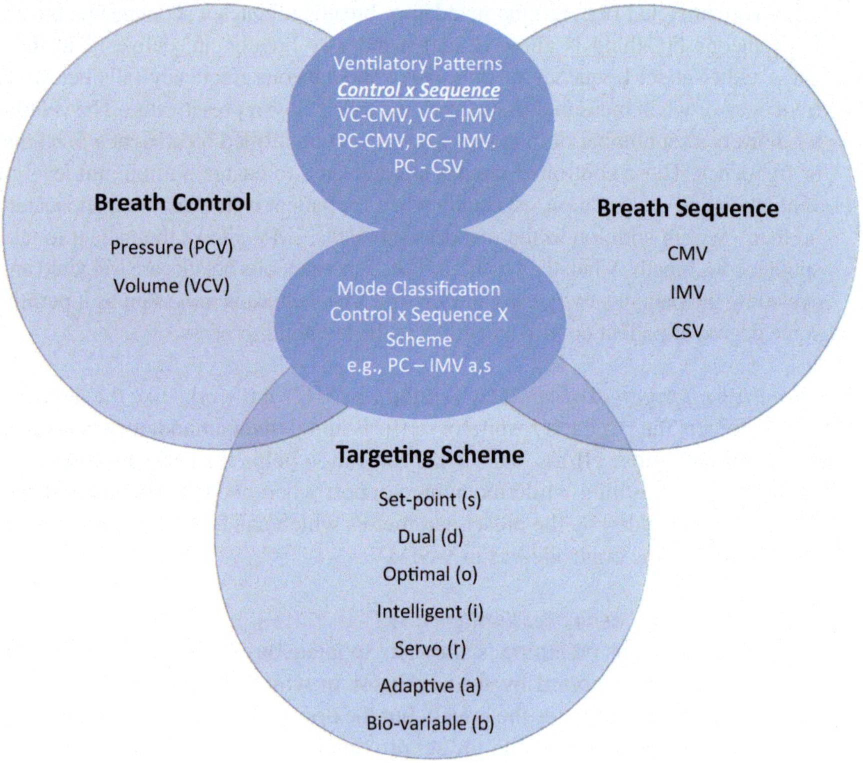

Fig. 5 Nomenclature of mechanical ventilatory modes

4 Basic Modes of Mechanical Ventilation

The breath is the bridge which connects life to consciousness. (Thich Nhat Hanh)

The "mode" is the first selection that must be made when a patient is to be started on mechanical ventilation. The variable that controls the key function of delivery of the breaths during the respiratory cycles defines the mode of mechanical ventilation. As described in the last section, these control variables are mainly volume (flow) and pressure. Hence, the most common and basic modes of mechanical ventilation are forms of volume control (also called volume assist-control) and pressure control (also called pressure assist-control). The term volume controlled may be more appropriately called flow-control mode as flow is controlled to deliver a set volume. However, volume control is more commonly used instead of flow control. Another common and basic mode is the pressure support in which pressure is the control variable, but all breaths are patient triggered, hence its name is pressure support rather than pressure control.

The controlling system of the ventilator is given a different task as a target function depending upon the selected mode of ventilation, e.g., in pressure control mode, this function is the target airway pressure to be achieved and maintained during the set inspiratory time and in volume control mode, this function is the target flow as an integral of time, i.e., a set volume to be delivered during the inspiratory time. There is no clear evidence if one control mode is superior to the other one, in terms of patient outcomes, however, choice of a mode may have clinical implications which is explored in more details in the following sections.

4.1 Volume Control Ventilation (VCV)

The VCV has been the most common ventilatory mode used in critical care units and operating rooms, although in recent times, pressure control and pressure support modes are becoming more popular. The highlights of VCV are the delivery of a fixed tidal volume at a fixed rate which guarantees a set minute ventilation. The tidal volume and respiratory rates are set by the operator. The target or control variable is the flow rate and the flow waveform which can be a square flow waveform or a decelerating flow waveform (Fig. 6). The cycling variable is flow in VCV. The inspiratory time is also set indirectly when the tidal volume and flow is set (time = volume/flow) and for this reason inspiratory time cannot be changed by changes in the respiratory system or by patient's breathing efforts. The proximal airway pressure is the dependent variable, and the shape of the pressure waveform changes with the patient's breathing efforts or respiratory system characteristics as shown in Fig. 6a and b.

In short, VCV is a flow targeted, volume-cycled mode of ventilation with volume as an independent and proximal airway pressure as a dependent variable which is determined by the lung compliance and airway resistance. Pressure can increase as the resistance increases or compliance decreases, the flow, however, will remain constant.

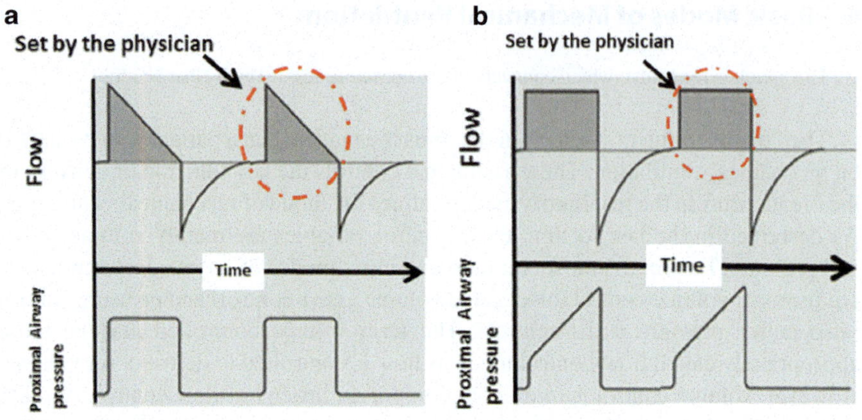

Fig. 6 Volume control ventilation flow and pressure waveforms. (**a**) Decelerating (ramp) flow (**b**) Constant (square) flow

4.2 Key Settings in VCV

The key operator setting in VCV is as following:

Tidal Volume
Respiratory Rate
Flow rate: depending on the ventilator type, operator may set the flow rate and tidal volume or flow rate and inspiratory time
PEEP
Fraction of inspired oxygen (Fio_2)

4.3 Advantages of VCV

The set tidal volume is guaranteed, so is the minute ventilation.

Over breathing by the patient is possible in the assist-control mode.

Breath delivery may be synchronized with patient's effort, which adds to patient's comfort.

VCV offers rest to the patient by unloading the respiratory muscles.

4.4 Disadvantages of VCV

Respiratory alkalosis may occur if the set respiratory rate is very high due to the rigid nature of the breathing schedule.

In case of poor lung mechanics, airway pressure can be high and may lead to barotrauma.

Dynamic hyperinflation may occur due to poor lung compliance.

Inappropriate flow settings or poor adjustment of trigger sensitivity may lead to increased work of breathing.

Atrophy of respiratory muscles is a risk factor due to prolong unloading of these muscles with VCV.

4.5 Different Modes of Volume-Controlled Ventilation

Volume-controlled ventilation (VCV) is a foundational mode of mechanical ventilation utilized in various clinical scenarios. While the basic principle of VCV remains constant across different ventilators, there are variations in modes designed to meet specific patient needs. Here are some different modes of VCV:

4.5.1 Assist-Control Volume-Controlled Ventilation (AC-VCV)

In AC-VCV, the ventilator delivers a set tidal volume with each breath, either initiated by the patient's own respiratory effort (assisted breaths) or triggered by the ventilator at a preset rate (controlled breaths). This mode ensures a minimum number of breaths per minute regardless of patient effort.

4.5.2 Synchronized Intermittent Mandatory Ventilation (VC-SIMV)

SIMV-VCV combines volume-controlled breaths with patient-triggered breaths. The ventilator delivers a set tidal volume at a preset rate (mandatory breaths), while allowing the patient to breathe spontaneously between mandatory breaths. The patient's spontaneous breaths are not assisted by the ventilator.

4.5.3 Pressure-Regulated Volume Control (PRVC)

PRVC is a hybrid mode that adjusts the inspiratory pressure to maintain a target tidal volume. The ventilator continuously monitors the patient's lung mechanics and adjusts the inspiratory pressure as needed to achieve the preset tidal volume. This mode aims to deliver consistent tidal volumes while minimizing the risk of barotrauma by adjusting the inspiratory pressure according to patient's respiratory mechanics.

4.5.4 Volume Support (VS)

Volume Support mode provides partial ventilatory support by delivering a set tidal volume during spontaneous breathing efforts. The ventilator calculates the required pressure needed to achieve the set tidal volume based on factors such as lung compliance and airway resistance of the previous breath. It adjusts the pressure support as needed to ensure the desired tidal volume is delivered. This mode is often used during weaning from mechanical ventilation.

4.5.5 Volume Control with Pressure Support (VC-PS)

VC-PS combines volume-controlled breaths with pressure support during spontaneous breathing efforts. The ventilator delivers a set tidal volume at a preset rate and provides additional pressure support during spontaneous breaths to facilitate patient comfort and reduce the work of breathing.

4.5.6 Pressure-Controlled Volume-Guaranteed (PC-VG)

PC-VG is a mode that combines pressure control with volume targeting. The ventilator delivers breaths with a set inspiratory pressure while ensuring that a minimum tidal volume is achieved. Unlike PRVC mode, where the ventilator adjusts inspiratory pressure (pressure is regulated) to maintain the tidal volume, in PC-VG maintains a consistent pressure (pressure is controlled) throughout the inspiratory phase. If the set pressure is not sufficient to deliver a set minimum tidal volume, then the ventilator increases the inspiratory time to ensure the minimum tidal volume delivery. PC-VG is particularly useful in patients with varying respiratory drive and in condition where achieving a set tidal volume would be challenging.

4.6 Pressure Control Ventilation (PCV)

The PCV has become more popular in recent years with more appreciation of risks associated with mechanical ventilation like barotrauma. The highlights of PCV are the application of a pre-set pressure and pressure waveform (most commonly square or trapezoid). The maximum airway pressure is the pressure set by the operator. The target or control variable is the pressure and the set pressure waveform (Fig. 7). The cycling variable is the time which is set as inspiratory time on the ventilator. Inspiration will end after the set inspiratory time is elapsed and this time cannot be changed by patient's breathing effort or by the changes in the respiratory mechanics, like in VCV. The volume (tidal volume) is the dependent variable in PCV and its value changes with changes in respiratory system resistance or lung compliance.

In short, PCV is a pressure-targeted, time-cycled ventilation mode in which proximal airway pressure is the independent variable and the tidal volume is dependent variable. It changes with the respiratory system resistance or lung compliance.

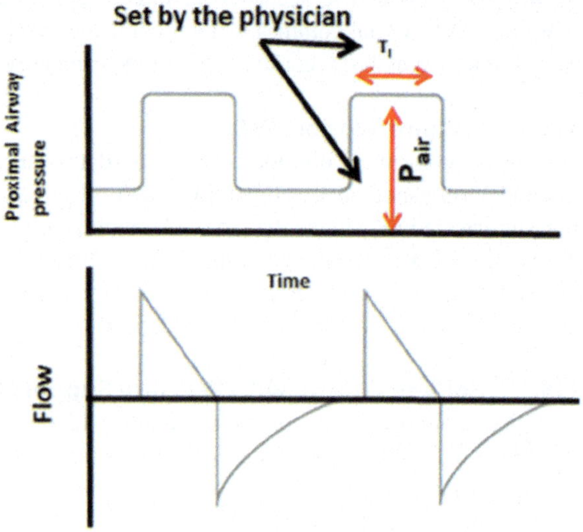

Fig. 7 PCV flow and pressure waveforms

The volume will decrease with the increase in the respiratory system resistance and decrease with the increase in lung compliance, the airway pressure will remain constant.

4.7 Key Settings in PCV

The key operator setting in PCV is as following:

Inspiratory pressure: depending on the ventilator type, operator may set the total inspiratory pressure or inspiratory pressure above the PEEP
Inspiratory time
Respiratory rate
PEEP
Fraction of inspired oxygen (Fio_2)

4.8 Advantages of PCV

The risk of barotrauma is minimized as the airway pressure does not exceed the set inspiratory pressure.

Patient can control their inspiratory flow rate as the air flow will increase in proportion to their inspiratory efforts.

Improved patient comfort due to the matching of inspiratory flow with patient's effort.

Less potential of patient-ventilator dyssynchrony as compared to VCV.

Compensation for air leaks in the ventilatory system.

4.9 Disadvantages of PCV

The main disadvantage of PCV is the variable tidal volume in response to changes in lung mechanics. If the resistance increases or compliance decreases, the same set pressure will deliver less tidal volume which may result in inadequate ventilation and CO_2 retention. On the other hand, if the resistance decreases or the compliance improves, the same set pressure will deliver larger tidal volume which may lead to volutrauma.

4.10 Different Modes of Pressure Control Ventilation

Pressure-controlled ventilation (PCV) is a foundational mode of mechanical ventilation utilized in various clinical scenarios. While the basic principle of PCV remains constant across different ventilators, there are variations in modes designed to meet specific patient needs. Here are some different modes of PCV.

4.10.1 Assist-Control—Pressure Control Ventilation (AC-PCV)

In AC-PCV, the ventilator delivers a set inspiratory pressure (Pinsp) with every breath. Patients can trigger breaths themselves, which are supported by the ventilator at the preset Pinsp. It is often used in patients who require full ventilatory support or those with varying levels of respiratory effort.

4.10.2 Synchronized Intermittent Mandatory Ventilation (PC-SIMV)

PC-SIMV combines pressure-controlled breaths with spontaneous breaths from the patient. The ventilator delivers mandatory breaths at a set inspiratory pressure and rate while allowing patients to take spontaneous breaths. It's commonly used when patients require a mix of controlled and spontaneous ventilation.

4.10.3 Intermittent Mandatory Ventilation (PC-IMV)

In PCV-IMV, the ventilator delivers mandatory breaths at a pre-set inspiratory pressure and rate. However, it does not synchronize with the patient's spontaneous breaths. PC-IMV is suitable for patients who require partial ventilatory support but do not necessarily need synchronization with their spontaneous efforts.

4.10.4 Airway Pressure Release Ventilation (APRV)

APRV is a variation of PCV that primarily uses two pressure levels: a high-pressure level (P_high) and a low-pressure level (P_low). Patients spend most of the time (T_high) of the respiratory cycle at P_high, which facilitates lung recruitment and oxygenation. During P_low, the ventilator releases the airway pressure to a lower level (P_low) for a brief duration known as the release phase or T_low. This release allows for passive exhalation and facilitates ventilation. The duration of the release phase can be adjusted based on the patient's respiratory mechanics and requirements. Patient is allowed to breath spontaneously during P_high and P_low phases.

4.10.5 BiLevel Positive Airway Pressure (BiLevel PCV)

BiLevel PCV delivers two different levels of pressures, i.e., a higher inspiratory pressure, P_high and a lower expiratory pressure, P_low. P_high helps the patient in overcoming the airway resistance ad expanding the lungs. It is set according to patient respiratory needs based on lung compliance, airway resistance, and desired tidal volume. P_low is set to maintain PEEP and to prevent alvoloar collapse and improving gas exchange in expiratory phase. In BiLevel PCV, patient can breathe spontaneously during the inspiratory phase, but the expiratory phase is passive which helps with the exhalation.

4.10.6 Pressure Control with Pressure Support (PC-PSV)

This mode combines PCV with pressure support ventilation (PSV). The inspiratory pressure is set for the mandatory breaths, and pressure support is applied during spontaneous breaths. It provides support for patients with varying levels of respiratory effort and can improve patient comfort.

4.11 Volume Control Vs. Pressure Control Ventilation

In Summary (Figs. 8 and 9), the VCV and PCV are similar that both use assist-control as the trigger, and both have predetermined inspiratory time which does not change with changes in respiratory mechanics or with changes in patient's efforts. However, in PCV, the inspiratory time is directly set while in VCV it is indirectly set by setting the flow (target) and the tidal volume (cycle). It is also noteworthy that in both, VCV and PCV, flow waveform is delivered which results in a pressure waveform and culminates in a tidal volume delivery. The flow and volume are set in the VCV which produce a proximal airway pressure while in PCV proximal airway pressure and inspiratory time are set which produces a flow and volume. If respiratory system resistance and compliance remain unchanged, switching between VCV & PCV will not change the ventilator output.

4.12 Pressure Support Ventilation (PSV)

Pressure support ventilation is another basic and commonly used mechanical ventilation mode. It is mostly used as a weaning mode or as an adjunct in volume or pressure control modes to improve patient comfort during spontaneous breathing efforts. The highlight of PSV is the control of the inspiratory pressure while all breaths, flow and inspiratory time are defined by the patient's respiratory effort. So, there are no control ventilator breaths. The control or target variable in PSV is the pressure. The ventilator augments the inspiratory effort according to this set pressure. The cycling variable in PSV is flow and is set as a percentage of peak inspiratory flow. In most ventilators this percentage is 25%. The time-cycling is used as a backup only, e.g., in case of leak the ventilator may fail to cycle from inspiration to expiration, the breath will be automatically switched from inspiration to expiration at a set time interval, usually 3–5 s in most ventilators.

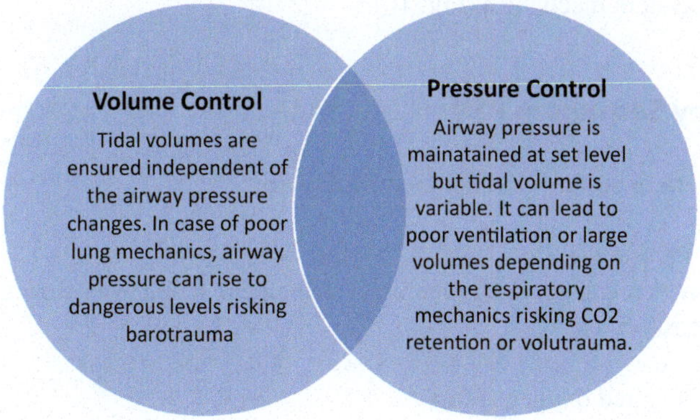

Fig. 8 Summary of VCV and PCV

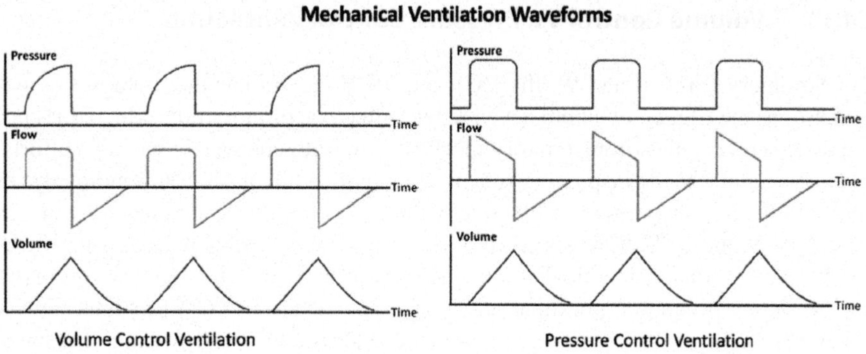

Fig. 9 Waveforms in VCV & PCV

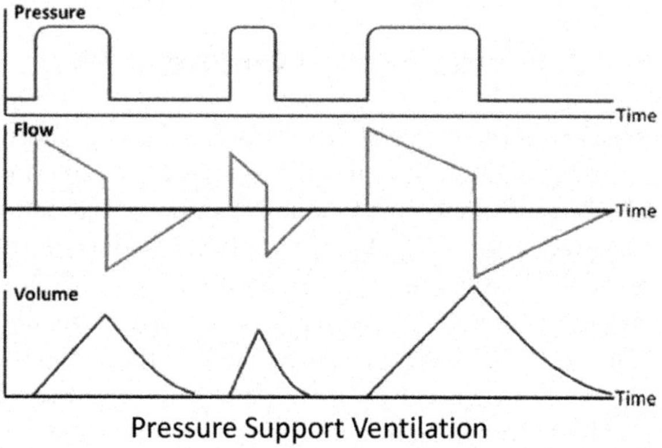

Fig. 10 Waveforms in PSV

In short, PSV is a pressure-targeted, flow cycled in which all breaths are triggered by the patient. There is no ventilator triggered breaths. The flow and volume waveforms and inspiratory time (in contrast to VCV and PCV where inspiratory time remains unchanged) vary depending upon the patient's respiratory effort and respiratory system mechanics (Fig. 10).

4.13 Key Settings in PSV

The key operator settings in PSV are as following:

Inspiratory Pressure (PS)
Cycling flow percentage, i.e., percentage of the peak inspiratory flow rate to terminate inspiratory phase
PEEP
Fraction of inspired oxygen (Fio_2)

There is not set respiratory rate or the inspiratory time. Both varies with patient's respiratory efforts.

4.14 Advantages of PSV

PSV is most used as a weaning mode as the inspiratory flow rate, inspiratory time, and respiratory rate are controlled by the patient.

4.15 Disadvantages of PSV

PSV cannot be used for patients with high oxygen consumption, with high airway resistance or for patients with decreased respiratory drive for any reason.

4.16 Pressure Control Vs. Pressure Support Ventilation

PCV and PSV, both have pressure as the control or target variable, i.e., flow is delivered in both at a set pressure. The trigger in the PCV can be either patient or ventilator trigger (assist-control) while in PSV there is only patient triggering. However, the patient triggering in both, PCV and PSV, can be flow or pressure trigger which means, a patient on PCV, triggering the ventilator at a higher than set rate, switching to PSV will not have any change in the triggering mechanism.

4.17 Summary of Basic Modes of Mechanical Ventilation

In summary (Table 2), each of the fundamental mode or its variable form offers unique advantages and is selected based on the patient's clinical condition, respiratory mechanics, and therapeutic goals. The choice of mode should be tailored to the individual patient's needs to optimize ventilation and promote successful weaning from mechanical ventilation. Close monitoring and adjustment of ventilator settings are essential to ensure patient safety and effective respiratory support.

Table 2 Summary of basic modes of mechanical ventilation

		Trigger			Types of breaths		
Mode	Target	Ventilator	Patient	Cycling	Mandatory	Assisted	Spontaneous
CMV	Volume (VCV)	Yes	No	Volume	Yes	No	No
	Pressure (PCV)	Yes	No	Time	Yes	No	No
AC	Volume (AC-VCV)	Yes	Yes	Volume	Yes	Yes	No
	Pressure (AC—PCV)	Yes	Yes	Time	Yes	Yes	No
IMV	Volume (S) IMV—VC)	Yes	Yes	Volume	Yes	Yes	Yes
	Pressure (S) IMV—PC)	Yes	Yes	Time	Yes	Yes	Yes
PSV	Pressure	No	Yes	Flow	No	Yes	No

5 Conclusion

In conclusion, this chapter offers an examination of fundamentals of mechanical ventilation nomenclature. It breaks down a mode into its constitutional components which is breath control, breath sequence, and target scheme. This makes it easier to understand any mode, basic or advanced. It also outlines basic foundational modes alongside their various names, aiding in a clearer understanding. By simplifying complex concepts and terminology, it facilitates comprehension, thereby simplifying the process of selecting the most appropriate mode according to the needs of the patient.

Bibliography

1. Hidalgo J, et al., editors. Personalized mechanical ventilation. Cham: Springer; 2022. https://doi.org/10.1007/978-3-031-14138-6_2.
2. Brochard LJ. Mechanical ventilation: negative to positive and back again. Crit Care Clin. 2023;39:437–49. https://doi.org/10.1016/j.ccc.2022.12.002.
3. Bellani G, editor. Mechanical ventilation from pathophysiology to clinical evidence; 2022. https://doi.org/10.1007/978-3-030-93401-9_2.
4. H. Poor, Basics of mechanical ventilation, 2018. https://doi.org/10.1007/978-3-319-89981-7_1.
5. MacIntyre NR. Indications for mechanical ventilation. In: Webb A, editor. Oxford textbook of critical care, Oxford textbook. 2nd ed. Oxford: Oxford Academic; 2016; online edn. https://doi.org/10.1093/med/9780199600830.003.0091.
6. Hickey SM, Giwa AO. Mechanical ventilation. [Updated 2023 Jan 26]. In: StatPearls [Internet]. Treasure Island: StatPearls Publishing; 2024. Available from: https://www.ncbi.nlm.nih.gov/books/NBK539742/
7. Mora Carpio AL, Mora JI. Ventilator management. [Updated 2023 Mar 27]. In: StatPearls [Internet]. Treasure Island: StatPearls Publishing; 2024. Available from: https://www.ncbi.nlm.nih.gov/books/NBK448186/
8. Chatburn RL, El-Khatib M, Mireles-Cabodevila E. A taxonomy for mechanical ventilation: 10 fundamental maxims. Respirat Care. 2014;59(11):1747–63. https://doi.org/10.4187/respcare.03057.
9. Poor H. Phase variables. In: Basics of mechanical ventilation. Cham: Springer; 2018. p. 11–27. https://doi.org/10.1007/978-3-319-89981-7_2.
10. Hasan A. Understanding mechanical ventilation: a practical handbook. London: Springer; 2010.
11. Hasan A. Understanding mechanical ventilation. London: Springer; 2010. https://doi.org/10.1007/978-1-84882-869-8_4.
12. Bellani G, editor. Mechanical ventilation from pathophysiology to clinical evidence. Cham: Springer; 2022. https://doi.org/10.1007/978-3-030-93401-9_4.
13. Poor H. Basics of mechanical ventilation. Cham: Springer. https://doi.org/10.1007/978-3-319-89981-7_2.
14. Ward J, Noel C. Basic modes of mechanical ventilation. Emerg Med Clin N Am. 2022;40:473–88. https://doi.org/10.1016/j.emc.2022.05.003.

Non-traditional Modes of Ventilation

Mohammed Shafee Shaikh, Muhammad Shakeel Riaz,
Abdul Gafoor Tharayil, Arshad Chanda,
Siddhartha Banerjee, and Wael Khalaf

1 Introduction

Progress lies not in enhancing what is, but in advancing towards what will be. (Khalil Gibran)

In this chapter, we will deal with non-traditional or unconventional modes of mechanical ventilation. As we have seen from the history of mechanical ventilation in the preceding chapters (chapters "Conventional Mechanical Ventilation—I *History, Mechanics, and Indications*" and "Conventional Mechanical Ventilation—II *Nomenclature and Basic Modes*"), there has been progressive advancement in the field since the advent of mechanical ventilation. The progress continues and indeed seems to be accelerating forward over the past three decades, with new modes being developed at an exponential rate.

The impetus for development has been an understanding of the limitations of basic modes and a greater understanding of the deleterious effects and complications associated with these modes.

This progress has been facilitated by technological advancement, with the starting point being ventilators as purely mechanical devices, e.g., Manley ventilator. This has progressed from ventilators limited by the mechanics of their engineering to modern microprocessor-controlled devices which are capable of processing input data sensed from patients, interpreting such data, and producing complex patterns of air flow and hence ventilatory support.

M. S. Shaikh (✉) · M. S. Riaz · A. G. Tharayil · A. Chanda · S. Banerjee · W. Khalaf
Surgical ICU, Department of Anesthesia, ICU and Perioperative Medicine, Hamad Medical Corporation, Doha, Qatar
e-mail: mshaikh10@hamad.qa; MRiaz2@hamad.qa; atharayil@hamad.qa; achanda@hamad.qa; SBanerjee1@hamad.qa; WKhalaf1@hamad.qa

N. A. Shallik (ed.), *Flow Controlled Ventilation Mode Through a Straw Size Tube*, https://doi.org/10.1007/978-3-031-77477-5_4

Table 1 Non-traditional modes of Ventilation addressing specific limitations of traditional modes

Disadvantages of traditional modes	How is it overcome?	Modes of ventilation
Pressure vs. pure volume modes Each with distinct advantages and disadvantages	Dual modes combining Volume and pressure modes	Volume-assured pressure support (VAPS) Pressure-regulated volume-controlled ventilation (PRVC)
Desynchrony, poor patient-ventilator interaction	Synchrony enhancing modes. Closed-loop systems	Neurally adjusted Ventilatory assist (NAVA) Proportional assist ventilation (PAV) ASV (adaptive support ventilation) Smartcare
Propensity to induce lung injury	Lung recruitment and protection modes	Airway Pressure release ventilation (APRV) High-frequency oscillation modes (HFJV)
Non-physiological nature of Positive pressure ventilation	Modern negative pressure ventilation	Biphasic cuirass ventilator (BCV)

These advancements represent progress on not only on the basic functions of ventilators, namely oxygenation and carbon dioxide removal but especially on some of the key associated goals of mechanical ventilation, namely patient safety, comfort, and ultimately facilitating the liberation from mechanical ventilation.

Based on the advantages associated with these novel modes of ventilation, non-traditional modes can be divided into:

1. Modes which address the limitations of traditional modes; Table 1 delineates these limitations how they are addressed and specific examples of modes which achieve this;
2. Modes with utility in specific patient populations
   (a) High-frequency jet ventilation (HFJV): used in surgical airway management and perioperative care of specific patient groups.
   (b) Cuirass ventilation: Applications include long-term ventilation to perioperative or periprocedural use.
   (c) Continuous positive airway pressure (CPAP)/Auto titrating (adjustable) positive airway pressure (APAP) Bilevel positive airway pressure (BiPAP) as non-invasive modes of ventilation for patients with obstructive sleep apnoea.

2 Benefits of Non-traditional modes of Ventilation Include the Following

1. *Improved Oxygenation and CO_2 Removal*: Advanced modes incorporate sophisticated algorithms to optimize the delivery of oxygen and removal of carbon dioxide, helping to maintain appropriate blood gas levels.
2. *Patient-Ventilator Synchrony*: Advanced modes are designed to enhance synchronization between the patient's respiratory efforts and the ventilator support. This can improve patient comfort, reduce the work of breathing, and decrease the risk of complications.
3. *Adhering to Lung Protection*: Many advanced modes incorporate lung-protective strategies, such as lower tidal volumes and optimal positive end-expiratory pressure (PEEP) settings. This helps to prevent ventilator-induced lung injury and minimize barotrauma.
4. *Adaptability to Patient Condition*: Advanced modes often have the capability to adapt to changes in the patient's respiratory condition.
5. *Automated Weaning Protocols*: Some advanced modes include automated weaning protocols, which help in the gradual reduction of ventilatory support as the patient's condition improves. This can contribute to faster liberation from mechanical ventilation.
6. *Enhanced Monitoring and Feedback*: Advanced modes typically come with advanced monitoring capabilities, providing real-time data on various parameters. This allows for the rapid assessment of the patient's response to ventilation and making informed adjustments as needed.
7. *Reduction of Sedation Requirements*: Improved patient-ventilator synchrony and comfort leads to a reduced need for sedation.
8. *Individualized Ventilation Strategies*: Advanced modes often allow for individualized ventilation strategies based on the specific needs of the patient, considering factors such as lung compliance, resistance, and the underlying pathology.
9. *Remote Monitoring and Telemetry*: Some advanced ventilation systems offer remote monitoring and telemetry capabilities, allowing healthcare providers to assess and adjust ventilator settings from a distance.

3 Dual Mode Ventilation

In the last chapter, we discussed the contrasting benefits and indeed limitations of pressure and volume modes, respectively. If one were to reap the benefits of each mode, while minimizing their disadvantages, the ideal solution would be a hybrid mode incorporating the best of both modalities. Dual modes represent precisely this attempt.

Simply put this "best of both" principle can be approached by using either basic mode as a foundation then making appropriate adjustments, e.g., start with an essentially volume-controlled mode, and then automatically adjust flow to produce a pressure/time waveform akin to that produced by a pressure-controlled mode. Conversely one can base it on a pressure-controlled mode, and consequently automatically adjust the pressure waveform to assure that a pre-set volume is achieved.

Alternatively, the ventilator can achieve this by a dual mode which works by switching form from one mode to another within a single inspiratory cycle to achieve both pre-set volume and pressure targets.

These adjustments can be made either by monitoring breath parameters and adjusting in subsequent breaths or by making the adjustments within a given breath.

3.1 Breath to Breath, Pressure Limited, Time Cycled

This is a mode where the clinician pre-sets a tidal volume that it requires the ventilator to deliver. The ventilator then delivers flow, which is adjusted to ensure that the associated pressure is limited (Controlled), until the pre-set volume is delivered. These are used both in theatre and critical care areas. Pressure-regulated volume-control (PRVC), adaptive pressure ventilation, auto-flow, volume-control plus, or variable pressure control ventilation are manufacturer specific examples of modes which rely on this principle.

The ventilator achieves this by monitoring for every breath, the tidal volume delivered in contrast to the set volume and the pressure required to achieve this volume. It consequently adjusts these in subsequent breaths to match the pre-set volume, while delivering the volume using the minimum pressure requires to do so. This mode it therefore able to adapt to changes in the patient's compliance and airway resistance, while assuring that a minimum pre-set tidal volume is delivered using lowest peak airway pressure possible.

3.2 Breath to Breath, Pressure Limited, Flow Cycled

This mode is flow cycled, so triggered by the patient akin to pressure support ventilation, however, unlike classical pressure support where the pressure support level is fixed at a set rate, in this mode, the pressure support is adjusted up or down, depending on the patients' lung compliance and airway resistance to ensure that a pre-set tidal volume is delivered. This is otherwise known as Variable Pressure Support or Volume Support Ventilation (VSV).

As the breath initiating trigger is flow, crucially this mode can only be delivered when the patient initiates the breath and hence can only be used in spontaneously breathing patients. Crucially this is where it differs from the breath to breath, pressure limited, time cycled modes described previously.

Hence it is used primarily as a weaning mode and has the advantage over classical Pressure Support Ventilation (PSV), in that pressure is titrated down as patients' compliance improves while maintaining a consistent title volume.

3.3 Dual Control Within a Breath

This is a mode which can switch from a pressure support to a volume-controlled mode within a single breath cycle. In this mode, a patient triggered breath results in variable flow delivered rapidly to generate a pre-set pressure support level. At the same time, the tidal volume being delivered is measured and if it is not being achieved by the set pressure support level, then the ventilator switches to a volume-controlled mode, with a constant flow rate, within that breath cycle to assure that a set tidal volume is delivered. This mode is otherwise known as pressure augmentation or volume-assured/ guaranteed pressure support ventilation (VAPS).

4 Closed-Loop Systems

In the field of mechanical ventilation, the combined factors of heavy workloads, staff shortages, and deficiency of expertise can lead to reduced incorporation of existing knowledge into clinical practice, leading to negative consequences for patient outcomes.

Modern technology provides a solution in the form of closed-loop systems of ventilation which automates the adjustment of ventilator parameters using continuous monitoring of patient's respiratory mechanics, blood gases, and other relevant physiological parameters. This real-time data allows the ventilator to adapt its settings dynamically, providing individualized respiratory support tailored to the patient's changing needs.

In essence a closed system requires

- Sensors to monitor parameters such as airway pressure, flow, volume, oxygenation, and sometimes even neurological signals.
- Control algorithms to process sensor data and determine optimal ventilator settings.
- The ventilator equipped with software to execute the instructions provided by the control algorithms.

As with all technological advancements, these have been achieved by continuum of advancement which progresses into the future.

4.1 Early Closed-Loop Systems—Semi-open Systems

Early iterations started closing the loop with the ventilator sensing patients' respiratory efforts and responding to these both with respect to timing and size of breath being delivered. These can be regarded as semi-open systems as they still require clinician input in terms of the magnitude of support to be delivered. Examples of these include proportional assist ventilation (PAV) and neurally adjusted ventilatory assist (NAVA).

4.2 Proportional Assist Ventilation (PAV)

This is a mode which has as the primary function to assist with the liberation of patients from mechanical ventilation. It works on the premise that a spontaneously breathing patient attached to a ventilator is essentially a system of two oscillatory pumps working in tandem. Proportional assist ventilation aims to optimize the way in which these pumps interact.

In PAV, the ventilator synchronizes with the patient's efforts to breath and generates flow and thus a consequent volume which is in proportion to the patient's effort. Additionally, this assistance varies in proportion to the patient's effort throughout the course of an inspiratory period.

Unlike other traditional modes where one can set the tidal volume or pressure, this mode allows the patient to determine their own tidal volume and inspiratory flow rate.

This mode uses pressure and flow data which is continuously measured throughout the respiratory cycle to determine the compliance and resistance and hence the work of breathing required for each breath.

These calculations are based on the law of equation on motion which can be simplified to the following: (neglecting Inertia).

$$\text{Pmus} = E \, \text{x} \, V + R \times Q$$

Pmus = Pressure generated by muscles
E = Elastic force
R = Resistive force (Airway resistance)
V = Volume displacement rate
Q = Flow Rate

The clinician then sets the ventilator to provide a percentage of the work of breathing for the patient. The ventilator provides this ventilatory assistance in terms of Volume assistance (cmH20/L) and flow assistance (cmH20/L/s).

This is typically set at 80%, hence will provide 80% Proportional Support to generate the work that is required to overcome both elastic and resistive forces.

As the patient's efforts which are determined by the patients' respiratory drive change, so are the volume and flow generated by the ventilator, thereby effectively bringing the ventilator under the control of the patient's respiratory drive.

However, despite the very promising theoretical benefits of PAV, and while demonstrating benefits of better oxygenation, carbon dioxide removal, greater variation in tidal volume in the face of increasing respiratory demand and the offloading of respiratory muscles, no studies have conclusively demonstrated a superiority of PAV over traditional PSV modes.

4.3 NAVA Ventilation

First described by Sinderby et al. in 1999, Neurally Adjusted Ventilatory Assist (NAVA) is a form of ventilation which focuses on optimizing the ventilator - patient synchrony. This form of ventilation does so by an enhanced form of triggering. Traditional modes of triggering rely on the ventilator sensing pneumatic variables, i.e., the ventilator sensing either a change in pressure or the detection of flow once the patient initiates a spontaneous breath. There is in this system, an innate delay from when the patient initiates muscular activity at the start of a breath, to this being translated to a pneumatic variable measured by the ventilator. This delay opens the potential for false and mis-triggering resulting in ventilator patient asynchrony.

NAVA represents a significant advancement on the traditional mechanism of triggering in that the ventilator can respond to the patient's respiratory drive by measuring the Electrical Activity of the Diaphragm (EADi). By measuring the time and amplitude of the EADi signal, the ventilator can respond by synchronizing to not only timing but also magnitude of the patients' respiratory effort and in so doing it is able to adapt to a patient's changing respiratory efforts.

4.3.1 How Does NAVA Work?

EADi is measured using a specially adapted nasogastric tube which has inbuilt electrodes which measure electrical activity in the crural diaphragm. It is imperative for this mode to function, for this signal, which is monitored by way of a tracing on the ventilator monitor screen, to be of sufficient quality. Therefore, an absence of this signal is a contraindication to the use of NAVA. In simple terms, ventilatory support commences at the onset of EADi is proportional to the magnitude if EADi and ceases when EADi ceases.

The triggering of the ventilator at the onset of EADi represents a more responsive trigger than pneumatic triggers. The proportionality of ventilatory support to the EADi, which is measured in μV, is achieved by setting a NAVA level which determines the level of pressure support above PEEP which the ventilator delivers for each μV sensed. NAVA level is therefore a proportionality factor and denoted as cmH20/μV.

The ventilator cycles to expiration when the EADi reaches 40–70% of flow value for a particular breath.

There is no clear consensus on ideal initial setting for NAVA, but the sensitivity is set to provide the minimum pressure support that is associated with the absence of respiratory distress, and which generate tidal volumes within the limits of 6–8 ml/Kg.

Usual NAVA Initial settings are in the range of 0.5–2 μV/cmH20. Setting levels lower than 0.5 μV/cmH20 risk being too sensitive and can result in auto-triggering or false triggering.

Once the NAVA level and the consequent pressure required to achieve the desired tidal volume in the absence of distress reaches 5cmH20, weaning from the ventilator should be considered.

The use of NAVA can also be extended to non-invasively ventilated patients where it has been shown to improve patient-ventilator synchrony and is especially useful for facilitating triggering in the presence of air leaks.

Overall evidence suggests that the use is NAVA may reduce duration of mechanical ventilation, however, has no impact on overall patient survival outcomes.

5 Closed-Loop Ventilation: Progress to Full Automation

Progression of closed-loop systems has led to automated ventilation, also known as ventilation autopiloting. The ventilator operates as a closed-loop system in which the ventilator in addition to sensing patient variables, interprets the data from these variables and consistently applies automated protocols which incorporating user-provided knowledge to automatically adjust ventilator settings. This approach can yield improved results, expedited weaning, and liberation from mechanical ventilation, decreased duration of ventilator usage, lower staff workload, and ultimately reduced cost. The level of automation may be partial or full.

Notable developments in this regard in the recent past are SmartcareTM (Dräger), Adaptive support VentilationTM and intellivent TM (Hamilton) and we will discuss them in some detail here.

6 Smartcare™

NeoGanesh/SmartCare™ consistently administers a weaning protocol in pressure support (PS) mode. The goal is to keep patients within a "comfort zone" of breathing by adjusting the level of PS for those breathing spontaneously. Additionally, the system automatically commences spontaneous breathing trials (SBT) for patients who meet specific predefined criteria. The system monitors three parameters, i.e., respiratory rate, tidal volume, and end-tidal CO_2. The system measures and calculates average values over 2–5 min and arrives at a conclusion as to whether patient needs more or less pressure support. Reference ranges for these parameters are built into the system to determine whether the support is adequate or not. A respiratory rate of 15–30 breaths/min (34/min in neurological disease), tidal volume (VT) of 250 ml below 55 kg body weight and 30 0 ml above 55 kg body weight, $ETCO_2$ maximal threshold of 55 mmHg (65 mmHg in Chronic Obstructive Pulmonary Disease) are the set threshold ranges in SmartCare.

Fig. 1 shows a schematic representation of this strategy employed by SmartCare. The system initiates weaning and transitions to SBT when the parameters fall within an acceptable range.

Research has demonstrated that SmartCare can reduce the time required for weaning, the overall duration of mechanical ventilation, and the length of stay in the

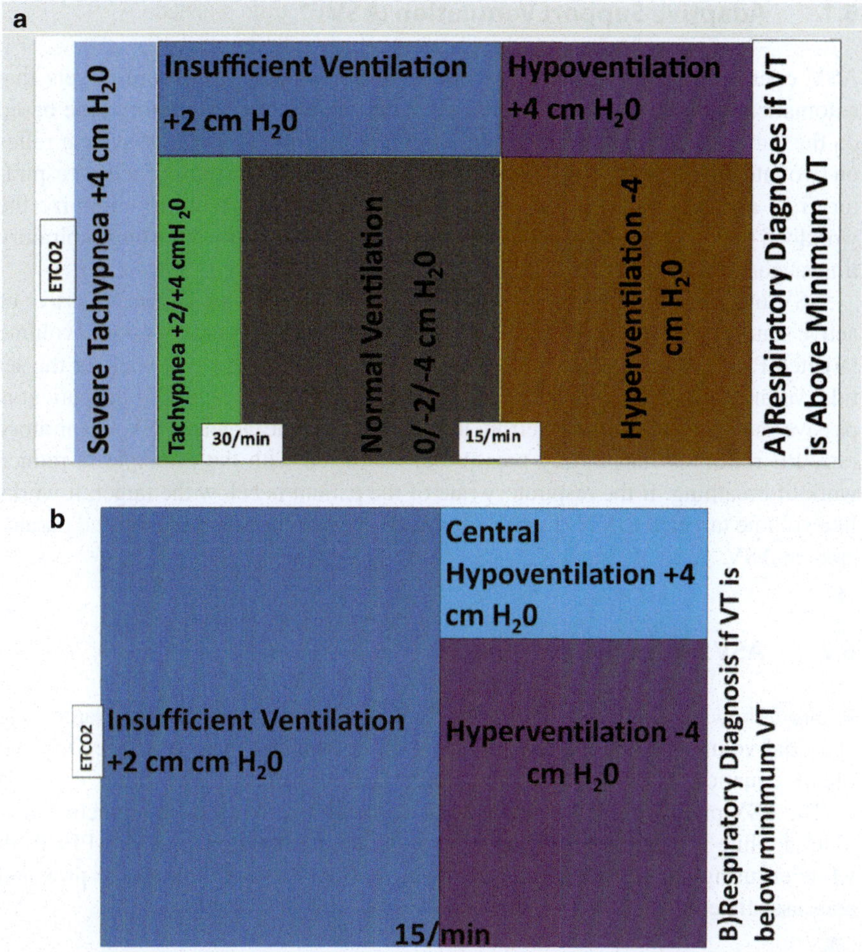

Fig. 1 Scheme used by SmartCare for respiratory diagnosis and modification of PS level in (**a**) Above minimum acceptable VT and (**b**) below acceptable VT

ICU. Lellouche et al. conducted the first randomized controlled trial (RCT) comparing standard care to the closed-loop system using SmartCare™. They observed a reduction in weaning duration from 5 to 3 days ($p < 0.01$), a decrease in mechanical ventilation duration from 12 to 7.5 days ($p < 0.003$), a shorter ICU stay from 15.5 to 12 days ($p < 0.02$), and no statistically significant difference in reintubation rates ($p = 0.4$). In another RCT conducted by Rose et al. at a single centre, it was found that with SmartCare™, the time to successful extubation was comparable to nurse-led weaning, with a tendency towards delayed liberation from mechanical ventilation. Furthermore, in the WEAN study, patients allocated to receive Smartcare™ experienced shorter durations of weaning and ICU stay. Generally, most of the studies are in favour of Smartcare™ system for early weaning, days on mechanical ventilation and ICU stay.

6.1 Adaptive Support Ventilation (ASV)™

ASV operates as a closed-loop system featuring adaptable pressure targets that automatically modify the respiratory rate, tidal volume, and inspiratory time based on the patient's exertion and closely monitored lung mechanics. The system relies on two integrated equations (Otis and Meads) to establish the most efficient respiratory rate and tidal volume, breath by breath, ultimately striving to minimize the workload of breathing. Dynamic hyperinflation is prevented by adjusting expiratory time according to the monitored expiratory time constant.

ASV utilizes Pressure targeted ventilation depending on the patient's passive or active state. If patient's respiratory rate is higher than the target, it works as volume targeted PSV (volume support) by adjusting the pressure support to deliver the set tidal volume with the least inspiratory pressure and respiratory rate. If the patient is passive and has no spontaneous effort, it works like volume targeted PCV. Respiratory rate, I:E ratio, and inspiratory pressure are adjusted with the principle to reduce work of breathing. If the respiratory rate of the patient is below the target, it works like volume targeted SIMV. Table 2 illustrates the set, derived, and adjusted parameters in ASV.

6.2 ASV Boundaries

Figure 2 shows the boundaries at which ASV strives to optimize the respiratory rate and tidal volume by minimizing the work of breathing derived from the Otis and Meads equation, most suitable for the lung mechanics of the patient.

The ASV principle employs an optimal approach to provide lung-protective ventilation while minimizing the risks of volutrauma, barotrauma, and auto-PEEP, all while ensuring the most efficient energy utilization. Table 3 outlines the pros and cons associated with ASV.

Table 2 Set, derived, and adjusted parameters in ASV

Set parameters	Derived parameters	Adjusted parameters
Minute ventilation percentage (25–300%)	Compliance	Respiratory rate
PEEP	Resistance	Tidal volume
FiO_2	Expiratory time constant	Inspiratory time
Maximum Pressure alarm (P max)	Dead space	Expiratory time
Gender, height, and body weight	Minute ventilation	1:E ratio
Trigger		Inspiratory pressure
Tube resistance compensation		

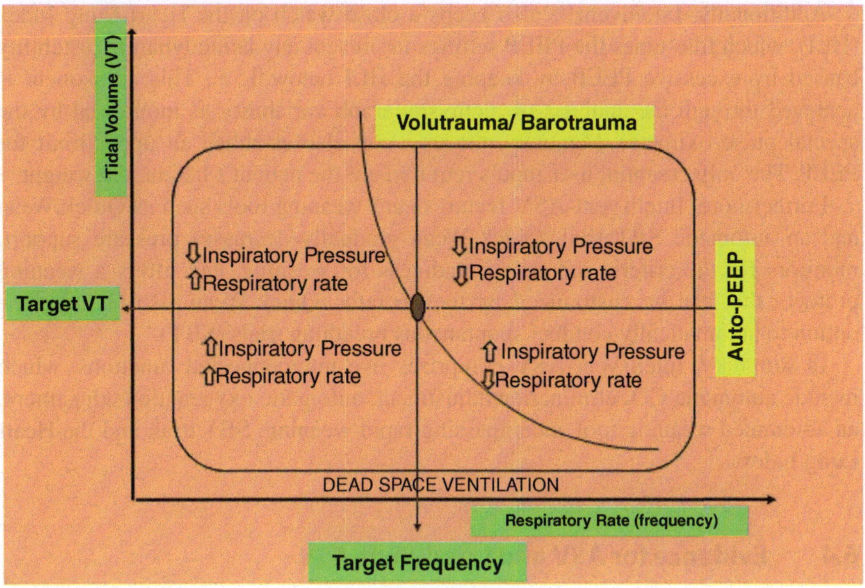

Fig. 2 ASV boundaries

Table 3 Advantages and Limitations of ASV

Advantages of ASV	Limitations of ASV
It adapts to the active and passive state of the patient	Low tidal volume is guaranteed at the expense of high respiratory rate to maintain minute ventilation
Adapts to the patient effort	Tidal volume, respiratory rate, and I:E ratio cannot be customized
Prevents Volutrauma, barotrauma, and dynamic hyperinflation	Limited to Hamilton ventilators
Reduce number of days on mechanical ventilator	Limited data in paediatric ventilation
Reduces staff dependence	Limited understanding among staff

6.3 IntelliVent-ASV™

IntelliVent™ represents a cutting-edge automated ventilation system that incorporates additional factors such as $ETCO_2$ and SpO_2. It adjusts the minute ventilation to either increase or decrease, aiming to keep ETCO2 levels within a predefined range, which can be tailored to the patient's condition. Furthermore, the oxygenation controller regulates PEEP and FiO_2 settings to maintain SpO_2 levels within an acceptable range, following the PEEP-FiO_2 table recommended by the ARDS network. The system requires capnograph and pulse oximeter.

Additionally, Intellivent™ also keeps a close watch on the Heart Lung Index (HLI), which fine-tunes the PEEP settings to prevent any hemodynamic instability caused by excessive PEEP by keeping the HLI below 15%. This adjustment is achieved through the analysis of plethysmograph variability as monitored by the special pulse oximeter. Manually, the user can also establish an upper limit for PEEP. The only essential user inputs required are the patient's height and weight.

Furthermore, IntelliVent-ASV features auto-weaning tools such as Quick Wean and an automatic SBT trial. Quick Wean gradually decreases pressure support, monitors for the criteria indicating readiness for weaning, and offers a weaning protocol that can be customized by the operator. Quick Wean also includes the option to automatically conduct spontaneous breathing trials (SBT).

In summary, IntelliVent-ASV comprises five interconnected functions, which include automatic CO_2 elimination adjustment, automatic oxygenation adjustment, an automated weaning tool encompassing rapid weaning, SBT trial, and the Heart Lung Index.

6.4 Evidence for ASV and IntelliVent-ASV

In 2012, Morato et al. compared three modes of closed-loop ventilation, namely ASV, Smartcare, and mandatory rate ventilation (MRV). The study was done on lung simulator and the comparison was in terms of weaning success, weaning failure, weaning success with extreme anxiety, weaning success with Cheyne-Stokes, weaning success with irregular breathing, and weaning failure with ineffective efforts. The three modes accurately identified successful and failed weaning scenarios, even in the presence of anxiety or irregular breathing. However, they erroneously identified weaning success in cases of Cheyne-Stokes breathing. MRV, on the other hand, mistakenly identified weaning failure in cases of ineffective efforts. The time required for pressure support (PS) to stabilize was shorter for ASV and MRV (1–2 min for all situations and 1–7 min, respectively) than for Smartcare (8–78 min). ASV exhibited a higher frequency of PS oscillations per 5 min (ranging from 4 to 15), as opposed to Smartcare (0-1) and MRV (0-12), except when extreme anxiety was present.

Kamel and colleagues conducted a study to investigate the effectiveness of adaptive support ventilation (ASV) compared to pressure support ventilation (PSV) for weaning COPD patients. After these patients had recovered with medical therapy and assist control ventilation, they were randomly assigned to undergo weaning with either ASV or PSV. The results indicated that weaning with ASV was more rapid and led to significant reductions in both ICU and hospital length of stay.

In a randomized controlled trial led by Pascale C. Gruber and her team, they compared adaptive support ventilation (ASV) to pressure-regulated volume control in the auto mode for 50 patients who had undergone uncomplicated cardiac surgery. The study examined the duration of intubation, mechanical ventilation, and the frequency of physician interventions during the weaning process. The findings revealed that ASV led to earlier extubation without an increase in clinician interventions.

In a randomized controlled trial conducted by Ritesh Agarwal and colleagues, they compared adaptive support ventilation (ASV) to volume-controlled ventilation in 48 patients diagnosed with acute respiratory distress syndrome. Their study revealed that both ventilation modes demonstrated similar outcomes across various aspects of mechanical ventilation, including the duration of mechanical ventilation, organ dysfunction, and mortality rates.

In another study by Laura A Buitman et al., mechanical power was compared with ASV and nonautomated PCV. In contrast to pressure-controlled ventilation, the mechanical power of ventilation with adaptive support ventilation was reduced (15.1 [10.5–25.7] compared to 22.9 [18.7–28.8] J/min; $p = 0.04$). There was no significant difference in tidal volume, but Pmax ($p = 0.012$) and respiratory rate ($p = 0.012$) were both lower when using adaptive support ventilation.

Closed-loop ventilation represents an advanced approach to ICU ventilation, guaranteeing lung-protective ventilation tailored to the individual lung mechanics of the patient. It also facilitates quicker, mostly automated weaning with minimal user involvement. By minimizing human intervention, these systems alleviate the workload for healthcare staff, particularly in resource-constrained settings. This is particularly valuable during pandemics when the volume of ventilated patients' surges, placing a strain on healthcare systems. This is an evolving frontier in mechanical ventilation, which combined with the rapid growth in artificial intelligence (AI), set the scene to the next leap of progress in mechanical ventilation.

7 Recruitment Enhancing/Lung Protection Modes

7.1 Airway Pressure Release Ventilation (APRV)

Airway Pressure Release Ventilation (APRV) is a relatively newer mode of ventilation and essentially a variation of conventional pressure control ventilation (PCV). It was first described by Stock et al. in 1987. The control variable in APRV is pressure and cycling from inspiration to expiration is time-based which makes it pressure-limited, time cycled mode of ventilation. However, the interplay of pressure and time is different from conventional PCV.

APRV mode primarily uses two pressure levels: a continuous positive airway pressure (CPAP) at a high-pressure level (P_high) for a longer period (inspiratory time) denoted as T_High. This inspiratory phase behaves like a constant recruitment manoeuvre as it maintains a high mean airway pressure. This is also in contrast to conventional ventilation where inspiration is relatively shorter than the expiration with usual Inspiratory: Expiratory (I:E) ratio of 1:2. This high-pressure phase is followed by low pressure (P_Low) for a brief expiratory phase (release time). This brief expiratory phase is denoted as T_Low (Fig. 3). This release phase allows for passive exhalation and facilitates ventilation.

It is important to understand the nomenclature of the APRV as there is no clear definition of this mode and the terms used in this mode are different from the conventional modes. The terms used in APRV are explained below with usual settings:

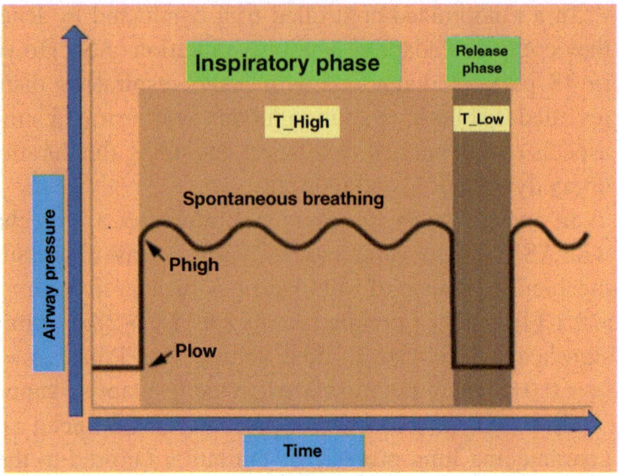

Fig. 3 Airway pressure release ventilation

P_High: This describes the highest level of pressure applied to the respiratory system. It can initially be set at plateau pressure and usually kept ≤30 cm of H2O. The usual range is 20–30 cm of H2O.

P_ Low: This describes the lowest pressure applied to the respiratory system. It can initially be set at zero cm of H2O with usual range of 0–5 cm of H2O.

T_High: This is the time in seconds which is spent at P_High. This accounts for most of the respiratory cycle. It can initially be set at 5 s with a usual range of 3–8 s.

T_Low: This is the time in seconds which is spent at P_Low. This is brief and titrated in such a way that intrathoracic pressure does not reach to atmospheric pressure and the lungs do not fully empty. It can initially be set at 0.5 s with usual range of 0.3–0.8 s.

It is important to remember while setting the ventilator for APRV mode, the P_ High is kept below the high inflection point (HIP) on the static pressure-volume curve (PV Curve) to avoid overdistention. P_Low is kept above the low inflection point (LIP) to avoid de-recruitment (Fig. 4). T_High is kept long enough to allow full inflation of the lungs and is indicated by no flow at end-inspiratory phase. T_ Low is brief to prevent de-recruitment but long enough to allow complete exhalation with no gas flow at the end of expiration to avoid building of intrinsic or auto-PEEP.

The physiological rationale of APRV is based on an open lung model as most of the respiratory cycle is at P_high level for the T_High duration which mimics to a continuous recruitment manoeuvre. This minimizes the stress and strain usually observed in the conventional ventilation with frequent inflation-deflation cycles. The stress is the applied force to the lungs and the strain is the resultant deformation and both are related to the initial lung volumes. In APRV, as the lungs are mostly in an open state and therefore the stress and strain are minimal. This open state with a brief release time increases the functional residual capacity (FRC) and maintains a relatively higher mean airway pressure which improves oxygenation. The Patient is allowed to breath spontaneously throughout APRV which helps in maintaining

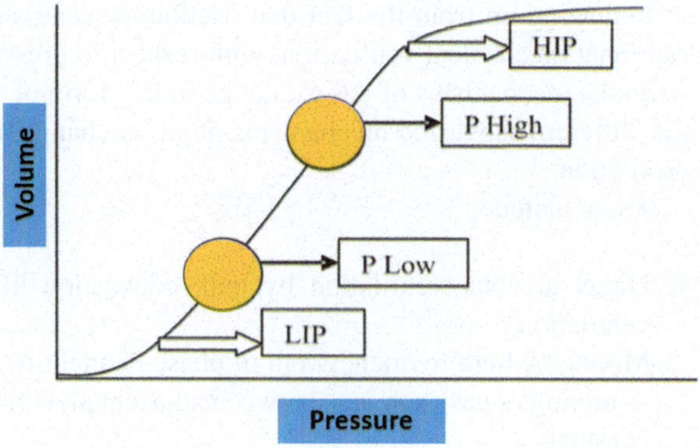

Fig. 4 Pressure–volume curve. *LIP* low inflection point, *HIP* high inflection point

respiratory muscles relatively active while requiring less sedation and less patient-ventilator asynchrony.

The physiological basis of APRV makes it a favourable mode in conditions of severe persistent hypoxemia due to a diffuse pathology like in ARDS, multifocal pneumonia, etc. It can particularly be useful in patients who are recruitable or in whom prone ventilation has failed or is contraindicated. Due to relatively lower potential of APRV for inducing or worsening lung injury, it is also potentially useful in patients whom lung-protective ventilation with low tidal volumes has failed. It is also noteworthy that APRV behaves like inverse ratio ventilation when there is no spontaneous breathing. It is a less favoured choice in patients with cardiovascular instability, right ventricular dysfunction, pulmonary hypertension, chronic lung disease, obstructive or restrictive, etc.

In short, APRV is a versatile mode of ventilation with a mechanism particularly helpful in improving oxygenation due to a homogenous lung pathology. It has relatively fewer ventilation related side effects as compared to other conventional modes of ventilation. However, it requires a relatively stable cardiovascular status of the patient and an ability to tolerate a degree of permissive hypercapnia.

7.2 High-Frequency Oscillation Ventilation (HFOV)

In contrast to conventional ventilation (CVV) where relatively large pressure and volume changes are produced to move air in and out of the lungs, High-Frequency Oscillation Ventilation (HFOV) utilizes a sustained mean airway pressure, with small oscillations, around this mean, at very high frequencies (up to 900 cycles per minute). These generate small tidal volumes which are typically less than the dead space volume. In avoiding the large pressure and volume changes of conventional ventilation, one avoids the associated forms of ventilator-induced lung injury, namely barotrauma and volutrauma. The use of sustained airway pressure allows the maintenance of recruitment, while the use of small tidal volumes is in keeping with protective ventilation. Both these principles constitute the fundamental components of an open lung strategy.

Following on from the fact that oscillatory ventilation differs vastly from conventional mechanical ventilation, with respect to pressure and flow characteristics, so do the mechanisms of gas exchange in this form of ventilation. They are at least five different suggested mechanisms of gas exchange in high-frequency oscillation ventilation.

These include:

1. Direct alveolar ventilation by bulk convection like conventional mechanical ventilation.
2. Mixing by high frequency (out of phase Pendelluft) which can also be described as mixing or gas exchange between adjacent alveoli and units with different time constants.
3. Convective change due to asymmetrical velocity profiles.
4. Taylor dispersion which is the mixing that occurs along the front of a high-velocity flow profile.
5. Molecular diffusion that occurs within alveolar units.

The primary indication of high-frequency oscillation ventilation is its use it as rescue therapy in patients with severe respiratory failure, typically caused by ARDs, who are either failing to be managed by conventional mechanical ventilation or where mechanical ventilation settings are approaching levels which have the potential to result in lung injury. High-frequency oscillation ventilation is also used as second line therapy in ventilated patients who have a bronchopleural fistula. Additionally, it is also used in the neonatal population in patients with air leaks syndromes, persistent pulmonary hypertension, and meconium aspiration.

In high-frequency oscillation ventilation, the operator set the following parameters:

- Mean airway pressure
- Frequency Hz (Oscillations per second)
- Pressure amplitude or peak to peak pressure
- Fraction of inspired oxygen

To optimize oxygenation, one can either manipulate the FiO_2 or manipulate the mean airway pressure as it is the mean airway pressure achieved which results in recruitment of alveoli and therefore oxygenation. To optimize ventilation, one adjusts the amplitude of oscillations as well as the frequency of these oscillations. Similar, to conventional mechanical ventilation, an increase in amplitude results in, an increase in tidal volume and therefore carbon dioxide clearance. However, in contrast to conventional mechanical ventilation, during high-frequency oscillation ventilation, to blow off CO_2 one must reduce the frequency of oscillations. This is explained by the operating frequency of high-frequency oscillation ventilation which is in the range of 3–15 Hz. In this range of oscillatory frequency, a reduction in frequency results in greater volume displacement and therefore tidal volume. Another parameter which is used to monitor ventilation during HFOV is the wiggle factor, which is the visually perceivable oscillatory movement of the chest wall. To ensure adequate ventilation setting are adjusted to achieve a state where this chest movement is just perceivable.

In terms of outcome data, there have been three notable studies comparing oscillation ventilation to conventional ventilation in patients with ARDS, namely the OSCILLIATE, OSCAR and RESTORE studies. These studies disappointingly produced less than favourable outcomes for patients receiving HFOV.

- OSCILLATE: This multinational trial enrolled adults with moderate to severe ARDS. Patients in the high-frequency oscillation ventilation protocol received recruitment manoeuvres and high mPAW according to the patient's severity of hypoxemia while the control group received conventional ventilation using low tidal volumes. This trial found the patients in the high-frequency oscillation group had significantly impaired hemodynamic, including cardiac output which may have worsened their overall condition. The study was stopped early due to mortality in the high-frequency oscillation group being significantly higher than in the conventional ventilation group.
- OSCAR: this UK-based trial enrolled patients with severe ARDS. A complex algorithm was used to titrate high-frequency oscillation ventilation to improve oxygenation while adjusting frequency as needed to improve CO_2 clearance. This study found no difference in mortality between the HFOV and conventional ventilation.
- RESTORE: This study found the use of HFOV in ARDS patients required an increased amount of sedation, and increased their hospital stay, hence yielding an overall negative impact on patients.

Despite the disappointing data described above high-frequency oscillation ventilation remains a potential therapeutic option as it improves oxygenation severely hypoxic ARDS patients especially in situations, where alternative approaches to improve oxygenation such as prone ventilation or extracorporeal membrane oxygenation are contraindicated or unavailable.

8 Negative Pressure Ventilation

Until the 1960s negative pressure ventilation remained a prominent modality of ventilatory support. However, with technological developments in delivering positive pressure ventilation and due to the relative cumbersome nature and complexity of the early devices used to deliver negative pressure ventilation, it was overtaken by positive pressure ventilation. This dominance of positive pressure ventilation was particularly facilitated by the successful use of positive pressure ventilation during the Poliomyelitis epidemic in the 1950s in Copenhagen where Bjorn Ibsen successfully used positive pressure ventilation to manage respiratory insufficiency in patients on a large scale.

However, with the use of modern innovations such as lightweight materials and technology advancements, his modality has seen somewhat of a resurgence of late.

The modern Cuirass ventilator consists of cuirass shell which is sealed around the patient's torso. A vacuum pump removes air from within the cuirass, creating a negative pressure environment. This negative pressure causes the chest and abdomen to expand, drawing air into the lungs during inspiration. Exhalation occurs passively as the negative pressure is released, allowing the chest and abdomen to return to their resting position. It is, however, fundamentally the same principle as the original Iron lung.

The modern Cuirass ventilator in current use is the Hayek RTX Biphasic Cuirass Ventilator (BCV) which can deliver a variety of modes of ventilation. These modes are negative pressure ventilation equivalents of positive pressure ventilation as well as some novel modes (Fig. 5).

These include the following:

1. Controlled biphasic cuirass ventilation: This is the Cuirass version of intermittent mandatory ventilation. However, the patient is still able to take spontaneous breaths between the mandatory breaths.
2. Continuous negative pressure this is akin to CPAP and can be set at any pressure below baseline and is used to enhance functional residual capacity.
3. Non-invasive synchronized Biphasic Cuirass Ventilation BCV. This mode is BCV version of synchronized intermittent mandatory ventilation (SIMV).
4. High-frequency oscillation can be applied in frequencies up to 1200 oscillations per minute to achieve oxygenation and CO_2 removal it has the added benefit of mobilizing secretions from the periphery of the lung.
5. Cardiac synchronized this is a relatively new mode of cuirass ventilation with the ability to time the ventilatory cycle to coincide with the cardiac cycle. This is done by sensing the ECG signals to drive the rate and timing of negative pressure cycles. This new mode of BCV has reported benefits in cardiac disease by

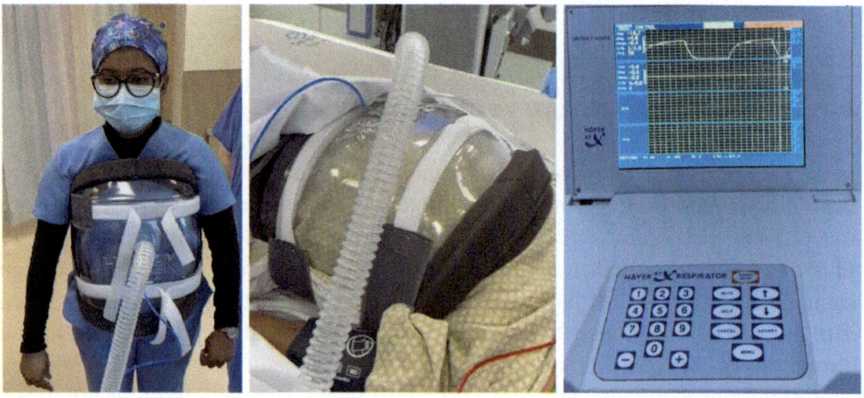

Fig. 5 Hayek RTX Biphasic Cuirass Ventilator (BCV)

enhancing cardiac output. Additionally, this has utility in cardiac imaging where movement artefacts can negatively affect cardiac imaging quality. With the use of this mode ventilatory activity can be timed to coincide with the cardiac cycle thereby decreasing motion artefact.

The modern Cuirass has several novel advantages over conventional positive ventilation and can be used in the context of acute and chronic respiratory failure as well as the perioperative and periprocedural setting.

In acute respiratory failure, it can provide respiratory support for patients with conditions such as acute respiratory distress syndrome (ARDS), pneumonia, or exacerbations of chronic obstructive pulmonary disease (COPD).

In chronic neuromuscular disorders, e.g., patients with conditions like muscular dystrophy or spinal cord injury may benefit.

In the post-operative care, BCV cuirass ventilation can be used in the post-operative period to support ventilation while minimizing the need for invasive mechanical ventilation.

With the use of the modern Cuirass ventilator, it is possible to ventilate a patient under general anaesthesia and with full neuromuscular block during airway surgery without any airway equipment such as the tracheal tube or other devices that might interfere with access to the surgical field.

BCV brings with it the advantage of being non-invasive, unlike invasive mechanical ventilation methods which require an endotracheal intubation or tracheostomy which in turn can be associated pneumonia or airway injury.

BCV cuirass enhances patient comfort by allowing patients to maintain oral communication, eat, drink, and expectorate more easily when compared to intubated patients.

Patients can remain mobile and perform activities of daily living while receiving BCV cuirass ventilation, enhancing their quality of life during ventilation therapy.

The non-invasive and comfortable nature also means that there is reduced need for sedation compared to invasive ventilation, potentially shortening ICU stays and improving patient outcomes.

The caveat to all these potential advantages is that this remains a departure from the more familiar positive pressure ventilation that clinicians are accustomed to and therefore requires additional clinician training and familiarization prior to use as well as careful patient selection and appropriate monitoring during its use.

9 High-Frequency Jet Ventilation (HFJV)

This form of ventilation was originally developed in the 1960s, as a conventional manual (not high frequency) jet ventilation technique that allowed uninterrupted patient ventilation to occur simultaneously with an unhindered surgical access throughout an open rigid bronchoscopy procedure (Fig. 6). Prior to this development, the only way to ventilate a patient undergoing rigid bronchoscopy was to temporarily withdraw instruments and stop surgery, following which the patient

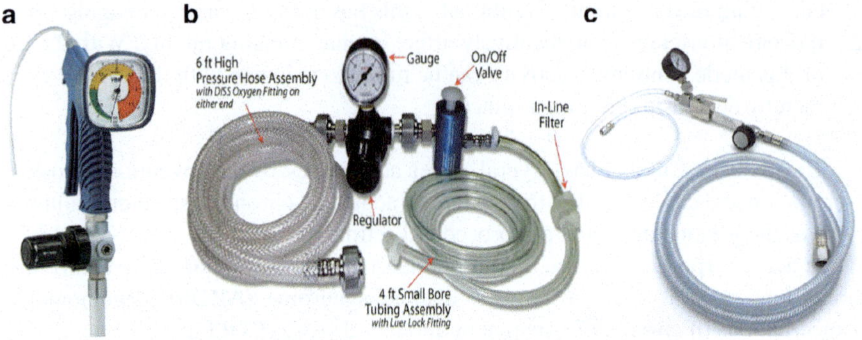

Fig. 6 (**a**) Manujet III, (**b**) Manual jet ventilator, (**c**) Sanders' injector

was manually ventilated through the side port of the bronchoscope while the surgeon occluded the proximal end with a thumb. The first version of this jet ventilation consisted of an adapter attached to the proximal end of the bronchoscope and connected to an oxygen supply by means of a pressure regulator and a handheld on/ off valve that allowed control of frequency of ventilation. The oxygen was delivered at high pressure, 50 lb. per square inch, in a jet through a nozzle inside the lumen of the bronchoscope and parallel to its long axis. The basic principle is that each jet of oxygen entrains air into the bronchoscope contributing to the tidal volume and each successive pause between the jet delivery allows passive expiration.

Subsequently this was developed into a ventilatory modality in the 1970s, capable of being delivered via an automated system. A HFJ ventilator incorporates a gas source with jet generator and control systems to regulate frequency, inspiratory time, and other parameters. Ventilation is delivered via small-diameter catheter or endotracheal tube inserted into the airway to deliver the gas jets directly into the trachea or main bronchi (Fig. 7).

The mechanisms of gas exchange in HFJV include amongst others, convective ventilation or bulk flow (i.e., the mass flow of gases into and out of the lung) in a similar manner to spontaneous respiration.

However, convectional rules for bulk flow do not apply at these high frequencies and therefore cannot ensure adequate ventilation via this mechanism and hence other mechanisms must come into play.

These include laminar flow which occurs in small airways where Reynolds number is low and the consequent velocity profile of airflow is parabolic, where air closest to the wall of the airway has a lower velocity than air in the centre of the airway. The difference in flow rates becomes more exaggerated with each breath such that HFJV produces a spike of rapidly moving gas travelling down the axis of the airway, while gas in the margins moves out of the lung.

Further mixing of air occurs by Taylor-type dispersion also known as enhanced molecular diffusion. This is the result of the interaction of the axial parabolic velocity profile seen in laminar flow and the radial concentration gradient producing

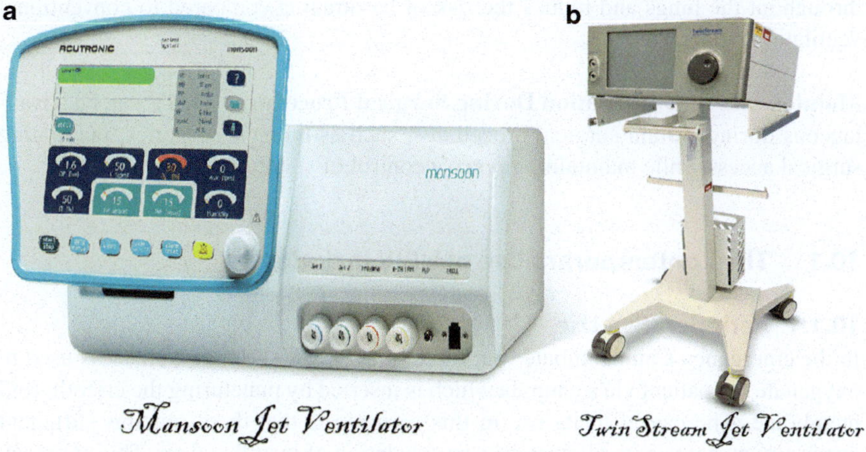

Fig. 7 Automatic jet ventilator; (**a**) Mansoon, Accutronic Medical Systems AG in Baar, Switzerland). (**b**) Superimposed high-frequency jet ventilation. (TwinStream, Carl Reiner GMBH, Vienna, Austria)

further mixing of gases. In larger airways, where flow is turbulent, eddies produced by the turbulence precede the bulk flow and produce a similar radial-mixing effect.

Pendelluft, or collateral ventilation, occurs because of regional variation in airway resistance and compliance causing some areas of the lung to fill or empty more rapidly than others. Such variation in time constants (resistance × compliance) leads to a phase lag between neighbouring lung units and causes gas to flow from one alveolus to another. This effect is exaggerated by high-frequency breaths and facilitated by the higher mean airway pressures seen in HFJV leading to extensive pendelluft with recirculation of gas between regions. This results in smaller gas volumes effectively reaching more respiratory units than similar volumes generated during conventional ventilation. Other mechanisms that may contribute to gas exchange during HFJV are molecular diffusion and cardiogenic mixing which occurs as a result of mechanical agitation of lung units in close proximity to the heart.

10 The Main Benefits of HFJV Include

Improved Gas Exchange: Delivering small, high-velocity gas jets into the airway jets create oscillations within the airspaces, enhancing ventilation and oxygenation of the lungs. This can be particularly beneficial in conditions such as acute respiratory distress syndrome (ARDS).

Lung Protection HFJV may have lung-protective effects by minimizing alveolar overdistension and reducing the risk of ventilator-induced lung injury. The small-volume, high-frequency nature of HFJV may help distribute ventilation more evenly throughout the lungs and reduce the risk of barotrauma compared to conventional ventilation strategies.

Maintenance of Oxygenation During Surgical Procedures HFJV can be advantageous during certain surgical procedures, such as thoracic surgeries, facilitating surgical access while maintaining precise control of ventilation.

10.1 The Contemporary Use of HFJV Includes

10.1.1 Perioperative Use

In the emergency Can't Intubate Can't Ventilate (CICV) scenario, HFJV is used to oxygenate the patient via a cannula which is inserted by puncturing the cricothyroid membrane. The caveat to its use in this scenario is that there remains sufficient upper airway patency to allow egress or exhalation of insufflated air. This approach has largely been superseded by the promotion of the open surgical front of neck access approach to these airway emergencies in modern CICV algorithms.

The elective use of jet ventilation includes management of the anticipated difficult airway where pre-emptive placement of a transtracheal jet cannula may be used, as well as direct laryngoscopy, and vocal cord surgery where unimpeded access the larynx and vocal cord is required. Furthermore, HFJV is utilized in major airway surgery such as carinal resections, resection of tracheal stenosis, and tracheal reconstruction as well as thoracic surgery.

As HFJV employs an open breathing system (there is no need for an airtight connection between the airway and the breathing system), the trachea can be open while still maintaining ventilation. HFJV also has the added benefit in that the degree of bronchial and mediastinal excursion is minimal when compared with conventional ventilation thereby improving surgical conditions. The relatively fine jet catheter can be passed through the surgical field and manipulated by the surgeon during the operation. This allows the surgeon to bridge the airway defect with the catheter and airway resection and end-to-end anastomosis can be accomplished around the relatively fine catheter.

In thoracic surgery, during single lung ventilation, HFJV is applied to the non-dependent in order to aid CO_2 elimination and improve oxygenation thereby reducing the ventilatory stresses on the dependent lung. Furthermore, HFJV is utilized in the management of bronchopleural fistulae and tracheo-bronchial tree disruptions where HFJV results in a smaller gas leak through pathological low-resistance pathways, because peak and mean airway pressures are smaller than with conventional positive pressure ventilation.

10.1.2 Intensive Care

In the management of patients with acute respiratory distress syndrome (ARDS), ventilator associated lung injury (VALI) is associated with increased morbidity.

HFJV may have lung-protective effects in these patients by minimizing alveolar overdistension and reducing the risk of ventilator-induced lung injury. The small-volume, high-frequency nature of HFJV may help distribute ventilation more evenly throughout the lungs and reduce the risk of barotrauma compared to conventional ventilation strategies.

In being a rather unconventional mode of ventilation special attention need to be paid to,

staff training in the setup, operation, and troubleshooting of HFJV equipment to ensure safe and effective use. An additional factor is the inability to monitor End-tidal CO_2 levels requiring alternative strategies to achieve this.

Patient selection, HFJV may not be suitable for all patients, and therefore careful consideration of individual patient factors and clinical indications are necessary before initiating therapy.

11 Continuous Positive Airway Pressure (CPAP) and Automatic Positive Airway Pressure (APAP) and Bilevel Positive Airway Pressure (BIPAP)

These are treatment options primarily used for obstructive sleep apnoea (OSA), where they provide positive airway pressure therapy, aimed at keeping the airway open during sleep to prevent episodes of apnoea and hence the associated symptoms such as snoring and daytime fatigue. While (APAP) in used exclusively for this indication, CPAP and BiPAP are also additionally used as a forms of respiratory therapy in the acute hospital setting.

11.1 Continuous Positive Airway Pressure (CPAP)

CPAP therapy involves delivering a flow of air through a mask worn over the nose or both the nose and mouth to provide a constant positive airway pressure throughout all phases of respiration. This continuous airflow acts as a pneumatic splint, preventing the collapse of the airway.

11.2 Automatic Positive Airway Pressure (APAP)

APAP, also known as Auto CPAP, varies the air pressure automatically in response to the individual's changing breathing patterns. APAP machines are equipped with algorithms that monitor breathing and adjust the air pressure in real time based on the severity of airway obstruction detected. Unlike CPAP, APAP machines have a prescribed pressure range rather than a fixed pressure setting. The machine adjusts the pressure within this range as needed, providing the minimum necessary pressure to maintain airway patency.

APAP machines can be beneficial for patients with varying degrees of airway obstruction as well as those who experience positional changes that affect their breathing during sleep. APAP offers the advantage of automatic adjustment, potentially increasing comfort, and compliance for some patients.

11.3 Bilevel Positive Airway Pressure (BiPAP)

BiPAP delivers two different levels of airway pressure: a higher pressure when the individual inhales (inspiratory positive airway pressure, IPAP) and a lower pressure when they exhale (expiratory positive airway pressure, EPAP).

This dual-pressure system can be more comfortable for some patients and may be better tolerated by those who have difficulty exhaling against a continuous pressure, as with CPAP.

BiPAP is commonly prescribed for individuals with certain types of sleep-disordered breathing, such as central sleep apnoea (CSA) as well as for those who require higher pressures to maintain airway patency.

12 Conclusion

The modern modes of ventilation represent a continuous spectrum of the evolution of mechanical ventilation. This evolution is driven both by our understanding of respiratory physiology as well as technological advancements in ventilators. While it is somewhat disappointing that there is a paucity of evidence that these newer modes of ventilator have resulted in clear benefits in terms patient outcomes such as an improvement in mortality, the overall trajectory of progress has resulted in improvement in multiple aspects of ventilator use.

In this this search for optimal ventilation strategies the advent of flow-controlled ventilation (FCV) represents one such advancement and as such, a paradigm shift in respiratory therapy. As opposed to conventional ventilators which rely on active inspiration to deliver tidal volume and a passive expiratory phase, flow-controlled ventilators employ active processes for both inspiration and expiration.

In chapter "The Respiratory Physics and Mechanics of Flow-Controlled Ventilation", we embark on a comprehensive exploration of flow-controlled ventilation including an understanding of the physical principles involved as well as clinical applications of this novel mode of mechanical ventilation.

Bibliography

1. van der Staay M, Chatburn RL. Advanced modes of mechanical ventilation and optimal targeting schemes. ICMx. 2018;6:30. https://doi.org/10.1186/s40635-018-0195-0.
2. Singh PM, Borle A, Trikha A. Newer nonconventional modes of mechanical ventilation. J Emerg Trauma Shock. 2014;7(3):222–7. https://doi.org/10.4103/0974-2700.136869.
3. Jackson CD, et al. Mechanical ventilation. 2020; https://emedicine.medscape.com/article/304068-overview#a1
4. Swindin J, Sampson C, Howatson A. Airway pressure release ventilation. BJA Educ. 2020;20(3):80–8. https://doi.org/10.1016/j.bjae.2019.12.001. Epub 2020 Jan 23. PMID: 33456934; PMCID: PMC7808079
5. Daoud EG. Airway pressure release ventilation. Ann Thorac Med. 2007;2(4):176–9. https://doi.org/10.4103/1817-1737.36556. PMID: 19727373; PMCID: PMC2732103

6. Barbas CSV, Nogueira Nemer S. Advanced modes of mechanical ventilation. Mechanical Ventilation; 2022. IntechOpen Available at https://doi.org/10.5772/intechopen.100283.e.
7. Ambrosino N. Rossi AProportional assist ventilation (PAV): a significant advance or a futile struggle between logic and practice? Thorax. 2002;57:272–6.
8. Sinderby C, Navalesi P, Beck J, Skrobik Y, Comtois N, Friberg S, Gottfried SB, Lindström L. Neural control of mechanical ventilation in respiratory failure. Nat Med. 1999;5(12):1433–6. [PubMed] [Reference list]
9. Ferrer M, Pelosi P. New developments in mechanical ventilation. European Respiratory Society; 2012, p 217–28.
10. Hidalgo J, Hyzy RC, Taha AMR, Tolba YYA. Personalized mechanical ventilation. Cham: Springer; 2022. p. 65–82.
11. Lellouche F, Mancebo J, Jolliet P, et al. A multicenter randomized trial of computer-driven protocolized weaning from mechanical ventilation. Am J Respir Crit Care Med. 2006;174:894–900.
12. Rose L, Presneill JJ, Johnston L, et al. A randomised, controlled trial of conventional versus automated weaning from mechanical ventilation using SmartCare/PS. Intensive Care Med. 2008;34:1788–95.
13. Burns KE, Meade MO, Lessard MR, et al. Wean earlier and automatically with new technology (the WEAN study): a protocol of a multicentre, pilot randomized controlled trial. Trials. 2009;10:81.
14. Morato JB, Sakuma MT, Ferreira JC, Caruso P. Comparison of 3 modes of automated weaning from mechanical ventilation: a bench study. J Crit Care. 2012;27(6):741.e1–8. https://doi.org/10.1016/j.jcrc.2011.12.021. Epub 2012 Mar 28. PMID: 22459160
15. Mohamed KAE, El Maraghi SK. Role of adaptive support ventilation in weaning of COPD patients. Egypt J Chest Dis Tuberc. 2014;63(2):449. https://doi.org/10.1016/j.ejcdt.2013.12.017.
16. Gruber PC, Gomersall CD, Leung P, Joynt GM, Ng SK, Ho KM, Underwood MJ. Randomized controlled trial comparing adaptive-support ventilation with pressure-regulated volume-controlled ventilation with automode in weaning patients after cardiac surgery. Anesthesiology. 2008;109(1):81–7. https://doi.org/10.1097/ALN.0b013e31817881fc. PMID: 18580176
17. Agarwal R, Srinivasan A, Aggarwal AN, Gupta D. Adaptive support ventilation for complete ventilatory support in acute respiratory distress syndrome: a pilot, randomized controlled trial. Respirology. 2013;18(7):1108–15. https://doi.org/10.1111/resp.12126. PMID: 23711230
18. Buiteman-Kruizinga LA, Mkadmi HE, Schultz MJ, Tangkau PL, van der Heiden PLJ. Comparison of mechanical power during adaptive support ventilation versus nonautomated pressure-controlled ventilation-a pilot study. Crit Care Explor. 2021;3(2):e0335. https://doi.org/10.1097/CCE.0000000000000335. PMID: 33604578; PMCID: PMC7886404
19. Meyers M, Rodrigues N, Ari A. High-frequency oscillatory ventilation: a narrative review. Can J Respir Ther. 2019;55:40–6. https://doi.org/10.29390/cjrt-2019-004. PMID: 31297448; PMCID: PMC6591785
20. Bouchut J-C, Godard J, Claris O, Weiskopf RB. High-frequency oscillatory ventilation. Anesthesiology. 2004;100:1007–12. https://doi.org/10.1097/00000542-200404000-00035.
21. Kristensen MS, Hesselfeldt R, Schmidt JF. Modern cuirass ventilation for airway surgery: unlimited access to the larynx and trachea in anaesthetised patients. Br J Anaesth. 2023;131(4):e106–9. https://doi.org/10.1016/j.bja.2023.07.010. Epub 2023 Aug 14. PMID: 37587006
22. Linton D. Cuirass ventilation: a review and update. Crit Care Resusc: Journal of the Australasian Academy of Critical Care Medicine. 2005;7:22–8. https://doi.org/10.1016/S1441-2772(23)01566-1.
23. Evans E, Biro P, Bedforth N. Jet ventilation. Continuing Education Anaesthesia Crit Care Pain. 2007;7(1):2–5. https://doi.org/10.1093/bjaceaccp/mkl061.
24. Lee KB, Lee W. Titration of positive airway pressure therapy for adults with obstructive sleep apnea. In: Connor RF, editor. UpToDate. Wolters Kluwer. Accessed on May 6, 2024.

The Respiratory Physics and Mechanics of Flow-Controlled Ventilation

Aneesha Thankamony, Shakeel Moideen, Anas N. Shallik, Regan B. Lloyd, Hany A. Zaki, and Nabil A. Shallik

1 Introduction

Understanding respiratory physiology and respiratory mechanics in mechanical ventilation by any mode is crucial for various reasons. It helps optimize patient care and improve outcomes. It is essential to refresh one's understanding of this science when embarking on a newer mode of ventilation for the following reasons:

1. Optimizing ventilatory settings: knowledge of respiratory mechanics allows clinicians to tailor ventilator settings to the individual needs of the patient. By understanding parameters such as compliance, resistance, and airway

A. Thankamony · S. Moideen
Anaesthesia, ICU and Perioperative Medicine Department, Hamad Medical Corporation, Doha, Qatar
e-mail: Athankamony@hamad.qa; smoideen@hamad.qa

A. N. Shallik
Royal College of Surgeons in Ireland Medical University of Bahrain, Manamah, Bahrain

R. B. Lloyd
Emergency Medicine, Aster hospital, Doha, Qatar

H. A. Zaki
Emergency Medicine, Hamad General Hospital, Doha, Qatar

N. A. Shallik (✉)
Anaesthesia, ICU and Perioperative Medicine Department, Hamad Medical Corporation, Doha, Qatar

Clinical Anaesthesiology Department, Weill Cornell Medical College in Qatar, Doha, Qatar

Clinical Anaesthesiology Department, College of Medicine Qatar University, Doha, Qatar

Anaesthesia and SICU Department, Tanta University, Tanta, Egypt
e-mail: nshallik@hamad.qa

N. A. Shallik (ed.), *Flow Controlled Ventilation Mode Through a Straw Size Tube*, https://doi.org/10.1007/978-3-031-77477-5_5

pressures, ventilator settings can be adjusted to ensure adequate ventilation and oxygenation while minimizing the risk of ventilator-induced lung injury (VILI).
2. Understanding synchrony between the patient and the ventilator: Understanding respiratory mechanics is essential for recognizing and managing asynchronies between the patient and the ventilator. Patient-ventilator asynchrony can lead to increased work of breathing, discomfort, and potentially prolonged mechanical ventilation. Identifying the underlying mechanics can guide adjustments in ventilator settings to improve synchrony.
3. Management of specific conditions: In conditions like acute respiratory distress syndrome (ARDS), where lung mechanics are significantly altered, a deep understanding of respiratory mechanics is vital. It guides the application of lung-protective ventilation strategies, such as the use of lower tidal volumes and higher positive end-expiratory pressure (PEEP), to improve gas exchange and reduce the risk of further lung injury [1].
4. Monitoring disease progression or response: Changes in respiratory mechanics can indicate the progression of lung disease or the response to therapeutic interventions. Regular assessment of these mechanics can help in timely decision-making regarding the escalation or de-escalation of support [2].
5. Prevention of iatrogenic injury and VILI: Understanding respiratory mechanics and physiology is critical to help avoid strategies that lead to overdistension or repetitive opening and closing of alveoli, both of which are risk factors for VILI. This includes the judicious use of tidal volume, PEEP, and understanding the implications of driving pressure.
6. Educational value: A thorough understanding of respiratory mechanics is not only essential for clinical practise but also for the education of healthcare professionals. It forms the basis for research into new ventilation strategies and technologies aimed at improving patient outcomes.

Flow-controlled ventilation (FCV) represents a significant advancement in the landscape of mechanical ventilation, offering a novel approach to managing patients undergoing general anaesthesia and supporting patients with respiratory failure. Unlike traditional modes of ventilation that primarily focus on pressure or volume control, FCV emphasizes the regulation of flow to optimize gas exchange and reduce the potential for ventilator-induced lung injury.

Flow-controlled ventilation represents a promising advancement in mechanical ventilation, offering potential benefits in terms of gas exchange, lung protection, and patient comfort [3]. Its relevance in clinical settings is increasingly recognized, particularly for managing patients with complex respiratory conditions where traditional ventilation strategies may fall short [4]. As research and clinical experience with FCV continue to grow, it is poised to become an integral part of the ventilatory management arsenal, offering a more tailored and physiologically sound approach to respiratory support.

2 Fundamentals of Respiratory Mechanics

The basic principles of lung mechanics, which are crucial for understanding respiratory physiology and the management of patients requiring mechanical ventilation, include compliance, resistance, and elasticity. These principles are fundamental to the assessment of lung function and the optimization of ventilatory support.

Compliance refers to the lung's ability to stretch and expand in response to applied pressure. It is defined as the change in lung volume per unit change in transpulmonary pressure (the difference between the pressure inside the lungs and the pressure in the pleural space). High compliance indicates that the lungs can easily expand, as seen in conditions like emphysema where the lung tissue loses elasticity. Low compliance suggests stiff lungs, which require more force to expand, as observed in conditions such as acute respiratory distress syndrome (ARDS) or pulmonary fibrosis. Compliance is influenced by the elastic properties of the lung and chest wall and can be affected by factors such as lung volume, age, and disease states [5].

Resistance in lung mechanics refers to the opposition to airflow within the respiratory system. It is primarily determined by the diameter of the airways and is influenced by both the airway's intrinsic properties and the dynamic changes that occur during breathing, such as bronchoconstriction or bronchodilation. High resistance is encountered in conditions like asthma or chronic obstructive pulmonary disease (COPD), where airway narrowing or obstruction increases the effort required to move air in and out of the lungs. The measurement of resistance helps in assessing the work of breathing and is critical in managing patients with obstructive lung diseases [6].

Elasticity describes the lung's tendency to return to its original size after being stretched or filled with air. It is a property that allows the lungs to recoil during exhalation, aiding in the expulsion of air. Elastic forces in the lung are provided by the elastic fibres in the lung parenchyma and the surface tension at the air–liquid interface within the alveoli. Surfactant, a substance produced by the alveolar cells, plays a crucial role in reducing surface tension, thereby increasing lung compliance and decreasing the work of breathing. Loss of elasticity, as seen in emphysema, leads to difficulty in expelling air and results in hyperinflation of the lungs.

Airflow through the respiratory system can be either laminar or turbulent, depending on the velocity of airflow and the characteristics of the airways. Laminar flow, which is smooth and orderly, typically occurs in the smaller airways, while turbulent flow, which is chaotic, occurs in the larger airways and during high-velocity airflow. Turbulence increases airway resistance and the work of breathing [7].

3 Flow-Controlled Ventilation: Concept and Principles

Flow-controlled ventilation (FCV) is a mode of mechanical ventilation where the primary controlled variable is the flow of gas into (and with newer devices, out of) the patient's lungs. This mode ensures a constant flow throughout the inspiratory (and expiratory) phase, potentially leading to a more uniform distribution of gas and improved alveolar ventilation. The concept behind FCV is to enhance the synchrony between the ventilator and the patient's respiratory efforts, thereby improving the efficiency of gas exchange and reducing the work of breathing [8].

It is important to understand the impact of the chosen mode of ventilation on lung mechanics. Conventional modes like volume-controlled ventilation (VCV) can lead to higher peak airway pressures, especially in the presence of decreased lung compliance or increased airway resistance, potentially increasing the risk of lung injury. Pressure-controlled ventilation limits the maximum pressure exerted on the lungs, reducing the risk of barotrauma but may result in variable tidal volumes, especially if lung mechanics change. Flow-controlled ventilation aims to optimize lung mechanics by ensuring a steady flow, potentially reducing peak airway pressures and improving alveolar ventilation. Therefore, potential benefits of FCV over conventional modes include improved oxygenation and ventilation efficiency as the constant inspiratory flow and controlled expiration can lead to a more uniform and efficient gas exchange, and reduced risk of ventilator-induced lung injury (VILI) by avoiding high peak inspiratory pressures and controlling expiratory flow [9].

The core principles governing FCV include the delivery of a constant inspiratory flow and the innovative management of expiration, through techniques that enhance expiratory flow control:

Constant Inspiratory Flow FCV delivers a constant flow of gas during the inspiratory phase. This constant flow is designed to improve gas exchange by ensuring a more uniform distribution of gas within the lungs. Unlike volume-controlled ventilation (VCV), which focuses on delivering a set volume, or pressure-controlled ventilation (PCV), which delivers gas until a certain pressure is reached, FCV's constant flow aims to maintain optimal gas distribution and lung recruitment throughout the entire inspiratory phase [10].

Enhanced Expiratory Flow Control FCV systems incorporate mechanisms to control expiratory flow. This technique can help in maintaining lung recruitment by preventing rapid de-recruitment that can occur with uncontrolled expiration [11].

Utilization of the Bernoulli Principle In FCV systems, the Bernoulli principle is exploited to facilitate expiration. A flow reversal device generates a negative pressure at the ventilator side of the endotracheal tube, effectively sucking gas out and aiding in the removal of CO_2. This principle is used to enhance the efficiency of gas exchange and to support the active control of expiratory flow.

4 Mechanics of Flow-Controlled Ventilation

Flow-controlled ventilation influences respiratory mechanics in several ways:

1. *Improved Alveolar Ventilation*: By providing a constant flow, FCV enhances the distribution of gas within the lungs. This leads to more uniform alveolar ventilation, improving gas exchange efficiency and reducing areas of ventilation-perfusion mismatch [12].
2. *Reduced Peak Airway Pressures*: FCV helps in minimizing peak airway pressures compared to traditional volume-controlled ventilation (VCV) or pressure-controlled ventilation (PCV). Since the flow is constant and can be adjusted to a lower rate, the build-up of pressure within the airways can be moderated, which is particularly beneficial in patients with compromised lung mechanics [13].
3. *Enhanced Patient-Ventilator Synchrony*: The constant flow characteristic of FCV improves synchrony between the patient and the ventilator. This is because the flow can be more closely matched to the patient's spontaneous breathing efforts, reducing the work of breathing and potentially decreasing the need for sedation [8].
4. *Impact on Respiratory Pattern*: FCV influences the respiratory pattern by allowing for a more physiological breathing cycle. Since the flow is constant, the inspiratory phase can be more closely aligned with the patient's natural inspiratory effort, potentially leading to a more comfortable and effective ventilation experience [12, 14].
5. *Lung Protection*: By avoiding high peak pressures and providing a more even distribution of ventilation, FCV may offer protective benefits against ventilator-induced lung injury (VILI). This is particularly relevant in patients with acute respiratory distress syndrome (ARDS) or other conditions characterized by fragile lung parenchyma.
6. *Adaptability to Patient Needs*: FCV allows for adjustments in flow to meet the specific respiratory mechanics and needs of the patient. This adaptability can be crucial in managing patients with varying degrees of lung compliance and resistance, ensuring that ventilation is both effective and minimally invasive.

The physics of flow-controlled mechanical ventilation (FCV) is fundamentally about managing the flow of gas into the patient's lungs in a way that optimizes ventilation while minimizing potential harm. This approach contrasts with traditional methods that focus primarily on controlling pressure or volume.

5 Physics of Flow-Controlled Ventilation

The key physical principles underlying FCV are as follows:

A. Constant Flow Delivery FCV delivers a constant flow of gas throughout the inspiratory phase. This constant flow is crucial for ensuring a steady and predictable gas delivery, which can lead to more uniform lung inflation. The physics behind this involves understanding how gas moves and distributes within the lung's complex structures and how a constant flow can promote more efficient gas exchange by reducing dead space ventilation and improving alveolar ventilation.

FCV can also incorporate constant negative expiratory flow (Fig. 1). It is important to note that in FCV the minute volume cannot be controlled by adjusting the tidal volumes or the respiratory rate. In fact, when the inspiration to expiration (I:E) ratio is set to 1:1, the minute volume is always half of the set flow. The respiratory rate, on the other hand, depends on the peak inspiratory pressure, the positive end-expiratory pressure (PEEP) that has been set, the inspiratory flow rate and the I:E ratio. It also depends on the compliance of the patient's lungs.

B. Pressure–Volume Relationships (PV loops) During flow-controlled ventilation (FCV), the respiratory system's pressure–volume relationship is influenced by the constant flow rate. In contrast to volume-controlled ventilation, where pressure

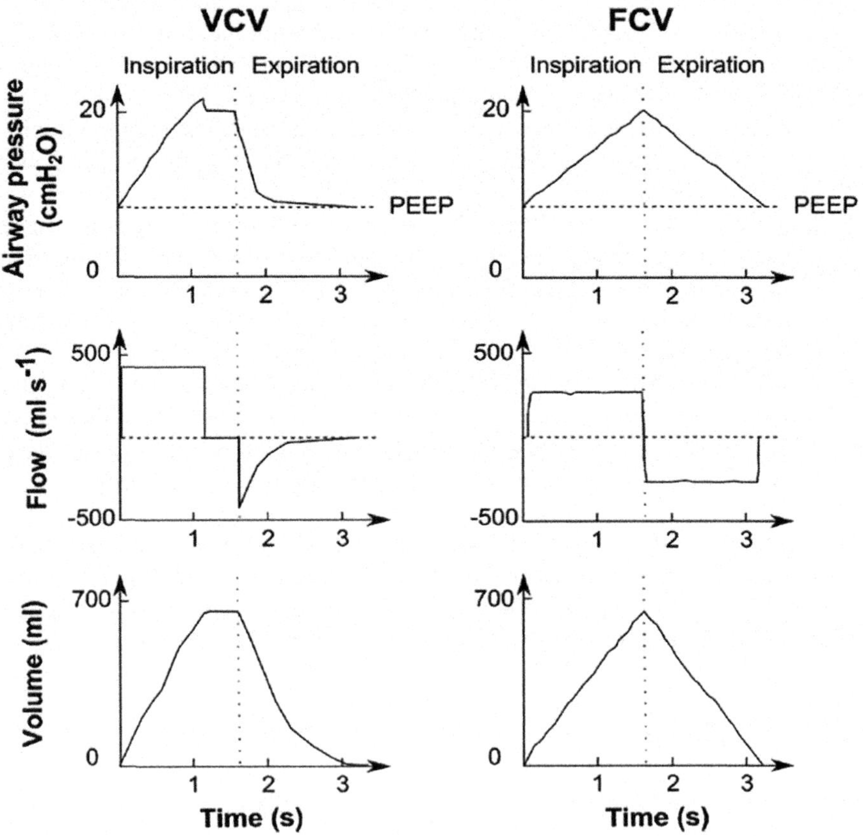

Fig. 1 Comparison of volume, flow, and pressure graphs during inspiration and expiration, during flow-controlled ventilation (with constant negative flow expiration) and conventional volume-controlled ventilation

fluctuates to deliver a predetermined volume, or pressure-controlled ventilation, where the delivered volume varies according to a set pressure, FCV seeks to strike a balance between these dynamics by maintaining a constant flow rate. This approach results in a more linear increase in pressure during inspiration, effectively reducing peak inspiratory pressures and the associated risk of barotrauma.

Idealized PV loops, shown in Fig. 2, represent a system consisting of a compliant reservoir (representing the lung) fed via a resistance (akin to the airway resistance). The pressure at the circuit end of the airway resistance is the pressure represented in this plot.

The PV loop of PCV is shown in Fig. 2 in red. In this mode, the pressure applied to the proximal end of the circuit alternates between the plateau pressure (P_{plat}) during inspiration and the positive end-expiratory pressure (PEEP) during expiration. The flow rate varies substantially, exhibiting highly dynamic behaviour, and is not truly controlled in either phase. This results in a characteristic pressure–volume loop. The horizontal (pressure) deviation of the plot from the static compliance curve connecting the PEEP and P_{plat} is related to the airway resistance and the flow rate. The (decelerating) flow rate is very high (typically greater than 40 l/min) immediately after the start of both inspiration and expiration phases, and consequently, the pressure deviations from the static compliance curve are most pronounced during these periods.

The PV loop in blue shown in Fig. 2 represents one that would be generated for the same patient using the VCV mode. In this mode, the flow rate is controlled and maintained at a constant value throughout the majority of the inspiration phase (until the set tidal volume is delivered, followed by a plateau pressure phase with minimal flow). However, during expiration, the flow rate is uncontrolled. The inspiratory flow rate is substantially lower than the peak flow observed in

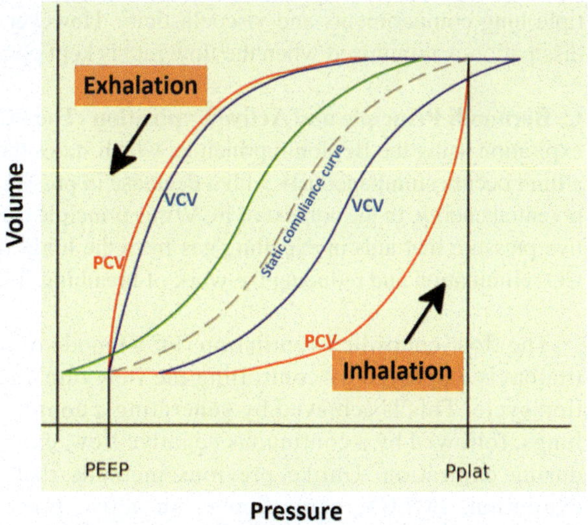

Fig. 2 Idealized PV loops during PCV (red), VCV (blue), and FCV (blue line for inspiration and green line for expiration). The dashed line represents the static compliance curve (of the chest and lungs), and the enclosed area of each loop is the dissipated energy

pressure-controlled ventilation (PCV), resulting in a constant pressure difference between the airway pressure and the static compliance curve (joining PEEP and P_{plat}) throughout inspiration. This manifests as a horizontal displacement of the inspiratory portion of the curve to the right, relative to the static compliance curve.

In both volume-controlled ventilation (VCV) and pressure-controlled ventilation (PCV), the energy dissipated within the patient per respiratory cycle is proportional to the area of hysteresis on the pressure–volume (PV) loop. Given the same positive end-expiratory pressure (PEEP), plateau pressure (P_{plat}), and respiratory rate, the energy dissipated during VCV is lower than that during PCV. The energy dissipation during the inspiration phase is minimized when the flow rate is maintained as a constant throughout the inspiratory period [15].

It is evident that energy dissipation can be further reduced by controlling the flow rate to remain constant during expiration as well, thereby minimizing the energy dissipated within the patient during this phase too. This modification would alter the expiratory portion of the pressure–volume (PV) loop in volume-controlled ventilation (VCV) to the shape depicted by the green trace. This curve is analogous to the optimal curve achievable during inspiration under VCV, but with the pressure on the lower side of the static compliance curve due to the reversal in the direction of flow.

If the flow rate is controlled during both inspiration and expiration, the overall lowest flow (and consequently the lowest overall energy dissipation) for a given minute volume is achieved, provided that the inspiratory and expiratory flow rates are equal. For a respiratory exchange ratio (RER) of unity, the inspiratory-to-expiratory (I:E) ratio necessarily becomes 1:1. It is worth noting that the RER has only a minor effect on the optimal I:E ratio. For instance, if oxygen uptake is 300 ml/min and carbon dioxide release is 210 ml/min (an RER of 0.7), the total expiratory volume over 1 min would be only 90 ml/min less than the inspiratory volume over 1 min. This difference is very small compared to typical minute volumes of 5 or 6 l/min. It is crucial to emphasize that the pressure–volume (PV) loops in Fig. 2 are for illustrative purposes only. Their detailed shape is influenced by the effects of multiple lung compartments and viscoelasticity. However, the conclusion that energy dissipation is minimized when the flow rate is kept constant remains valid [15].

C. Bernoulli Principle and Active Expiration The FCV system incorporate active expiration using the Bernoulli principle, which states that an increase in the speed of a fluid occurs simultaneously with a decrease in pressure or a decrease in the fluid's potential energy. In the context of FCV, this principle can be applied to create a negative pressure that aids in expelling gas from the lungs during expiration, enhancing CO_2 elimination and reducing the work of breathing (Figs. 3 and 4) [16].

The flow-controlled ventilation (FCV) mode of newer flow-controlled ventilators is employed by controlling the flow rate throughout the entire ventilation cycle. This is achieved by generating a continuous flow into the patient's lungs, followed by a continuous negative flow, extracting gases from the lungs during expiration. Unlike previous methods that applied resistance during expiration, in FCV, expiration is an active process. To efficiently control

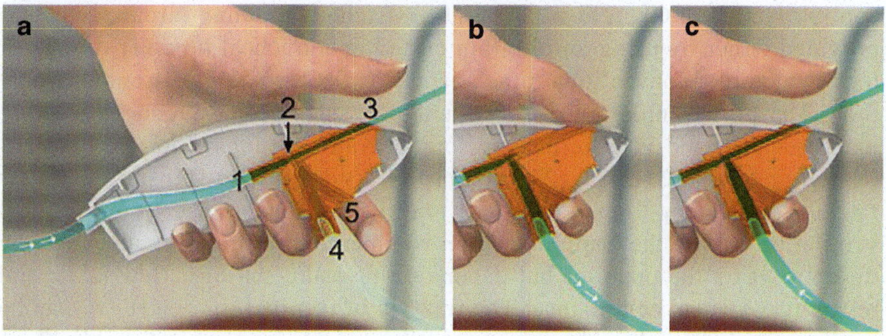

Fig. 3 The working mechanism of Ventrain® (Ventinova Medical BV, Eindhoven, The Netherlands) that uses the Bernoulli Principle for active expiration [16]. (**a**) High pressure oxygen inlet (1), the flow of oxygen is accelerated by a narrowing nozzle (2) and exits the device (Ventrain®) (3), creating a sub-atmospheric pressure at port (4). This outlet (4) is connecting to a small-bore lumen inside the patient's airway. A bypass port (5) is designed as an air inlet and will activate the device when this port is closed. (**b**) Closing port (3) creates an insufflation via (4). (**c**) Opening port (3) creates exhalation. (With written permission from Ventinova Medical, Eindhoven, the Netherlands)

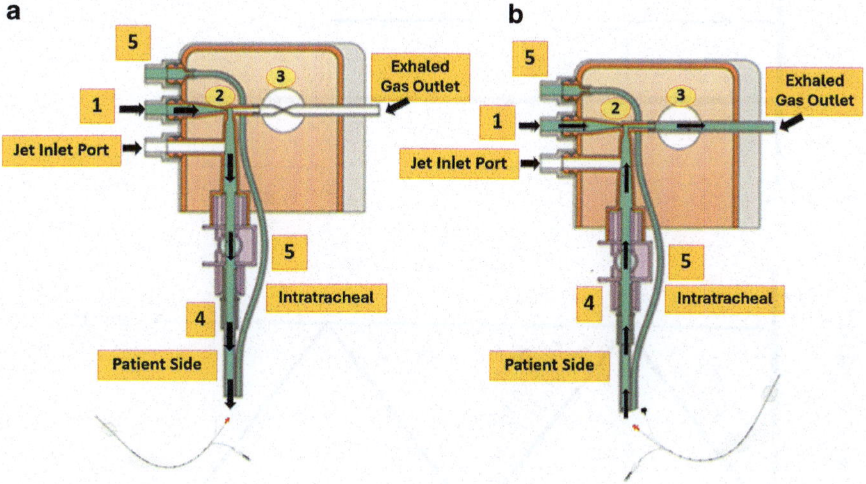

Fig. 4 Schematic representation of Evone® cartridge or flow-controlled ventilator (FCV) cartridge. 1 = gas inlet. 2 = narrow jet nozzle, 3 = exhaust pipe, 4 = port towards (inspiration) and from (expiration) Tritube® and patient. These components are equivalent to those depicted in Fig. 3 (schematic representation of Ventrain®) and represented by the same numbers. 5 = port for continuous intratracheal pressure measurement. (**a**): Closure of the exhaust pipe (3) leads to inspiration (gas flows from 1, via 2 to 4). (**b**): After opening of the exhaust pipe (3), driving gas flows through the jet nozzle (2) and exhaust pipe (3) to the outside. By Bernoulli's principle the flow entrains gas from the patient through port (4). (Courtesy of Dr. Nabil Shallik)

expiratory flow, FCV relies on a high-resistance breathing circuit, which is provided either by using an ultrathin cuffed endotracheal tube (Tritube®) or by connecting a conventional tube adapter (CTA®) to a regular endotracheal tube. The FCV ventilation cycle depends on accurate intratracheal pressure measurements and is governed by four operator settings (Fig. 5): (1) end-expiratory pressure (EEP), (2) peak inspiratory pressure, (3) inspiratory flow rate, (4) inspiratory-to-expiratory (I:E) ratio. Thus, in contrast to conventional ventilation modes, the inspiratory tidal volumes and respiratory rate cannot be directly set by the operator but depend on pressure settings, flow rates, and respiratory system compliance. The fraction of inspired oxygen (F_iO_2) can be set directly. FCV is based on a constant inspiratory and expiratory gas flow, whereby the desired ventilation pressures (PEEP and Peak) are pre-set by the user. The constant gas flows cause a linear rise and fall of intratracheal pressures (Fig. 5). There are no significant periods of no flow, as are known during volume-controlled ventilation (VCV) and pressure-controlled ventilation (PCV) [17]. The expiratory pressure drop in the airway is thus significantly milder with FCV than with VCV and PCV.

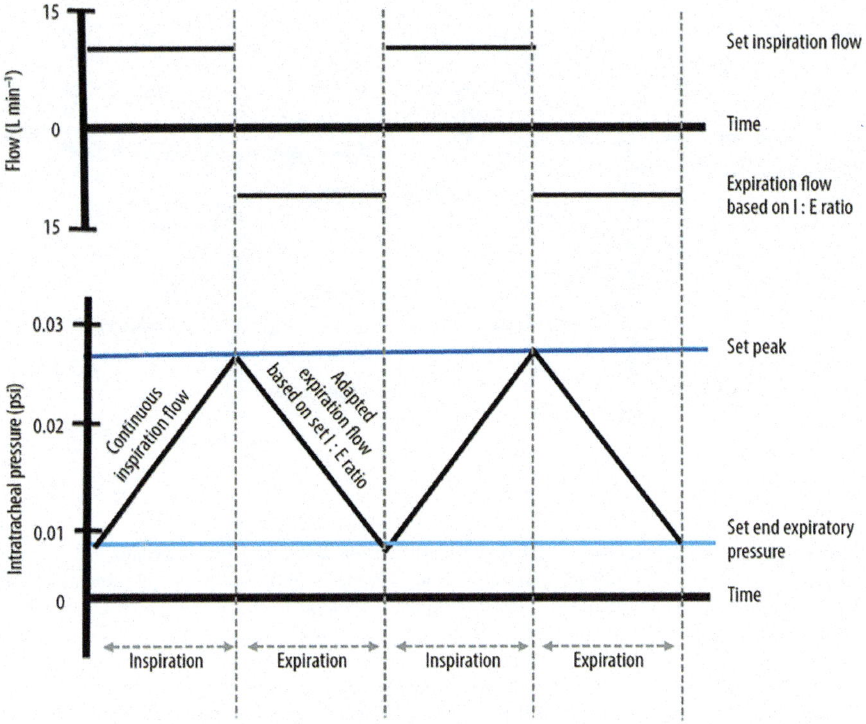

Fig. 5 During FCV gas is insufflated from end-expiratory pressure until it reaches the peak level. Then the flow is reversed and gas is sucked out at the rate to reach the set I:E ratio until the end-expiratory pressure is reached. This is followed by the next insufflation. (With written permission from Ventinova Medical, Eindhoven, the Netherlands)

D. Mechanical Power and Lung Protection The physics of FCV also involves considerations of mechanical power, which is the energy transferred to the respiratory system per unit time. By controlling flow and minimizing unnecessary pressure fluctuations, FCV can potentially reduce the mechanical power applied to the lungs, thereby decreasing the risk of ventilator-induced lung injury (VILI). This is particularly relevant in patients with compromised lung function, where traditional ventilation modes might exacerbate lung injury [18].

In a study by Van Oosten et al. in 2024, they showed that optimized FCV provided ventilation with significantly lower mechanical power. Their findings indicated that FCV can achieve stable gas exchange at lower minute volumes and with reduced dissipated energy compared to other modes. Additionally, FCV resulted in a more homogeneous spatial distribution of ventilation, with increased participation of the dorsal lung regions) [18].

E. Efficiency in Gas Exchange The continuous and controlled flow of gas in FCV can lead to improvements in gas exchange efficiency. This is because the constant flow can enhance the distribution of ventilation across different lung regions, improving the match between ventilation and perfusion. This efficient gas exchange is crucial for optimizing oxygen delivery and CO_2 removal, especially in critically ill patients.

F. Global Thoracic Electrical Impedance Electrical impedance tomography (EI_{Th}) enables dynamic visualization of the status of the lungs during ventilation. It allows for continuous monitoring of regional ventilation and thus a functional visualization of the lungs. Functional variables include regional compliance, regional lung volume, and regional changes in end-expiratory lung volume.

Weber et al. did a study to investigate the influence of FCV on respiratory mechanics and regional ventilation in obese and morbidly obese patients [19]. By employing the measurement of regional ventilation, they could demonstrate that the linearized expiratory flow during FCV provided better preservation of lung aeration with comparable tidal volume, plateau pressure (P_{plat}), and positive end-expiratory pressure (PEEP), when compared to volume-controlled ventilation (VCV).

They showed that during mechanical ventilation, end-expiratory lung volume decreased (Fig. 6). The difference between end-expiratory lung volumes between baseline ventilation and FCV was lower than between baseline and VCV. The difference between mean lung volumes between baseline and FCV was lower than between baseline and VCV (Fig. 7). (P_{mean} and $P_{mean\ expiration}$) was higher during FCV. No significant differences in tidal volume, ventilation frequency, (P_{plat}), SpO2, and CRS were found between FCV and VCV. All hemodynamic variables were comparable during FCV and VCV. FCV was characterized by a more even decay of impedance throughout the expiration phase (Fig. 8) [19].

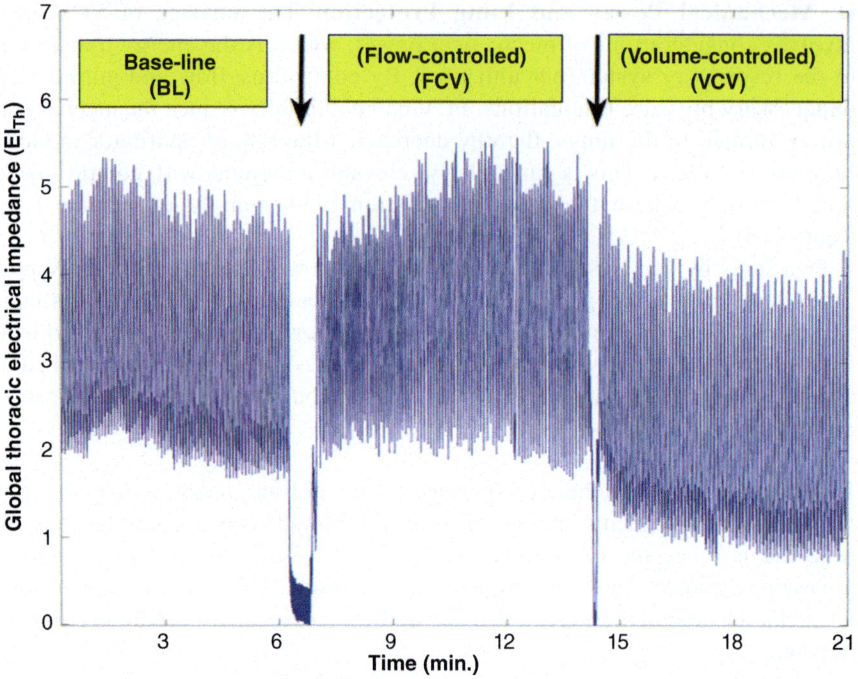

Fig. 6 A relative global thoracic electrical impedance (**EI$_{Th}$**) of one obese patient during the study procedure. Baseline (**BL**) (volume-controlled) ventilation; volume-controlled ventilation (**VCV**); flow-controlled ventilation (**FCV**)

They concluded that the recruiting effect caused by the linearized expiratory airflow and the elevated mean airway pressure (P_{mean}) during FCV might help prevent atelectasis and hypoxemia during mechanical ventilation in obese patients.

The first slope represents the insertion of the ultrathin tube (Tritube®) into the standard tracheal tube.

The second slope represents the remove of the ultra-thin tube (Tritube®) and reconnecting to the Dräger Fabius Tiro ventilator. Arrows indicate the switch between the respective ventilation modes (Published with written permission) [19].

6 Physiological effects of FCV on the respiratory system

To understand the physiology behind FCV mode, we need to understand the physiology of energy dissipation in the lung tissues.

A. *Energy dissipation*

As the lung expands and contracts with each ventilatory breath, both stress and strain change with time. As this happens, work is done on the lung system or in other words energy is applied. This energy is either stored and can partially be

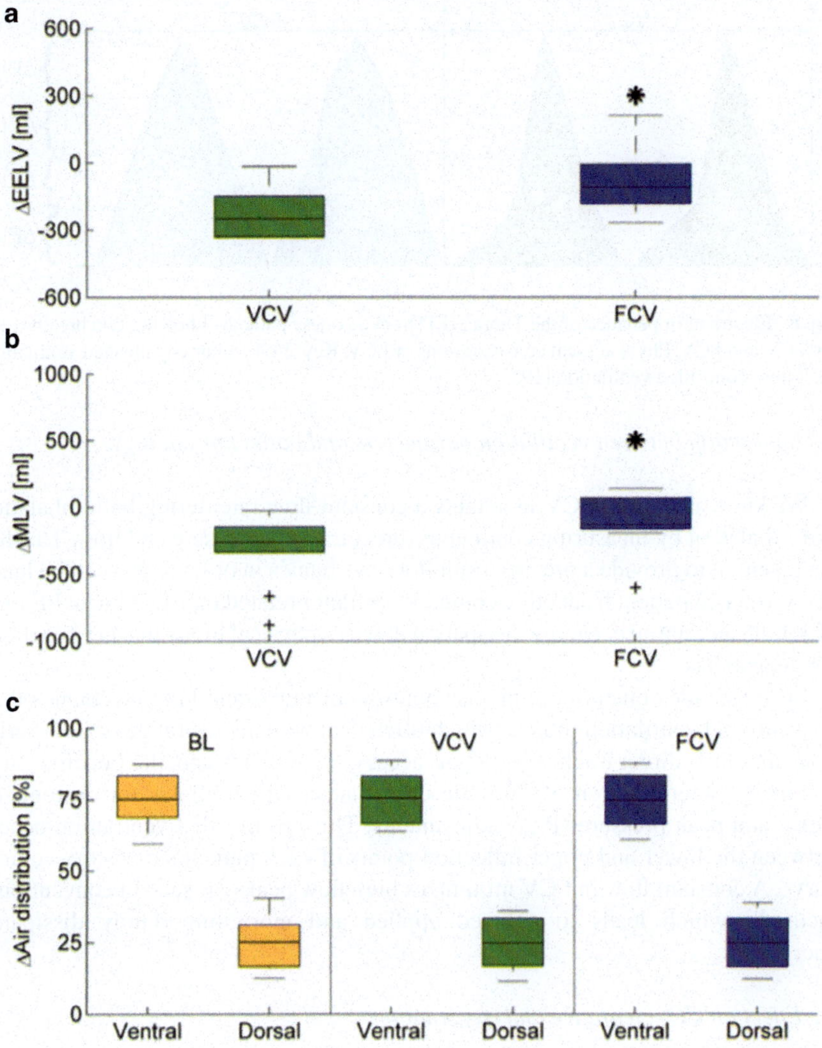

Fig. 7 (**a**) Changes in end-expiratory lung volumes, (**b**) Changes in mean lung volumes, (**c**) Change in air distribution between dorsal and ventral lung areas expressed as a percentage. Key: *BL* baseline for VCV, *VCV* volume-controlled ventilation, *FCV* flow-controlled ventilation [19]

recovered or is otherwise dissipated in the airways and lung tissue. Mechanical or thermal stresses, which can cause lung injury, occurs essentially by dissipating energy in the tissues at a rate above a certain threshold at which damage occurs [13]

This principle may also be applied to a ventilated lung. This can be achieved during ventilation by maintaining a constant flow rate during both inhalation and exhalation. In simpler terms, keeping the flow steady can help minimize lung damage caused by the ventilator.

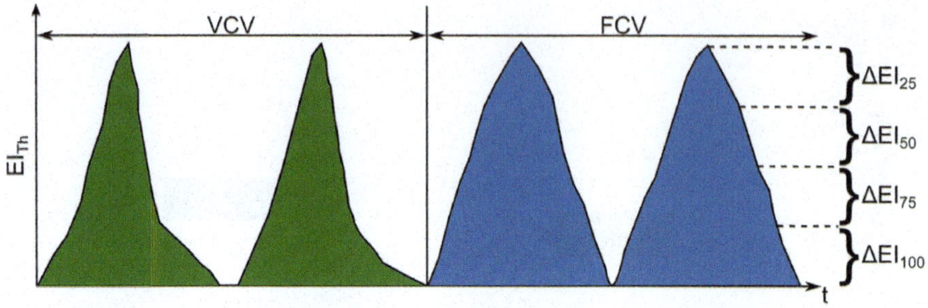

Fig. 8 Electrical impedance of the Thorax (EITh) in an obese patient—showing two breaths each for VCV and FCV. Physiological considerations of FCV. Key: *VCV* volume-controlled ventilation, *FCV* flow-controlled ventilation [19]

B. *Interaction between ventilation parameters and patient physiology.*

We know now that, FCV maintains a constant flow rate during both inhalation and exhalation by measuring continuous direct tracheal pressure and flow. This has the potential to provide a precise respiratory mechanics in order to protect the lungs of a ventilated patient from other common ventilator related injury. With an I:E ratio of 1:1, it can minimize energy dissipation down to physical limits that are beneficial for the patients.

FCV provides much more precise analysis of individual lung mechanics than conventional ventilation modes, which often deal with a wide range of flow variations and lack direct tracheal pressure access. FCV offers specific benefits, such as precise determination of dynamic compliance, which allows for customized PEEP and peak pressure (P_{peak}) adjustments. This ensures that ventilation occurs between the lower and upper inflection points of each patient's pressure–volume curve. A constant flow in FCV minimizes high flow peaks, as seen in conventional methods, which leads to reduced applied and more importantly dissipated energy [3].

C. *Effect on CO_2 clearance and oxygenation.*

Spraider et al. study demonstrates that normocapnia was sustained in individualized FCV even as the respiratory minute volume was reduced drastically by 50% in comparison to PCV. Moreover, individualized FCV resulted in substantially improved oxygenation and noticeably reduced non-aerated lung tissue. These results suggest an enhancement in ventilation efficiency and lung aeration. Individualized FCV, as shown in Spraider et al.'s study, has displayed advantages in maintaining normocapnia, improving oxygenation, and decreasing non-aerated lung tissue [10].

D. *Consideration of patient-specific factors influencing ventilation strategy selection.*

Mechanical ventilation carries the risk of a serious complication called ventilator-induced lung injury (VILI). This issue significantly impacts both the morbidity and mortality of critically ill patients. Over the past few years, there's been growing curiosity in the potential role of ventilator-delivered energy during inspiration in contributing to ventilator-induced lung injury (VILI). Research indicates that applying energy to lung tissue plays a significant role in ventilator-induced lung injury (VILI) development, with energy dissipation being tied to flow. When a patient is on a ventilator, the measured pressure is corrected for pressure drop in the ventilation system (i.e., intratracheal pressure) which is used to determine work done by the ventilator (the area within the loop). This represents the effort made by the ventilator on the patient's respiratory system during one breath (which is a quarter of the respiratory cycle). This energy, originating from the ventilator, can be a factor in the energy dissipated within the patient during the breathing process. This suggests that this ventilation strategy, with minimal energy dissipation in the patient, could have potential implications for lung-protective ventilation especially in ARDS patients.

Individualized flow-controlled ventilation (FCV) stands out by naturally linking tidal volume (TV) to individual lung compliance, reflecting the ventilation of the available aerated lung tissue. This can result in higher VT for lung-healthy individuals, but lower VT for injured lungs with reduced compliance. Improved lung aeration and less atelectasis were observed in FCV animals, despite lower PEEP levels compared to PCV [10].

E. *Haemodynamic and Cardiovascular system.*

It is a known fact that during positive pressure ventilation, there is increase in intrathoracic pressure which decreases the venous return and the cardiac output. Most studies have shown stable and comparable haemodynamic between FCV and other ventilation modes in otherwise healthy patients. The mean arterial pressure (MAP) is maintained at the patient's baseline or higher. But the heart rate can vary significantly depending on the patient profile. Figure 9 shows the physiological effects of FCV on the cardiovascular system. In one of the studies patients with acute lung injury or moderate acute respiratory distress syndrome were ventilated using FCV mode for 30 min, and subsequently in volume-control mode (VCV) for 30 min and oxygenation was measured using the PaO_2/FiO_2 ratio (mmHg) which was the primary outcome parameter. The secondary outcomes measured were ventilator parameters, $PaCO_2$ and haemodynamic data. Out of the 11 patients enrolled, two participants (20%) had an increase in heart rate of > 15% compared to baseline. There was no decrease in heart rate or MAP of > 15% and no increase of > 15% in MAP was noted [11].

It has been theorized that increased intrathoracic pressure which results from increased PEEP, mean airway pressures, and lung volumes may decrease venous return and pre-load thereby, impacting the cardiac output. However, since the EEP in FCV is not significantly different from PEEP in other modes of ventilation, it may not translate into significant changes in pre-load. Additionally, increases in

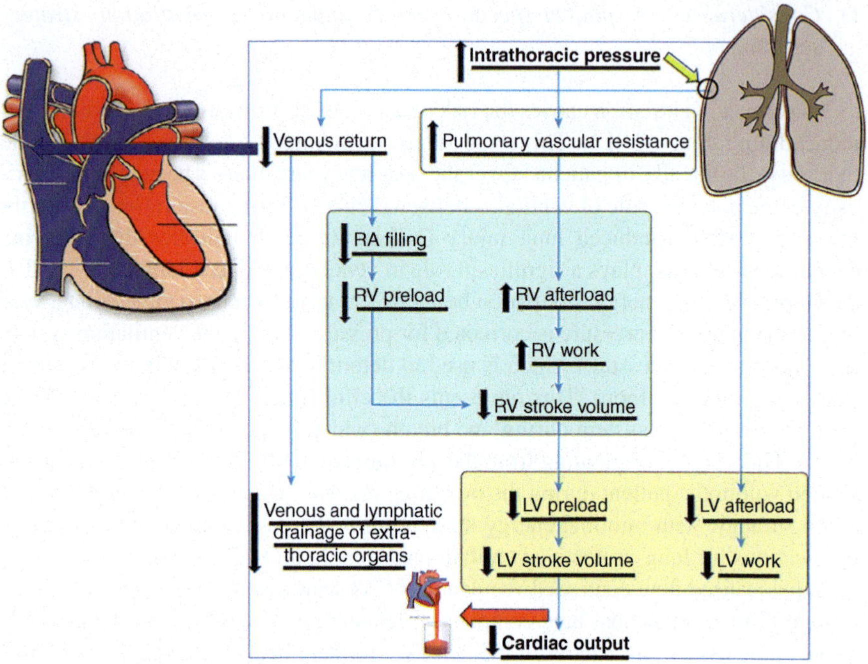

Fig. 9 The physiological effects of FCV on the cardiovascular system

mean airway pressures might not necessarily result in different haemodynamics in patients due to the relatively small difference in mean airway pressures between FCV and other ventilation methods. A study in a porcine model showed increased venous return, cardiac output and mean arterial pressure in FCV compared to other conventional ventilatory modes, because of the slow and stable mean increase/release intrathoracic pressure [20].

An unconventional application of the device involves the ability to establish a negative end-expiratory pressure (NEEP). Theoretically, leveraging NEEP's effect could aid in life-threatening hypovolemic shock situations by enhancing cardiac output through a reduction in intrathoracic pressure and subsequent elevation of the pressure gradient, facilitating improved venous return to the heart [20]. However, NEEP poses risks, including atelectasis. Balancing the risk of metabolic acidosis (during PEEP) against atelectasis (during NEEP) is crucial for hypovolemic patients [21].

F. *Arterial blood gas analyses.*

In FCV, arterial oxygenation (PaO_2) is higher, whereas partial pressure of carbon dioxide ($PaCO_2$) is lower.

In a randomized interventional cross over study done where the arterial blood gases were compared between volume-controlled ventilation (VCV) and FCV in 20 consecutive patients during and before they underwent abdominal surgery, it was observed that arterial oxygenation was higher with FCV [3].

The *alveolar–arterial oxygen* {(*A-a*) O_2} gradient was also significantly lower with FCV compared to baseline ventilation and volume-controlled ventilation (VCV). Partial pressure of carbon dioxide ($PaCO_2$) was lower with FCV when compared to baseline ventilation and VCV. In this study, the hemodynamic parameters did not differ with different ventilation modes [3].

7 Conclusion

Understanding respiratory physics and mechanics in the context of flow-controlled ventilation (FCV) is crucial for several reasons, particularly in optimizing patient care and enhancing the efficacy of mechanical ventilation strategies. It helps prevent lung injury, enhances patient comfort and synchrony, and helps in managing a diverse range of respiratory conditions. The significance of understanding respiratory physics and mechanics in the context of FCV lies in its direct impact on clinical outcomes through optimized patient management, prevention of complications, and contribution to the broader field of respiratory care and research.

Disclaimer Here we introduce the flow-controlled manual ventilator (FCmV), exemplified frequently by the Ventrain®, merely because there is no alternative of its kind on the market. You may also find a particular focus on the only commercially available FCV ventilator, the "Evone" ventilator. Moreover, using (Tritube®) instead of ultrathin or straw sized ETT terminology is due to the lack of other examples and not as a commercial endorsement of the products.

References

1. Grotberg JC, Reynolds D, Kraft BD. Management of severe acute respiratory distress syndrome: a primer. Crit Care. 2023;27:289. https://doi.org/10.1186/s13054-023-04572-w.
2. Larsson A, Guerin C. Monitoring of lung function in acute respiratory distress syndrome. Ann Transl Med. 2017;5(14):284. https://doi.org/10.21037/atm.2017.06.56. PMID: 28828359; PMCID: PMC5537117
3. Weber J, Schmidt J, Straka L, Wirth S, Schumann S. Flow-controlled ventilation improves gas exchange in lung-healthy patients- a randomized interventional cross-over study. Acta Anaesthesiol Scand. 2020;64(4):481–8. https://doi.org/10.1111/aas.13526. Epub 2019 Dec 30
4. Grassetto A, Pettenuzzo T, Badii F, Carlon R, Sella N, Navalesi P. Flow-controlled ventilation may reduce mechanical power and increase ventilatory efficiency in severe coronavirus disease-19 acute respiratory distress syndrome. Pulmonology. 2023;29(2):–154, 156. https://doi.org/10.1016/j.pulmoe.2022.05.006. Epub 2022 Jun 10. PMID: 35864057; PMCID: PMC9186429
5. Edwards Z, Annamaraju P. Physiology, lung compliance. [Updated 2023 Mar 13]. In: StatPearls [Internet]. Treasure Island: StatPearls Publishing; 2024 Jan-. Available from: https://www.ncbi.nlm.nih.gov/books/NBK554517/
6. Sarkar S, Jadhav U, Ghewade B, Sarkar S, Wagh P. Oscillometry in lung function assessment: a comprehensive review of current insights and challenges. Cureus. 2023;15(10):e47935. https://doi.org/10.7759/cureus.47935. PMID: 38034137; PMCID: PMC10685051

7. Hurley JJ, Hensley JL. Physiology, airway resistance. [Updated 2022 Nov 19]. In: StatPearls [Internet]. Treasure Island: StatPearls Publishing; 2024. Available from: https://www.ncbi.nlm.nih.gov/books/NBK542183/
8. Yang LY, Huang YC, Macintyre NR. Patient-ventilator synchrony during pressure-targeted versus flow-targeted small tidal volume assisted ventilation. J Crit Care. 2007;22(3):252–7. https://doi.org/10.1016/j.jcrc.2006.12.003. Epub 2007 Mar 30. PMID: 17869978
9. Ordies S, Orlitova M, Heigl T, Sacreas A, Van Herck A, Kaes J, Saez B, Vanstapel A, Ceulemans L, Vanaudenaerde BM, Vos R, Verschakelen J, Verleden GM, Verleden SE, Van Raemdonck DE, Neyrinck AP. Flow-controlled ventilation during EVLP improves oxygenation and preserves alveolar recruitment. Intensive Care Med Exp. 2020;8(1):70. https://doi.org/10.1186/s40635-020-00360-w. PMID: 33237343; PMCID: PMC7686942
10. Spraider P, Martini J, Abram J, Putzer G, Glodny B, Hell T, Barnes T, Enk D. Individualized flow-controlled ventilation compared to best clinical practice pressure-controlled ventilation: a prospective randomized porcine study. Crit Care. 2020;24(1):662. https://doi.org/10.1186/s13054-020-03325-3. PMID: 33239039; PMCID: PMC7686826
11. Van Dessel ED, De Meyer GR, Morrison SG, Jorens PG, Schepens T. Flow-controlled ventilation in moderate acute respiratory distress syndrome due to COVID-19: an open-label repeated-measures controlled trial. Intensive Care Med Exp. 2022;10(1):19. https://doi.org/10.1186/s40635-022-00449-4. PMID: 35608696; PMCID: PMC9127816
12. Spraider P, Abram J, Martini J, Putzer G, Glodny B, Hell T, Barnes T, Enk D, Flow-controlled versus pressure-controlled ventilation in cardiac surgery with cardiopulmonary bypass – A single-center, prospective, randomized, controlled trial. Journal of Clinical Anesthesia. Volume 91. 111279. ISSN 0952-8180. 2023; https://doi.org/10.1016/j.jclinane.2023.111279.
13. Barnes T, van Asseldonk D, Enk D. Minimisation of dissipated energy in the airways during mechanical ventilation by using constant inspiratory and expiratory flows—flow-controlled ventilation (FCV). Med Hypotheses. 2018;121:167–76. ISSN 0306-9877. https://doi.org/10.1016/j.mehy.2018.09.038.
14. Roehrig S, Ait Hssain A, Shallik NAH, Elsaid IMA, Mustafa SF, Smain OAM, Molokhia AA, Lance MD. Flow controlled ventilation in acute respiratory distress syndrome associated with COVID-19: a structured summary of a study protocol for a randomised controlled trial. Trials. 2020;21(1):781. https://doi.org/10.1186/s13063-020-04708-1. PMID: 32917259. PMCID: PMC7483072. https://pubmed.ncbi.nlm.nih.gov/32917259/
15. Barnes T, Enk D. Ventilation for low dissipated energy achieved using flow control during both inspiration and expiration. Trends Anaesth Crit Care. 2019;24:5–12. https://doi.org/10.1016/j.tacc.2018.09.003.
16. Bialka S, et al. Flow-controlled ventilation—a new and promising method of ventilation presented with a review of the literature. Anaesthesiol Intensive Ther. 2022;54(1):62–70. https://doi.org/10.5114/ait.2022.112889.
17. Enk D. Method and device for ventilating a patient. Available at: https://patentscope.wipo.int/search/en/detail.jsf?docId=WO2017148639.
18. Van Oosten JP, Francovich JE, Somhorst P, et al. Flow-controlled ventilation decreases mechanical power in postoperative ICU patients. ICMx. 2024;12:30. https://doi.org/10.1186/s40635-024-00616-9.
19. Weber *et al.* Flow-controlled ventilation (FCV) improves regional ventilation in obese patients—a randomized controlled crossover trial BMC Anesthesiol (2020) 20:24 doi:https://doi.org/10.1186/s12871-020-0944-y.
20. Böttinger L, van der Hoorn J. Negative pressure ventilation: a special application of expiratory ventilation assistance. ICMx. 2019;7:22. https://doi.org/10.1186/s40635-019-0248-z.
21. André Roggan, "EN instructions for use," 2014., https://ventinovamedical.com/wp-content/uploa6.15_IFUEvone_EN_Final.pdf.

Flow-Controlled Manual Ventilator (FCmV): A New Horizon in Elective and Emergency Airway Scenarios

Shawn D'Souza, Anas N. Shallik, and Nabil A. Shallik

1 Introduction

Continuous oxygenation through a small-bore device (transtracheal 18 G cannula = 1.02 mm) was first described in 1956 in patients with upper airway malignancies [1]. Hypercarbia and respiratory acidosis was a noted complication of this technique due to inadequate expiration [2]. In 1971, intermittent positive pressure ventilation through a 16 G (internal diameter 1.29 mm) transtracheal needle was conducted successfully in patients with patent upper airways. CO_2 retention was not an issue due to their patent upper airway [3]. Since then, various devices have been described to ventilate patients with small-bore tracheal catheters. However, a common issue of CO_2 retention and air trapping seemed to plague all of these devices if the patient had an upper airway obstruction. Since the 1950s, there have been several publications about aiding expiration in breathing circuits by utilizing the Venturi effect (i.e., increase in speed of gas flowing at a constriction corresponds to a

S. D'Souza
Anaesthesia, ICU and Perioperative Medicine Department, Hamad Medical Corporation, Doha, Qatar
e-mail: SDsouza4@hamad.qa

A. N. Shallik
Royal College of Surgeons in Ireland Medical University of Bahrain, Manamah, Bahrain

N. A. Shallik (✉)
Anaesthesia, ICU and Perioperative Medicine Department, Hamad Medical Corporation, Doha, Qatar

Clinical Anaesthesiology Department, Weill Cornell Medical College in Qatar, Doha, Qatar

Clinical Anaesthesiology Department, College of Medicine Qatar University, Doha, Qatar

Anaesthesia and SICU Department, Tanta University, Tanta, Egypt
e-mail: nshallik@hamad.qa

N. A. Shallik (ed.), *Flow Controlled Ventilation Mode Through a Straw Size Tube*, https://doi.org/10.1007/978-3-031-77477-5_6

decreased pressure which entrains air) [4, 5]. The early 1990s also saw some ideas for systems where expiration was assisted by active suction [6]. Ultimately, the Venturi effect has prevailed as the principle behind assisted expiration in the flow-controlled manual ventilator.

In 2008, an entrepreneur named Dirk van Asseldonk and an anaesthesiologist inventor, Prof. Dr. med. Dietmar Enk, began developing a manual ventilator that could overcome this issue of air trapping when ventilating through a narrow bore catheter. In 2010, the device received a CE Marking (The CE marking is an acronym for the French term "Conformite Europeenne" which certifies that a product has met EU health, safety, and environmental requirements). It was termed the Ventrain® (Ventinova Medical B.V., Eindhoven, the Netherlands) Flow-Controlled manual Ventilator (FCmV). The device is also referred to as a novel ejector-based device, expiratory ventilation assistance (EVA), and ejector ventilator.

2 Flow-Controlled Manual Ventilator (FCmV) (Ventrain®)

Expiration in most ventilators is a passive process. At airway diameters less than 4.5 mm, this time increases considerably. If the only conduit for expiration is a 14 G cannula (internal diameter 1.6 mm) perhaps because of an obstructed upper airway, more than 30 seconds may be required for a single expiration [7]. This can trigger air trapping within the lungs, potentially leading to pulmonary barotrauma and hypotension due to reduced venous return [8]. It would be advantageous to have a ventilating device that could actively assist expiration through small-bore airway catheters, especially for emergency situations.

The creators of the FCmV initially developed a purpose-built ventilator ejector that could achieve minute volumes of 7.5 L/min in vitro through a transtracheal catheter with an inner diameter of 2 mm (12 G). This device generated suction by using the Venturi principle to augment expiration, prevent air trapping and enhance minute volumes generated. In a hypoxic animal model with complete upper airway obstruction and a transtracheal catheter, this prototype ventilator was able to restore oxygenation and limit hypercarbia for over 15 min. Based on this preliminary model, the Ventrain® [Flow-Controlled manual Ventilator or novel ejector-based device or expiratory ventilation assistance (EVA) or ejector ventilator] was developed [9].

The expiratory ventilatory assistance (EVA) technology (which is the basic form of flow-controlled ventilation (FCV) as applied by Evone®, creates active expiration by suction, utilizing the Venturi principle). This shortens expiration time, increases the achievable minute volume and reduces the risk of air trapping, barotrauma and circulatory collapse, when compared to other small lumen ventilation techniques in obstructed airways (e.g., jet ventilation). The FCmV is a single-use ventilation device, dedicated to manage and prevent difficult or challenging airway situations. It allows adequate ventilation in any adult patient and paediatric emergency, in combination with any narrow bore lumen [e.g., transtracheal catheter Cricath® (Ventinova Medical B.V., Eindhoven, the Netherlands), airway exchange catheter, rigid bronchoscope, etc.] via any route of airway access [oral, nasal, front-of-neck airway (FONA)]. It is easy to use for inspiration, oxygenation, expiration, and washing out CO_2, by using just the thumb and index finger. The only requirement is O_2 from a high-pressure gas source, with a pressure-compensated flowmeter [10].

3 Flow-Controlled Manual Ventilator Device Specifications

The FCmV is a handheld, compact, single use, manually operated, portable ventilatory system or ejector ventilator which connects a pressurized oxygen source to any airway cannula, catheter or tube with a Luer-lock connection (Figs. 1 and 2). The device's inner component is an oxygen ejector driven by a high-pressure source (which could be an oxygen cylinder or a wall-mounted pressure-compensated flowmeter). Oxygen flow entering the device is accelerated by an internal jet nozzle and it leaves the exhaust port at a high speed. This creates a sub-atmospheric pressure by virtue of the Venturi effect and facilitates an active expiration by essentially suctioning pulmonary gases. Active expiration or equilibration of pulmonary and atmospheric pressures is performed by releasing the occlusion over one or both apertures of the device respectively [9, 11]. This technique has been termed expiratory ventilatory assistance (EVA) by the manufacturer (Ventinova Medical B.V., Eindhoven, the Netherlands) and is the basic form of the flow-controlled ventilation (FCV) used in their Evone® ventilators. The Tritube®, which is an ultrathin ventilation tube, has been developed to intubate and ventilate patients for laryngotracheal surgery and provide excellent surgical access to the glottis *(Please refer to chapters "Ultrathin Cuffed Endotracheal Tube (Tritube®)" and "Use of Tritube for Oropharyngeal and Laryngeal Surgery" for more details).* It has an inner diameter of less than 3 mm and outer diameter of 4.4 mm. It can be used exclusively with Ventrain® FCmV and Evone® ventilators (Fig. 2).

The device is basically a T-piece with gas inflow on one side and two outflow ports on the other. There are two connections: an inlet tube (length, 213 ± 20 cm; internal diameter, 3.0–4.5 mm) connected to the outlet of an oxygen source and a

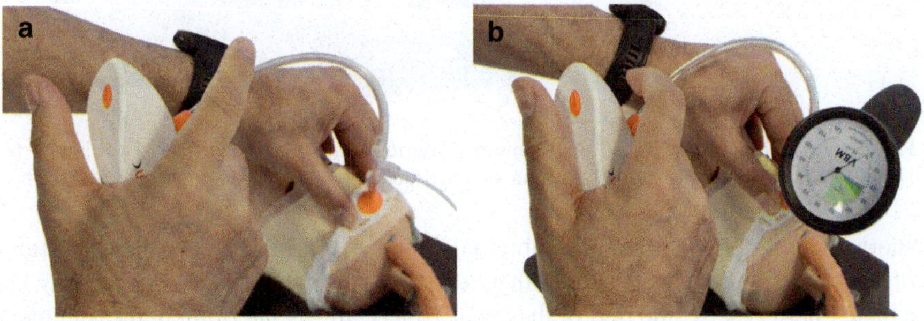

Fig. 1 Ventrain® with Cricath®, (**a**) $ETCO_2$ sample line. (**b**) Manometer®. (Courtesy, Dr. Shallik, Doha Airway Equipment Museum, Qatar)

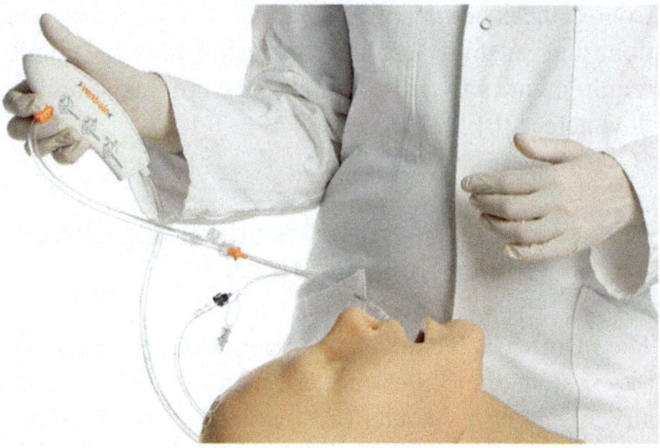

Fig. 2 Ventrain® with Tritube®. (Ventinova Medical, Eindhoven, the Netherlands)

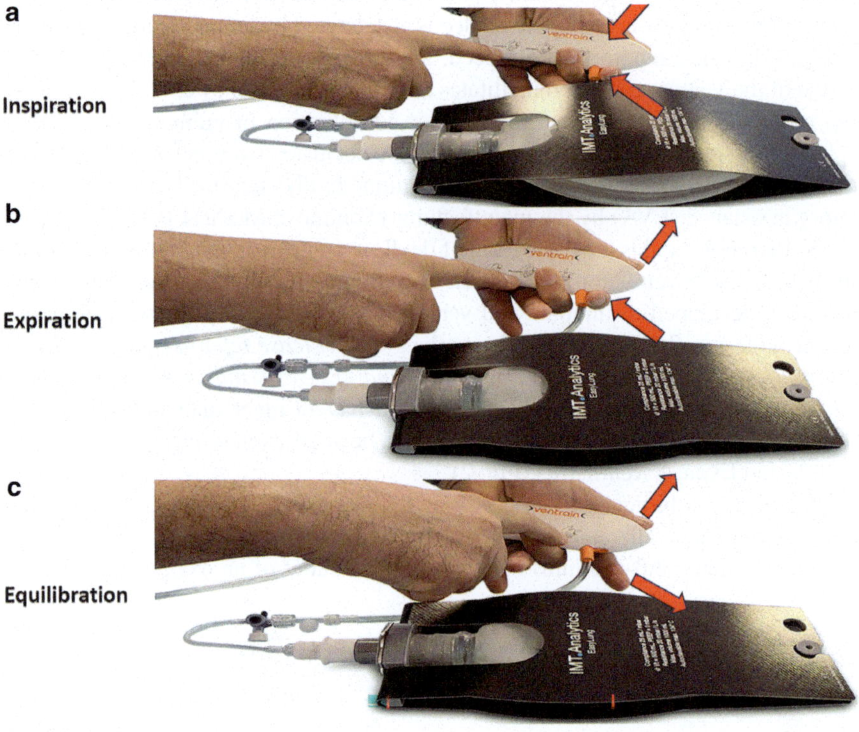

Fig. 3 Ventrain® attached to lung simulator during: (**a**) Inspiration. (**b**) Expiration. (**c**) Equilibration. (Courtesy, Dr. Shallik, Doha Airway Equipment Museum, Qatar)

short sidearm (length, 20 ± 1 cm; internal diameter, 5.20 ± 0.15 mm) at the bottom of the FCmV with a distal T-piece that connects the patient's small-bore airway via a male Luer Lock. A side port of the distal T-piece allows intermittent measurement of end-tidal CO2 concentration (Fig. 3). Inside the shell, the inlet channel narrows to a diameter of 0.75 mm before splitting into a T-shape and the gas will be directed

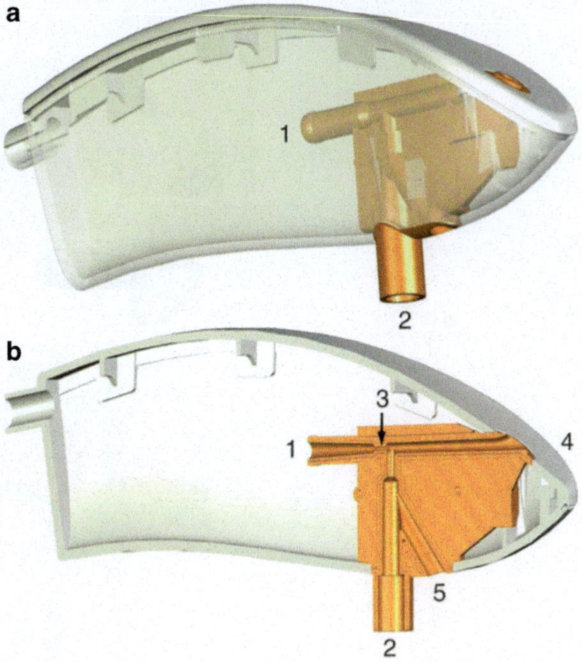

Fig. 4 The mechanism of EVA is shown by the cross of Ventrain® above: (Ventinova Medical, Eindhoven, the Netherlands). *1* Inlet hose connection to hospital O2 gas flow. *2* Connection to patient. *3* Narrow diameter to increase gas velocity. *4* Outlet gas flow. *5* Equilibration

either along the inspiratory/expiratory sidearm to the airway or along the exhaust channel to an opening on the upper surface. The internal dead space volume of the FCmV is 5 mL [12] (Figs. 4 and 5).

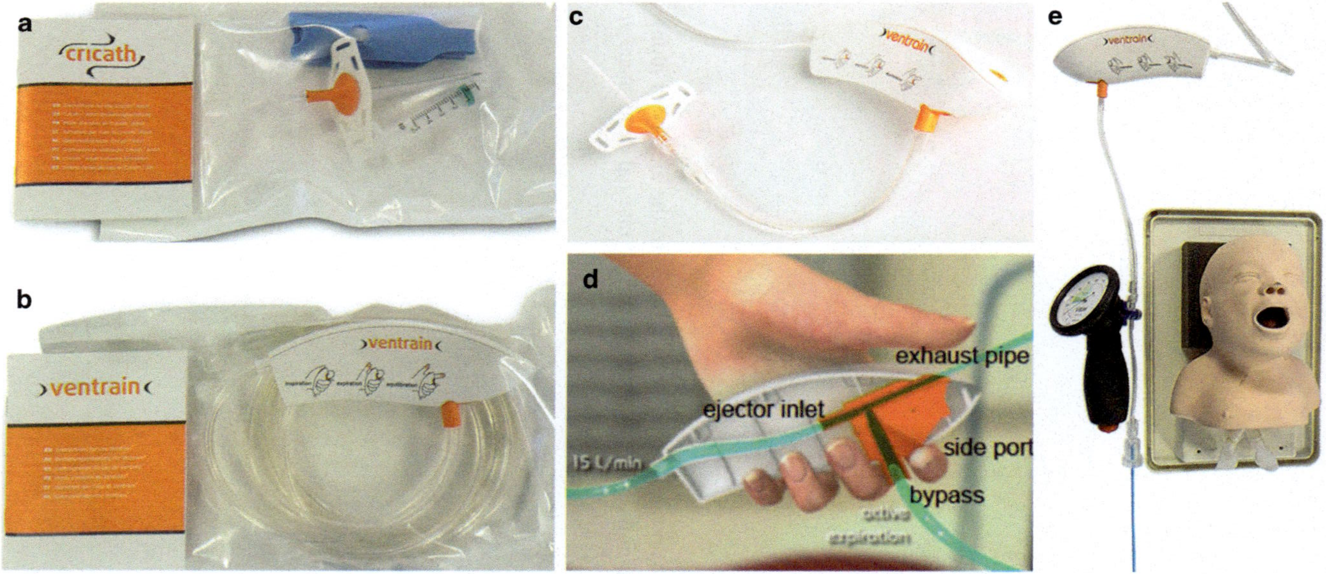

Fig. 5 (**a**)–(**c**) Ventrain® and Cricath® (size 12G). (**d**) Cross sectional area in Ventrain® and (**e**) Ventrain® connected to small bore tube and manometer in kid. (Ventinova Medical, Eindhoven, the Netherlands)®

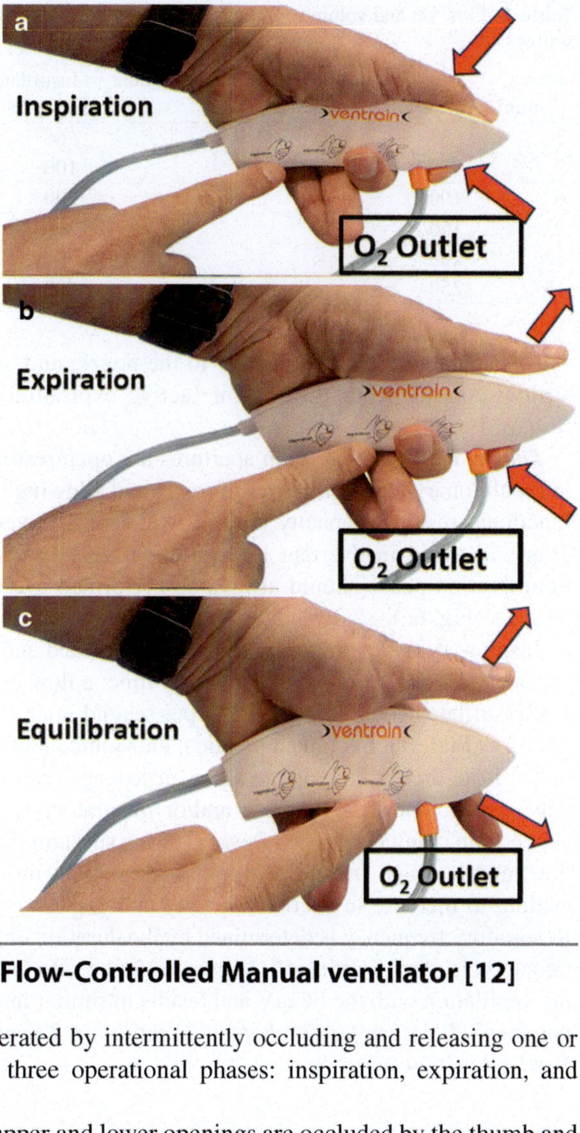

Fig. 6 Mode of action of flow controlled manual ventilator (Ventrain®). (**a**) During inspiration. (**b**) During expiration. (**c**) During equilibration. (Courtesy, Dr. Shallik, Doha Airway Equipment Museum, Qatar)

4 Operating the Flow-Controlled Manual ventilator [12]

The FCmV is manually operated by intermittently occluding and releasing one or two apertures resulting in three operational phases: inspiration, expiration, and equilibration.

During inspiration, the upper and lower openings are occluded by the thumb and index fingers, respectively. Oxygen flow accelerates under high proximal driving pressure across a narrow constriction and is diverted along the inspiratory channel, via the sidearm towards the patient's airway (Fig. 6a).

During expiration, the upper exhaust aperture is opened by lifting the thumb, while maintaining the lower opening closed. The gas, on its way through the ejector, passes through the 0.75 mm ID inlet constriction. This increases the velocity and therefore the dynamic pressure of the flowing gas and leads to a decrease in the static pressure of the gas surrounding the jet emerging from the nozzle (Bernoulli's principle). The acceleration of the oxygen flow creates a

Table 1 Flow set and volume administered per time or tidal volume at different inspiratory flow settings

Flow (L/min).	Insufflated volume (ml) or tidal volume after 1 s inspiration	Insufflated volume (ml) or tidal volume after 2 s inspiration
2	33	66
3	50	100
6	100	200
9	150	300
12	200	400
15	250	500

sub-atmospheric pressure distally to the nozzle and exerts a suction effect on the airflow coming from the patient (active expiration) due to the Venturi effect (Fig. 6b).

During equilibration, both apertures are open resulting in slow equilibration of intrapulmonary and ambient air pressure and allowing lung volume to stabilize near functional residual capacity (FRC), while fresh oxygen escapes via the exhaust. This will avoid inadvertent hyperinflation or excessive suctioning on the lungs. Equilibration pause should always be performed every 5-ventilation cycles for at least 5 s (Fig. 6c).

Inspiratory tidal volume can easily be estimated and controlled over time by setting an appropriate flow and inspiratory time: a flow of 6 L/min (=6000 ml in 60 s) will insufflate 100 ml tidal volume per second after 1 s of inspiration and 200 ml after 2 s (Table 1). In clinical practice, the volume delivered will be lower than estimated from the set flow due to some air leakage around the small-bore airway and may need to increase the flow and/or inspiratory time. Expiratory tidal volume depends on many factors: set flow, resulting sub-atmospheric pressure, resistance to flow, and leakage. Increasing the flow, results in more sub-atmospheric pressure leading to increase in suction capacity and expiratory volume per time unit [13]. Respiratory frequency is determined by the duration of the manual inspiratory/expiratory cycle. An I:E ratio of 1:1 is proven to be safe in most paediatric patients during ventilation with the FCmV and results in similar inspiratory and expiratory tidal volumes. [*Please refer to chapter "Ventilation Through Small Bore Catheter in Paediatrics" for more details.*]

5 Manufacturer's Recommendations for the FCmV Use [10]

A few points must be considered before using the FCmV.

- The patient must be on total intravenous anaesthesia (TIVA or TCI) for maintenance for elective procedure.
- All personnel should receive device-specific training. It can be used only with small-bore lumen catheters.

- While it can be used for all patients, the manufacturer recommends limiting it to emergency life-saving use only for patients weighing <40 kg (i.e., children and infants). While there are no absolute contra-indications, some potential complications include barotrauma to the lungs, pneumomediastinum, and aspiration.
- As stated previously, the FCmV is a manually controlled, single-use difficult airway ventilator to be used with a transtracheal or endotracheal small lumen catheters only. It consists of a handheld unit with tubing for connection to a flowmeter on one end and a male Luer-lock connector for the airway catheter on the other end (Figs. 2, 3 and 5).
- Additional equipment required for use are:

1. a high-pressure oxygen supply (3.5–5.0 bar, 100%). This could be a medical oxygen cylinder with a flow regulator or a pipeline medical oxygen supply with a pressure-compensated flow regulator.
2. It should not be connected to the flow output of an anaesthesia machine without a pressure-compensated flowmeter (Fig. 7).
3. Suitable airway catheter (described below) (Table 2).

- FCmV must only be used with the recommended catheter dimensions to ensure adequate ventilation. Using the device longer than 20 min is not recommended, as it can cause dehydration related complications.
- Caution must be exercised when high oxygen concentrations are used in flammable environments such as LASER surgery.
- Capnography should be used to confirm proper placement of the airway catheter and to observe overall trend in the end-tidal CO_2 concentration (applicable ide-

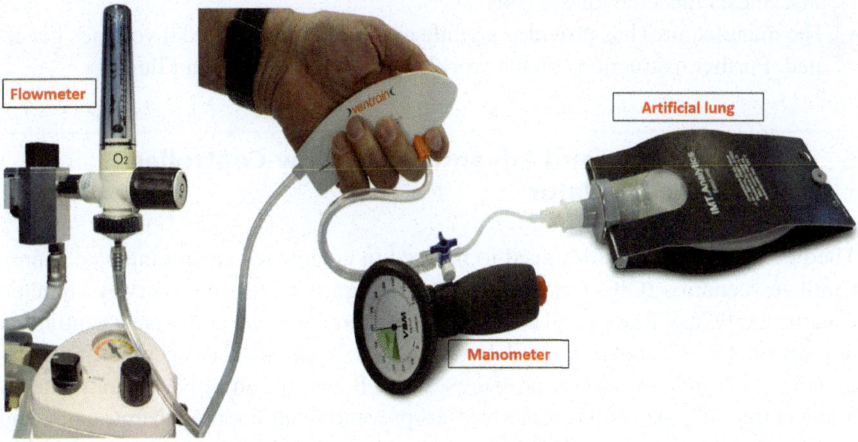

Fig. 7 Anaesthesia machine flowmeter connection with Ventrain®, manometer, and artificial lung. (Courtesy, Dr. Shallik, Doha Airway Equipment Museum, Qatar)

Table 2 Attainable minute volumes and proposed I:E ratios for recommended catheter dimensions in different situations

Patient group/ situation	Catheter type	Set inspiration flow (L/min)	Catheter ID (mm)	Length (cm)	I:E ratio	Minute volume (L/min)
Healthy adult patient	Transtracheal	15	2.0	7	1: 1.1	7
	Endotracheal	15	2.3	40	1: 0.9	7.5
		15	3.0	100	1: 1.0	7
Paediatric patient		6	1.6	40	1: 1.7	2
Collapsed adult lung	Bronchial blocker	6	1.7	78	1: 2.5	1.5

ally for closed airways, but also helpful to observe trend in partially closed airways if a side stream capnograph is used).

- Lastly, expiratory phase debris is ejected out of the thumb hole. So, it should either be pointed away from bystanders or covered without occluding the holes.
- A few more words of caution include closely observing the patient's chest excursion during ventilation and being aware that using the equilibration phase results in a lower overall respiratory rate and minute volume. In a total (or near total) obstructed upper airway, equilibration lasting 5 s must be performed every every ventilation cycles to prevent excessive positive or negative pressure from developing in the lungs. For low compliance states (paediatrics and collapsed lung) and/or catheters <2 mm ID or <12 G, a maximum O_2 flow of 6 L/min is set to avoid excessive pressure buildup in the oxygen tubing.
- In case of a failure in the flow-controlled ventilator (FCV) (Evone®), the FCmV (Ventrain®) works as a rescue device similar to an Ambu bag for a traditional anaesthesia machine failure (Fig. 7).
- The manufacturer has provided a guide correlating flows to tidal volumes generated. Further instructions on the workflow of Ventrain® are in (Table 1).

6 Clinical Uses and Advantages of Flow-Controlled Manual Ventilator

The FCmV was initially designed to be used in emergency cannot intubate cannot ventilate scenarios (CICO) and for using through a narrow bore airway catheter. Clearly, the FCmV has several advantages compared to other emergency ventilation devices such as a manual jet ventilator (Fig. 8a–c) or the ENK oxygen flow modulator (Fig. 9). FCmV uses lower pressures, stable flows, and an active expiration technique employing the venturi principle thus preventing air trapping, barotrauma, and overcoming the expiratory resistance of narrow bore tubes by keeping the inspiratory and expiratory tidal volumes (TV) equal (assuming the correct I:E ratio and

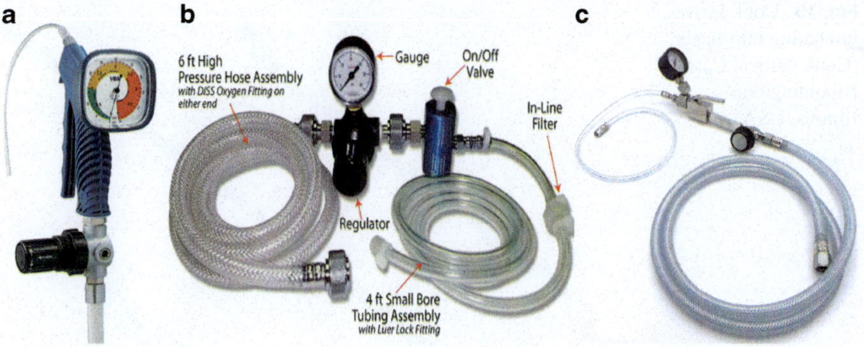

Fig. 8 (**a**)–(**c**): Different types of manual jet ventilators. (Courtesy, Dr. Shallik, Doha Airway Equipment Museum, Qatar)

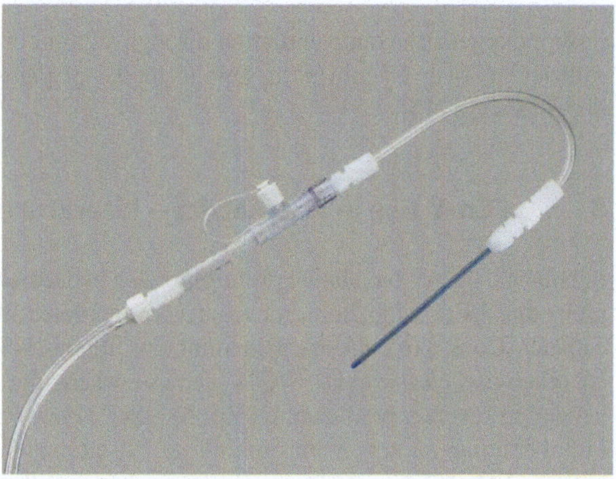

Fig. 9 Cook Enk oxygen flow modulator. (Cook Critical Care, Bloomington, Illinois, USA)

equilibration phase is used). It does not require a patent upper airway to ventilate a patient with a small-bore tracheal catheter. It can work with any tracheal catheter as long as it has a Luer-lock connector. It can provide oxygenation and full ventilation with ultrathin tubes (Tritube®) as small as <3 mm internal diameter and allows for side stream capnography [10].

7 Cannot Intubate Cannot Oxygenate (CICO) Situations

Cannot intubate cannot oxygenate (CICO) scenarios are potential anaesthetic catastrophes. Due to their rare and emergent nature, it would be unfeasible to conduct randomized clinical trials to compare different airway rescue techniques. So far, there have been several cases published in the literature about the use of FCmV in CICO situations (both in vitro and in vivo studies). In 2009, the technology that pioneered the current commercially available FCmV (Ventrain®) was used to

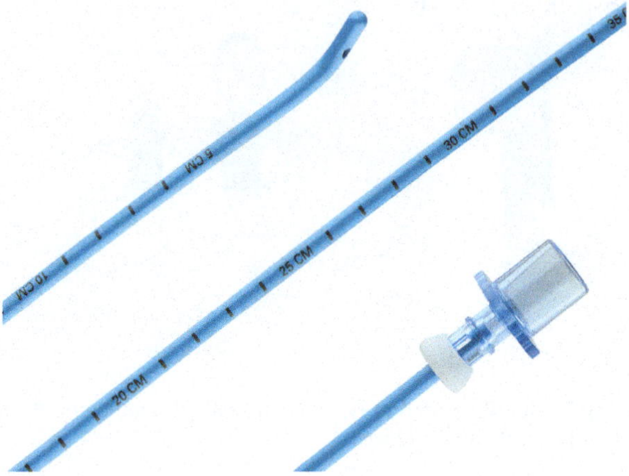

Fig. 10 Cook Frova intubating introducer. (Cook Critical Care, Bloomington, Illinois, USA)

restore oxygenation and ventilation through a 2 mm internal diameter transtracheal catheter for over 15 min in an animal model of pigs with completely obstructed upper airways [15].

8 FCmV Use in Paediatrics—Literature Review

In humans, FCmV has shown promise for use in paediatric CICO scenarios. A 2.1 kg premature baby with glottic oedema was ventilated through an 8 French Frova® catheter (Cook Critical Care, Bloomington, Illinois, USA) (Fig. 10) using FCmV in an otherwise catastrophic CICO scenario where the baby was desaturating and becoming severely bradycardic [16]. Another case involved a 4.3 kg baby undergoing abdominal surgery with multiple failed intubation attempts who was rescued with the FCmV connected to an airway exchange catheter (ID 1.66 mm) for ventilation [16]. FCmV has been used with rigid bronchoscopy for ventilation in a 7 month old baby with subglottic stenosis and again after intubation when conventional Paediatric Intensive Care (PICU) ventilators were unusable due to high peak pressures >50 cm H2O [17]. A study published in 2021 comparing various cannula insufflation devices used in emergency front-of-neck access (eFONA) (3-way stopcock, Rapid-O2, Manujet, Enk oxygen flow modulator, FCmV, and self-inflating bags) in test lung models with upper airway obstruction (adult, child, and infant) showed that FCmV was the only device which produced acceptable pressures (<35 cm H2O) and acceptable lung volumes (<7 ml/kg) in all airway models.[19] (Please refer to chapter "*Ventilation Through Small Bore Catheter in Paediatrics*" for more details.

9 FCmV Use in Adults—Literature Review

There have been several cases of FCmV being used successfully in adult CICO scenarios published in the literature. A 77-year-old lady presenting to the emergency department with airway obstruction due to tracheal stenosis secondary to

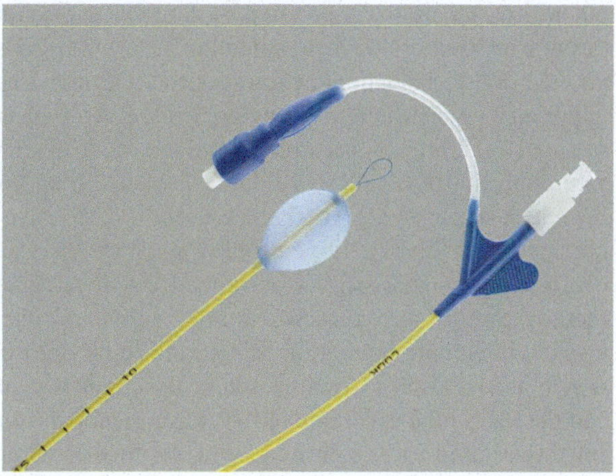

Fig. 11 Arndt® Endobronchial Blocker. (Cook Critical Care, Bloomington, Illinois, USA)

prior prolonged mechanical ventilation and tracheostomy could not be intubated with a size 5.0 mm internal diameter (ID) endotracheal tube under direct laryngoscopy. A 4.4 mm internal diameter tube exchanger ((VBM) Medizintechnik GmbH, Sulz am Neckar, Germany) was passed successfully and the patient was ventilated safely using FCmV until tracheal dilation and repeat tracheostomy was performed [19]. A 66-year-old lady with near complete upper airway obstruction due to oropharyngeal cancer presenting to the emergency department was ventilated using FCmV through a Cricath® (Ventinova Medical, Eindhoven, the Netherlands) tracheal cannula. It was a CICO scenario where the anaesthesiologist made the difficult but necessary decision of front-of-neck access and FCmV use, and this saved the patient's life [20]. Another case of successful emergency FCmV use involves a 71-year-old man with advanced vocal cord cancer and upper airway obstruction who failed an awake fibroscopic intubation. His airway was rescued by threading an Arndt® Endobronchial Blocker (Cook Critical Care, Bloomington, Illinois, USA) over a guidewire and ventilating with the FCmV for 40 minutes until a tracheal cannula was sited after the surgery (Fig. 11) [21]. Emergency cricothyrotomy with the Tritube® *and FCmV use* has been performed at our institution. A 34-year-old male patient with tracheal stenosis secondary to radiation therapy and a history of known difficult intubation was scheduled for a tracheal dilation. He refused an awake-fibreoptic intubation after the risks were explained. When intubation with a video laryngoscope proved unsuccessful, he had to undergo front-of-neck access with a Tritube® which saved the airway. The Tritube® was advanced using the needle-catheter-wire cricothyrotomy technique. The patient was ventilated with the aid of FCmV. He was successfully extubated at the end of the case.

10 FCmV Use in Elective Adult Surgeries

FCmV has been used electively for ventilating patients with upper airway obstruction via front-of-neck access. A 58-year-old man with squamous cell carcinoma of the vocal cords was successfully ventilated for the entire surgery lasting over

60 min (LASER excision of post-surgical supraglottic stenosis) using FCmV through a Cricath® tracheal cannula (ID 2.0 mm). His previous surgery had been aborted due to inadequate expiration with a high frequency jet ventilator due to upper airway obstruction. Flow-controlled ventilation through the FCmV with a rate of 10–12 breaths per minute and I:E ratio of 1:1 was able to maintain an O2 saturation of 100% and end-tidal CO_2 of less than 46 mmHg for the duration of the entire surgery [22] Another case report of elective FCmV use in upper airway obstruction involves a 49-year-old woman who was scheduled to undergo dilation of a C5 pharyngeal stricture. She had laryngeal fixation secondary to radiation therapy. She refused a tracheostomy for this specific procedure. After a difficult awake fibroscopic intubation using a micro-laryngoscopy (MLS) tube and induction of anaesthesia, a Cricath® tracheal cannula was inserted, connected to FCmV and the MLS tube was removed to aid surgical exposure. The patient was successfully ventilated for the entire case using FCmV without any complications [23]. Another instance of successful elective FCmV use involves a 60-year-old man with a glottic tumour scheduled for a diagnostic laryngo-tracheo-bronchoscopy. A 2.0 mm ID transtracheal airway catheter was inserted in the patient's cricothyroid membrane and he was successfully ventilated with FCmV for the 20 minute duration of the procedure [24].

A middle-aged woman with a 44-pack-year history of smoking presented with 4 weeks of hoarseness and intermittent obstructed breathing. A flexible endoscopic exam showed a large pedunculated left vocal cord mass that occluded the glottis and was mobile with respiration. For her surgery, a 14G ((VBM) Medizintechnik GmbH, Sulz am Neckar, Germany) transtracheal catheter was inserted through the cricothyroid membrane and she was ventilated with the FCmV device for the entire procedure while being maintained on TIVA. She was discharged home the same day. Another case reported by the same author involved a man in his 70s presenting 2 weeks after a coronary artery bypass graft surgery with increasing dyspnoea on rest. He was found to have supraglottic stenosis, which improved with humidified O2 and steroid therapy but needed definitive surgical treatment. For airway access intraoperatively, A 14 G Ravussin needle *((VBM) Medizintechnik GmbH, Sulz am Neckar, Germany)* (Fig. 12) was used for a cricothyrotomy. He was ventilated with FCmV for the

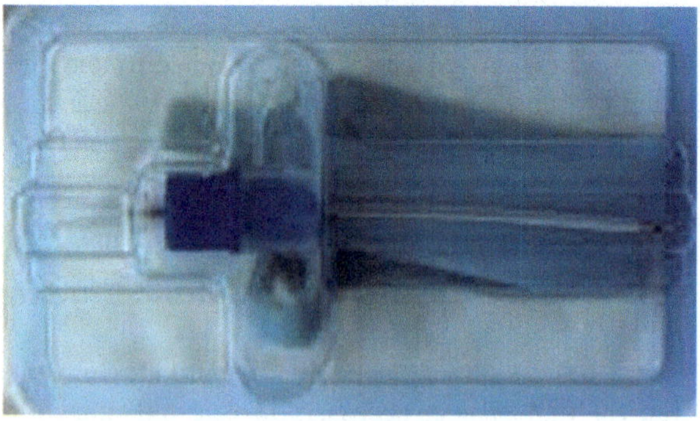

Fig. 12 Ravussin. [(VBM) Medizintechnik GmbH, Sulz am Neckar, Germany]

entire surgical procedure while being maintained on total intravenous anaesthesia [25].

In a case series of seven ENT surgical patients with airway narrowing, ventilation under general anaesthesia was successfully performed using FCmV with the Tritube® maintaining intratracheal pressures between 5 and 20 cm H2O. Five of the seven patients even had the Tritube® maintained comfortably after emergence from anaesthesia in the post-anaesthesia recovery unit (PACU) [26]. *Using CT 3D reconstruction and Virtual Endoscopy (VE) of the upper airway are very crucial steps in the management of tracheo-bronchial stenosis airway scenarios.* [27, 28] The Tritube® has been used for elective FONA at our institution. A 60-year-old man with a large parotid mass presented for surgical resection. The surgeons preferred neither oral nor nasal intubation. Thus, an elective FONA was performed using the needle-catheter-wire technique to place the Tritube® in the first tracheal ring interspace. The patient was successfully extubated at the end of the surgery. For the most part, however, the Evone® FCV has superseded the Ventrain® *FCmV* in elective surgeries where the Tritube® is employed as it avoids the inconvenience of manual ventilation [29]. Nevertheless, the Ventrain® remains as a plan B to manually ventilate the patient with a Tritube® in case of a failure in the Evone® ventilator (we reiterate the fact that it works as a rescue device similar to an Ambu bag in case of a traditional anaesthesia machine failure).

11 FCmV with One-Lung Ventilation

There has also been a case report published of FCmV being used for one-lung ventilation. A 52-year-old woman, with normal preoperative pulmonary function tests, undergoing video-assisted thoracoscopic surgery (VATS) under general anaesthesia with a left sided 37-Fr double-lumen tube (DLT) (Shiley Medtronic, Watford, UK) was facing refractory hypoxemia once one-lung ventilation was initiated. Despite confirmation of the DLT placement with a bronchoscope, alveolar recruitment, increasing FiO_2, and PEEP titration, her O2 saturation hovered around 89%. Only with insertion of an 11-Fr airway exchange catheter [(VBM) Medizintechnik GmbH, Sulz am Neckar, Germany] through the tracheal lumen and manual ventilation of the right lung with FCmV did O2 saturation improve to 98% after 1 min [30]. Another case involves a patient undergoing thoracoscopic esophagectomy and wedge resection of the right lower lung lobe, under general anaesthesia with a double-lumen tube. An iatrogenic lesion in the left main bronchus was identified by the surgeon after right lung wedge resection had been performed, which needed immediate repair. Positive pressure ventilation with a deflated right lung and left main bronchus tear would be impossible. The patient was managed by using FCmV through a small-bore catheter with a cuff (Arndt® Endobronchial Blocker, Cook Critical Care, Bloomington, Illinois, USA) inflated beyond the bronchial defect [31] (Fig. 11).

12 Flow-Controlled Manual Ventilator (FCmV) Use in Elective paediatric Surgeries

The manufacturer states that for patients weighing less than 40 kg (i.e., children and infants), FCmV should be used only for life-saving purposes. In children, it has been used for emergency ventilation through 8 Fr intubating catheters or airway exchange catheters only thus far [13]. The aforementioned cases noted under "Ventrain® use in Paediatrics—Literature" cover its emergency use in paediatrics. To our knowledge, there has been one case report of elective use of the Ventrain® in paediatric anaesthesia to date. *(Please refer to chapter Ventilation Through Small Bore Catheter in Paediatrics for more details).*

13 Future Plans

13.1 Evone® and Ventrain® FCV as an Option on the DAS Guidelines

As seen in this chapter, Ventrain® and Tritube® have shown promise in both elective and emergency use in patients with a difficult airway. However, they are yet to be incorporated into official difficult airway management guidelines. CICO scenarios are extremely rare (1 in 12,500 general anaesthetics) [32], so it would be both unfeasible and obviously unethical to conduct randomized controlled trials to compare their efficacy to the current standard of care (scalpel-bougie-tube for adults and needle cricothyrotomy in paediatrics). It may be particularly beneficial in narrow bore cricothyrotomy as compared to transtracheal jet ventilation, flow-controlled ventilation (FCV) generates lower peak pressures, enables active expiration, continuous monitoring, maintaining PEEP, controlled PEEP, cuffed secure airway, capnography monitoring, etc. The psychological component of performing a front-of-neck access cannot be understated, as a needle cricothyrotomy/needle-guidewire-Tritube® technique with flow-controlled ventilation would probably be more acceptable to a lot of physicians than a first time surgical cricothyrotomy. Nevertheless, further evidence is needed before the Ventrain® and Tritube® become a permanent fixture on difficult airway management guidelines [12]. Perhaps the Ventrain® could one day replace Plan D on difficult airway guidelines.

13.2 Ventrain® with Fibroscopic Intubation During Airway Management (Fig. 13)

Another very useful clinical trick is to use Ventrain® during fibroscopic airway management by connecting it via the Luer-lock port.

Flushing of low flow O_2 through the working channel of the scope will flush the airway with O_2 when closing both openings of the Ventrain®.

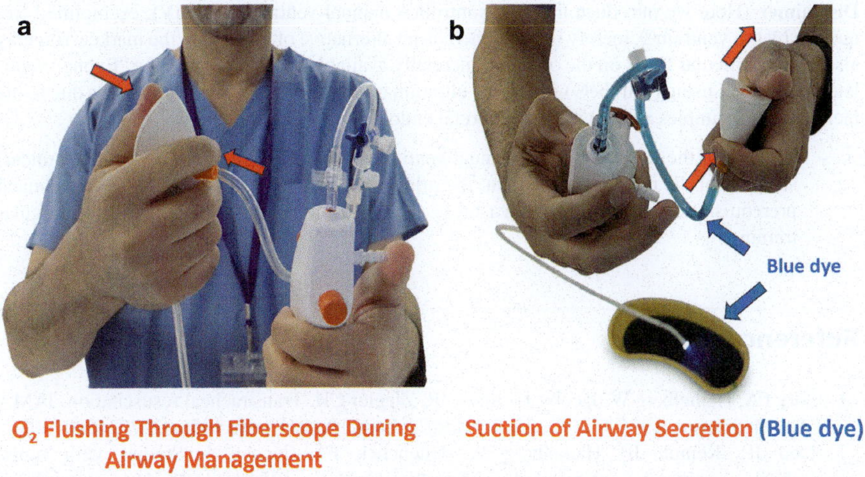

Fig. 13 (**a**) O_2 flushing through fiberscope during airway management. (**b**) Suction of airway secretion (blue dye). (Courtesy, Dr. Shallik, Doha Airway Equipment Museum, Qatar)

By closing the lower opening only, the Bernoulli principle can be utilized to suction out airway secretions, but this requires higher flows of O_2 from the flowmeter (Fig. 13).

14 Conclusion

Overall, the Ventrain® is a promising ventilation device for CICO scenarios and elective difficult airways. In paediatric patients aged 1–8, needle cricothyroidotomy is the recommended FONA technique by the Difficult Airway Society (DAS). Whereas in adults, surgical cricothyrotomy with the scalpel-bougie-tube technique is preferred for emergency FONA by DAS although needle cricothyrotomy still remains an option. When needle cricothyrotomy with small-bore cannulas is performed, Ventrain® is likely the best insufflation device when comparing lung volumes and pressures generated due to its EVA technology. Potential disadvantages include requirement for manual operation and lack of continuous airway pressure monitoring. This has been solved with the development of the Tritube® and Evone® flow-controlled ventilator. CICO scenarios are extremely stressful and the clinician will have to operate the flow ports of the Ventrain® device. Chest movements must be continuously assessed to minimize risk of air trapping and barotrauma. There is evidence in the literature for Ventrain® use in a wide variety of clinical situations as described in this chapter.

Acknowledgements A special thanks is extended to **Mr. Abil Luez** who artistically captured all images and video clips of this chapter.

Disclaimer Here we introduce the flow-controlled manual ventilator (FCmV), exemplified frequently by the Ventrain®, merely because there is no alternative of its kind on the market. You may also find a particular focus on the only commercially available FCV ventilator, the "Evone" ventilator. Moreover, using (Tritube®) instead of ultrathin or straw sized ETT terminology is due to the lack of other examples and not as a commercial endorsement of the products.

- The use of the flow-controlled manual ventilator (Ventrain®) demands a thorough understanding of the required equipment, the principle and function of the Ventrain®, technical prerequisites, clinical safety measures, and, most importantly, an appropriate regular training.

References

1. Flory FA, Hamelberg W, Jacoby JJ, Jones JR, Ziegler CH. Transtracheal resuscitation. JAMA J Am Med Assoc. 1956;162(7):625–8. https://doi.org/10.1001/jama.1956.02970240007003.
2. Reed JP, Kemph JP, Hamelberg W, Hitchcock FA, Jacoby J. Studies with transtracheal artificial respiration. Anesthesiology. 1954;15(1):28–41. https://doi.org/10.1097/00000542-195401000-00006.
3. Spoerel WE, Narayanan PS, Singh NP. Transtracheal ventilation. BJA Br J Anaesth. 1971;43(10):932–9. https://doi.org/10.1093/bja/43.10.932.
4. Eger EI, Hamilton WK. Positive-negative pressure ventilation with a modified Ayre's T-piece. Anesthesiology. 1958;19(5):611–8. https://doi.org/10.1097/00000542-195809000-00004.
5. Keuskamp DH. Automatic ventilation in paediatric anaesthesia using a modified Ayre's T-piece with negative pressure during expiratory phase. Anaesthesia. 1963;18:46–56. https://doi.org/10.1111/j.1365-2044.1963.tb13704.x.
6. Schapera A, Bainton CR, Kraemer R, Lee K. A pressurized injection/suction system for ventilation in the presence of complete airway obstruction. Crit Care Med. 1994;22(2):326–33. https://doi.org/10.1097/00003246-199402000-00026.
7. Dworkin R, Benumof JL, Benumof R, Karagianes TG. The effective tracheal diameter that causes air trapping during jet ventilation. J Cardiothorac Anesth. 1990;4(6):731–6. https://doi.org/10.1016/S0888-6296(09)90012-6.
8. Mora Carpio AL, Mora JI. Positive end-expiratory pressure. In: StatPearls. StatPearls Publishing; 2023. Accessed December 2, 2023. http://www.ncbi.nlm.nih.gov/books/NBK441904/
9. Hamaekers AEW, Borg PAJ, Enk D. Ventrain: an ejector ventilator for emergency use. BJA Br J Anaesth. 2012;108(6):1017–21. https://doi.org/10.1093/bja/aes033.
10. Ventrain | Ventinova. Accessed November 21, 2023. https://ventinovamedical.com/ventrain/
11. Dos Santos RA, Habre W, Albu G. Novel ventilation techniques in children. Paediatr Anaesth. 2022;32(2):286–94. https://doi.org/10.1111/pan.14344. Epub 2021 Dec 5. PMID: 34837438; PMCID: PMC9300098
12. Morrison S, Aerts S, Saldien V. The Ventrain device: a future role in difficult airway algorithms? Aa Pract. 2019;13(9):362–5. https://doi.org/10.1213/XAA.0000000000001084.
13. de Wolf M, Enk D, Jagannathan N. Ventilation through small-bore airways in children by implementing active expiration. Pediatr Anesth. 2022;32(2):312–20. https://doi.org/10.1111/pan.14379.
14. MSS138.02_IFUVentrain_EN-master_09092021.pdf. Accessed December 18, 2023. https://ventinovamedical.com/wp-content/uploads/2022/05/MSS138.02_IFUVentrain_EN-master_09092021.pdf
15. Hamaekers A, Theunissen M, Jansen J, Honig W, Enk D. Fast recovery from severe hypoxia through a 2 mm transtracheal catheter in pigs with a completely obstructed upper airway: 19AP1–9. Eur J Anaesthesiol EJA. 2010;27(47):247.
16. Willemsen MGA, Noppens R, Mulder ALM, Enk D. Ventilation with the Ventrain through a small lumen catheter in the failed paediatric airway: two case reports. Br J Anaesth. 2014;112(5):946–7. https://doi.org/10.1093/bja/aeu125.

17. Escribá Alepuz FJ, Alonso García J, Cuchillo Sastriques JV, Alcalá E, Argente NP. Emergency ventilation of infant subglottic stenosis through small-gauge lumen using the Ventrain: a case report. Aa Pract. 2018;10(6):136–8. https://doi.org/10.1213/XAA.0000000000000657.
18. Mann CM, Baker PA, Sainsbury DM, Taylor R. A comparison of cannula insufflation device performance for emergency front of neck airway. Pediatr Anesth. 2021;31(4):482–90. https://doi.org/10.1111/pan.14128.
19. Wahlen BM, Al-Thani H, El-Menyar A. Ventrain: from theory to practice. Bridging until re-tracheostomy. BMJ Case Rep. 2017;2017:bcr2017220403. https://doi.org/10.1136/bcr-2017-220403.
20. Heuveling DA, Mahieu HF, Jongsma-van Netten HG, Gerling V. Transtracheal use of the CriCath cannula in combination with the Ventrain device for prevention of hypoxic arrest due to severe upper airway obstruction: a case report. AA Pract. 2018;11(12):344–7. https://doi.org/10.1213/XAA.0000000000000823.
21. Failed awake intubation for critical airway obstruction rescued with the Ventrain device and an Arndt Exchange Catheter: a case report. Accessed November 22, 2023. https://oce.ovid.com/article/02054229-201907010-00008?relatedarticle=y
22. Elective use of the Ventrain for upper airway obstruction during high-frequency jet ventilation—ClinicalKey. Accessed November 22, 2023. https://www.clinicalkey.com/#!/content/playContent/1-s2.0-S095281801630040X
23. Onwochei DN, El-Boghdadly K, Ahmad I. Two-stage technique used to manage severe upper airway obstruction and avoid surgical tracheostomy: a case report. AA Pract. 2018;10(5):118–20. https://doi.org/10.1213/XAA.0000000000000645.
24. Borg PAJ, AEW H, Lacko M, Jansen J, Enk D. Ventrain® for ventilation of the lungs. Br J Anaesth. 2012;109(5):833–4. https://doi.org/10.1093/bja/aes366.
25. Rosenblatt WH, Popescu WM. Master techniques in upper and lower airway management. Philadelphia: Lippincott Williams & Wilkins; 2015.
26. Kristensen MS, de Wolf MWP, Rasmussen LS. Ventilation via the 2.4 mm internal diameter Tritube® with cuff—new possibilities in airway management. Acta Anaesthesiol Scand. 2017;61(6):580–9. https://doi.org/10.1111/aas.12894.
27. Moustafa AH, Shallik NA. Radiological evaluation of the airway: one-stop shop. In: Shallik NA, Moustafa AH, Marcus MAE, editors. Virtual endoscopy and 3D reconstruction in the airways. Cham: Springer; 2019. https://doi.org/10.1007/978-3-030-23253-5_3.
28. Kumar N, Dardeer A, Hammad Y, Shallik N, Shaikh N, Ganaw A, et al. Pushed away: how did 3D reconstruction solve this airway problem? Trends Anaesth Crit Care. 2020;30:e36–7.
29. Grassetto A, Pettenuzzo T, Badii F, et al. A new perspective during laryngo-tracheal surgery: the use of an ultra-thin endotracheal tube (Tritube®) and flow-controlled ventilation—a retrospective case series and a review of the literature. J Anesth Analg Crit Care. 2022;2(1):39. https://doi.org/10.1186/s44158-022-00066-3.
30. Piccioni F, Caccioppola A, Rosboch GL, Templeton W, Valenza F. Use of the Ventrain ventilation device and an airway exchange catheter to manage hypoxemia during thoracic surgery and one-lung ventilation. J Cardiothorac Vasc Anesth. 2021;35(12):3844–5. https://doi.org/10.1053/j.jvca.2021.06.023.
31. Evers VM, Immink RV, van Boven WJP, van Berge Henegouwen MI, Hollmann MW, Veelo DP. Intraoperative use of the Ventrain for single lung ventilation after iatrogenic trauma to the left main bronchus during thoracoscopy: a case report. Case Rep. 2017;9(4):116–8. https://doi.org/10.1213/XAA.0000000000000542.
32. Kheterpal S, Martin L, Shanks AM, Tremper KK. Prediction and outcomes of impossible mask ventilation: a review of 50,000 anesthetics. Anesthesiology. 2009;110(4):891–7. https://doi.org/10.1097/ALN.0b013e31819b5b87.

Specifications of the Flow-Controlled Ventilation Ventilator (Evone®)

Muhammad Firas Alhammad, Nada N. Shallik, and Nabil A. Shallik

1 Introduction

Upper airway surgeries pose challenges for both anaesthesiologists and surgeons. Ensuring adequate patient oxygenation while maintaining proper ventilation, alongside achieving optimal surgical field exposure, presents inherent difficulties in procedures involving laryngeal tumours, tracheal stenosis, vocal cord masses, epiglottic pathology, and oropharyngeal malignancies.

For an extended period, standard endotracheal intubation or high-flow jet ventilation (HFJV) has been customary in these surgeries. Nonetheless, these methods come with notable drawbacks, including potential compromise to surgical field exposure, heightened risks of aspiration, barotrauma hyperinflation or the possibility of losing airway control, and the need of emergency front-of-neck airway (eFONA).

Newly introduced Evone® (Ventinova Medical, Eindhoven, the Netherlands) flow-controlled ventilation (FCV) ventilator, employing an ultra-thin endotracheal tube (Tritube®) (Ventinova Medical, Eindhoven, the Netherlands), effectively

M. F. Alhammad
Anaesthesia, ICU and Perioperative Medicine Department, Hamad Medical Corporation, Doha, Qatar

N. N. Shallik
Faculty of Oral and Dental Medicine, Future University in Egypt, Cairo, Egypt

N. A. Shallik (✉)
Anaesthesia, ICU and Perioperative Medicine Department, Hamad Medical Corporation, Doha, Qatar

Clinical Anaesthesiology Department, Weill Cornell Medical College in Qatar, Doha, Qatar

Clinical Anaesthesiology Department, College of Medicine Qatar University, Doha, Qatar

Anaesthesia and SICU Department, Tanta University, Tanta, Egypt
e-mail: nshallik@hamad.qa

N. A. Shallik (ed.), *Flow Controlled Ventilation Mode Through a Straw Size Tube*, https://doi.org/10.1007/978-3-031-77477-5_7

address the previously mentioned limitations associated with conventional ventilation methods.

Evone® is a mechanical ventilator utilizing flow-controlled ventilation (FCV) for mechanical ventilation. The manufacturer recommends it for mechanical ventilation for less than a continuous 72 h [1] period. Evone® is typically used in operating theatres by anaesthesiologists or in intensive care units by intensivists. It differs from standard mechanical ventilators; volume-controlled ventilation (VCV) and pressure-controlled ventilation (PCV) and necessitates comprehensive training for proper operation. Evone® usage is restricted based on patient weight, with a recommendation against use in patients weighing less than 40 kg of ideal body weight to prevent barotrauma and patient harm [1].

In fact, there are certain procedures that may compromise Evone's functionality, including high-frequency electro-surgery equipment, short-wave therapy equipment, defibrillators, or magnetic resonance imaging (MRI) equipment, potentially leading to malfunction [2].

Disclaimer: The use of the flow-controlled ventilator (Evone®) (Ventinova Medical, Eindhoven, the Netherlands) demands a thorough understanding of the required equipment, the principle and function of the Evone®, technical prerequisites, clinical safety measures, and, most importantly, appropriate regular training.

2 Indications

The flow-controlled ventilator (FCV) offers outstanding ventilation for anesthetized patients by ensuring adequate oxygenation, preventing hypoxemia, and maintaining normocapnia.

The evidence surrounding the use of the flow-controlled ventilator is continuously developing. Presently, it is extensively employed in a diverse array of upper airway surgeries, showcasing its growing acceptance and utilization within the field. Including and not limited to; micro-laryngoscopy (MLS), transoral laser microsurgery (TLM), subglottic stenosis, tracheal stenosis [3], and other tracheal surgeries.

3 Flow-Controlled Ventilation: Advantages Over Conventional Ventilation

Throughout laryngeal surgery, flow-controlled ventilator enhances visibility at the surgical site. Additionally, FCV demonstrates enhanced lung aeration and respiratory system compliance.

Numerous studies have demonstrated the safety and efficacy of its application across various upper airway surgical procedures in patients categorized as ASA 1 or ASA 2 [4, 5]. However, additional research is required for other types of surgeries to establish a stronger evidential base.

FCV demonstrates efficacy in CO_2 elimination, with increased ventilation efficiency and improved alveolar recruitment even among patients with morbid obesity

[6]. Moreover, among patients with heightened susceptibility to compression atelectasis such as those in the Trendelenburg position or undergoing laparoscopy, FCV demonstrates the potential to reduce occurrences of hypercapnia or desaturation, consequently lowering the requirement for elevated ventilation pressures [3]. Additionally, individuals with diminished ventilation capacity (such as during one-lung ventilation) might experience improved ventilation and oxygenation during surgery [1].

The uninterrupted flow characteristic of FCV might leads to significantly lower shear stress in comparison to conventional ventilation modes VCV and PCV, consequently minimizing energy dissipation [7] (Fig. 1) for more details please refer to chapter "The Respiratory Physics and Mechanics of Flow-Controlled Ventilation".

In contrast to traditional ventilators that derive intratracheal pressures from measurements taken on the ventilator side, FCV directly measures intratracheal pressures. This approach enables reliable measurement of energy dissipation, represented by the area of the pressure–volume loop.

FCV has the capacity to mitigate or restrict lung injury in instances of severe stenosis. The ultra-thin endotracheal tube (Tritube®) has the potential to obviate the necessity for extracorporeal membrane oxygenation (ECMO) during surgery, as illustrated in a case involving critical tracheal stenosis [3].

An unconventional application of the device involves the ability to establish a negative end-expiratory pressure (NEEP). Theoretically, leveraging NEEP's effect could aid in life-threatening hypovolemic shock situations by enhancing cardiac output through a reduction in intrathoracic pressure and subsequent elevation of the pressure gradient, facilitating improved venous return to the heart [8].

In summary the benefits associated with FCV are:

- Decreases alveoli atelectasis.
- Enhances lung aeration.
- Improves gas exchange efficiency, resulting in enhanced oxygenation and CO_2 removal.
- Reduces dissipation of respiratory energy, contributing to more efficient ventilation.

In addition, incorporating a Tritube® with the Evone® ventilator may prove beneficial in unforeseen challenging airway situations, such as unexpected tracheal stenosis, potentially averting the necessity for emergent front-of-neck access and surgical airway interventions [9].

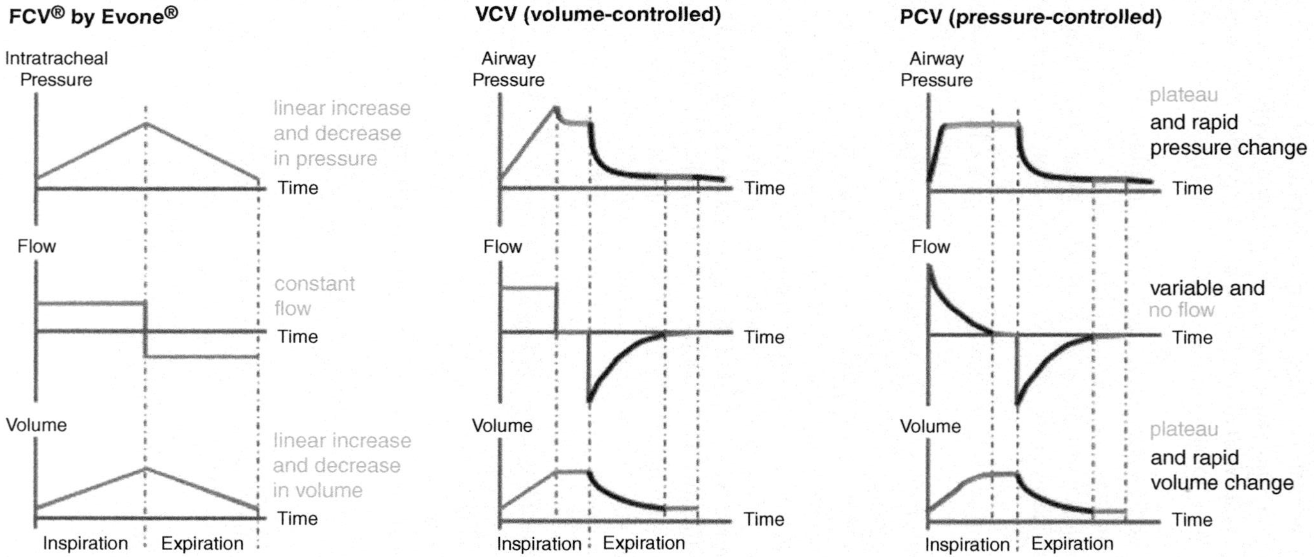

Fig. 1 Demonstrating the differences in airway pressure during volume control (middle), pressure control (right), and flow control ventilation (left) (courtesy of Ventinova Medical, Eindhoven, The Netherlands)

4 Mechanism of Action of Flow-Controlled Ventilator: The Bernoulli's Principle in Effect

Conventional ventilators rely on active inspiration to deliver tidal volume, with a passive mechanism during expiration. In contrast, the FCV ventilator employs active processes for both inspiration and expiration, facilitating inhalation and exhalation for patients under anaesthesia through active mechanisms. This essentially refers to the process of extracting air from the lungs during exhalation.

4.1 The Bernoulli's Principle in Effect

The advent of ultra-thin ETT was accompanied by an innovative mode of mechanical ventilation called FCV, which can accommodate the resistance to airflow caused by the tube's narrow diameter, in addition to; tackling the risk of air-trapping and lung hyperinflation given the presence of an inflated cuff. To fully understand how flow-controlled ventilation operates, it is worth revising Bernoulli's principle, the basis of how the hand-operated manual flow-controlled ventilator (Ventrain®) and the automatic flow-controlled mechanical ventilator (Evone®) function.

In essence, Bernoulli's principle describes the relationship between the velocity, pressure, and the flow of a fluid (liquid or gas). It states that, as the speed of a moving fluid increases, the pressure within the fluid decreases. During the inspiratory phase of the respiratory cycle, the air is insufflated from the air inlet of the flow-controlled mechanical ventilator to the patient through the narrow lumen Tritube®

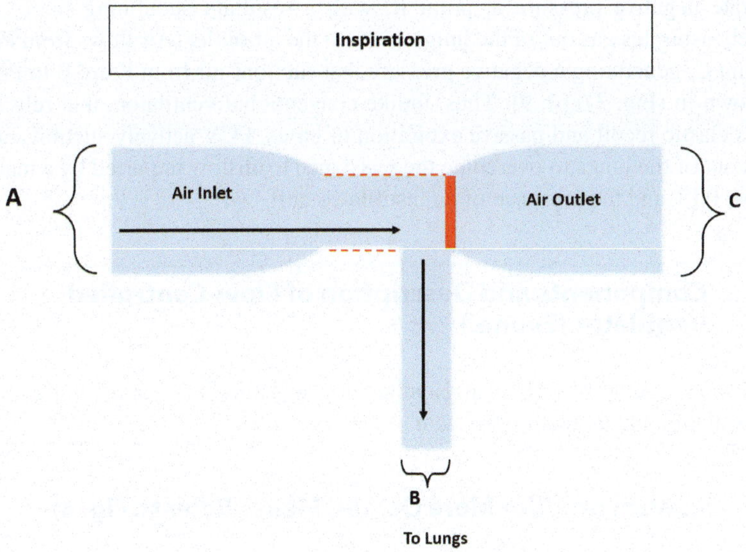

Fig. 2 Bernoulli's principle in the Evone® mechanical ventilator during the inspiratory phase

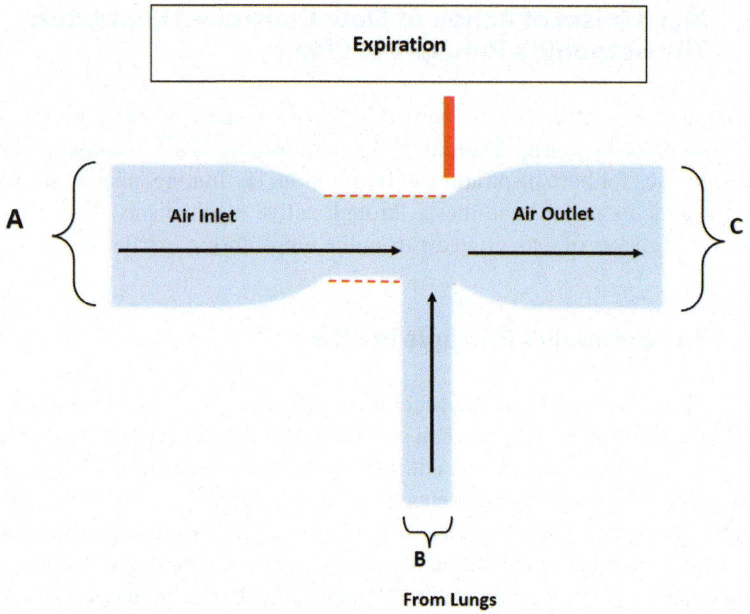

Fig. 3 Bernoulli's principle in the Evone® mechanical ventilator during the expiratory phase

(Ventinova Medical, Eindhoven, The Netherlands) (From point A to point B) in (Fig. 2) [4, 10]. The air stream has no alternative route as the air outlet is blocked. During the expiratory phase of the respiratory cycle, the blockage at point C is released, giving way to the high-velocity air that is injected through the air inlet to generate negative pressure at point B, with a resultant suctioning force, which actively aspirates gas out of the lungs and into the air outlet (Air flows from Point A to Point C, generating a negative pressure that suctions air from Point B to Point C, as shown in (Fig. 3)) [4, 9]. Thus, unlike conventional ventilators that rely on the lung's elastic recoil and passive expiration of gases, FCV actively suctions expired gases out of the lungs to overcome the resistance to airflow imparted by a markedly narrow ETT and the presence of an insufflated cuff.

5 Components and Description of Flow-Controlled Ventilator (Evone®)

The Evone® (Ventinova Medical, Eindhoven, the Netherlands) apparatus comprises a control unit and a breathing system,

5.1 Control Unit (for More Details, Please Refer to Fig. 4)

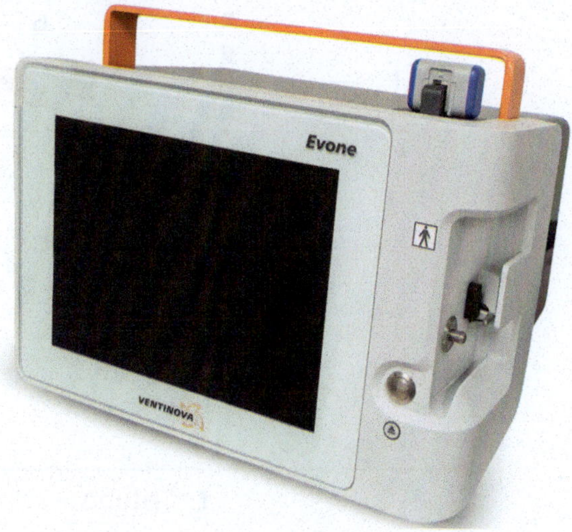

Fig. 4 All parts of the control unit (courtesy of Ventinova Medical, Eindhoven, the Netherlands)

5.2 Breathing System (for More Details, Please Refer to Figs. 5, 6, and 7)

5.2.1 $ETCO_2$ Measurement

EVONE ventilator utilizing a mainstream method for carbon dioxide measurements, a measuring cuvette positioned directly between the Cartridge and the Humid-Vent Filter Pedi efficiently assesses the absorption of infrared light. The measurement process in this method is instantaneous, without any time delay, and it effectively captures data across the entirety of the air volume. Evone mainstream End Tidal Carbon Dioxide ($ETCO_2$) capnometer and its position is illustrated in (Figs. 5, 6, and 7).

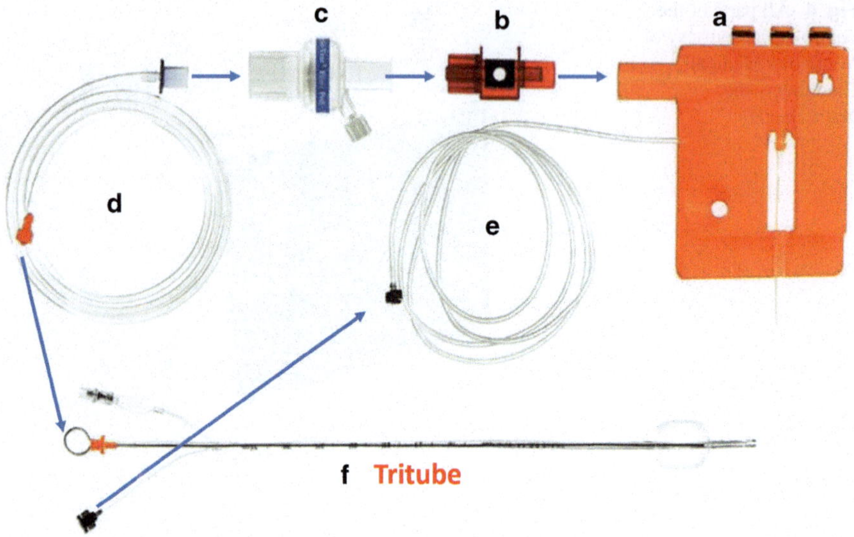

Fig. 5 All parts of the breathing unit for Tritube® connection. (**a**) Cartridge, (**b**) $ETCO_2$ measurement adaptor or airway adapter, (**c**) humid-vent filter pedi straight, (**d**) Evone breathing tubing, (**e**) Intra-tracheal (IT) tube measurement line, (**f**) Tritube® (courtesy of Ventinova Medical, Eindhoven, The Netherlands)

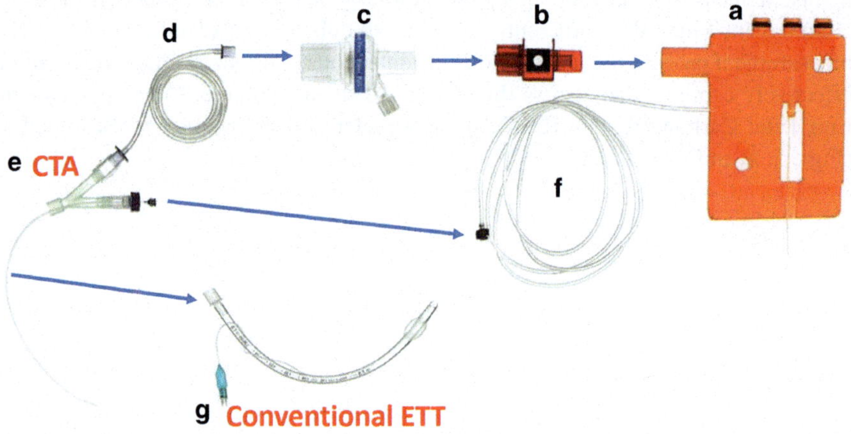

Fig. 6 All parts of the breathing unit for CTA® and conventional tube connection: (**a**) Cartridge, (**b**) $ETCO_2$ measurement adaptor or airway adapter, (**c**) humid-vent filter pedi straight, (**d**) evone breathing tubing, (**e**) conventional tube adaptor (CTA®), (**f**) intra-tracheal (IT) tube measurement line, (**g**) conventional ETT larger than 5 mm (courtesy of Ventinova Medical, Eindhoven, The Netherlands)

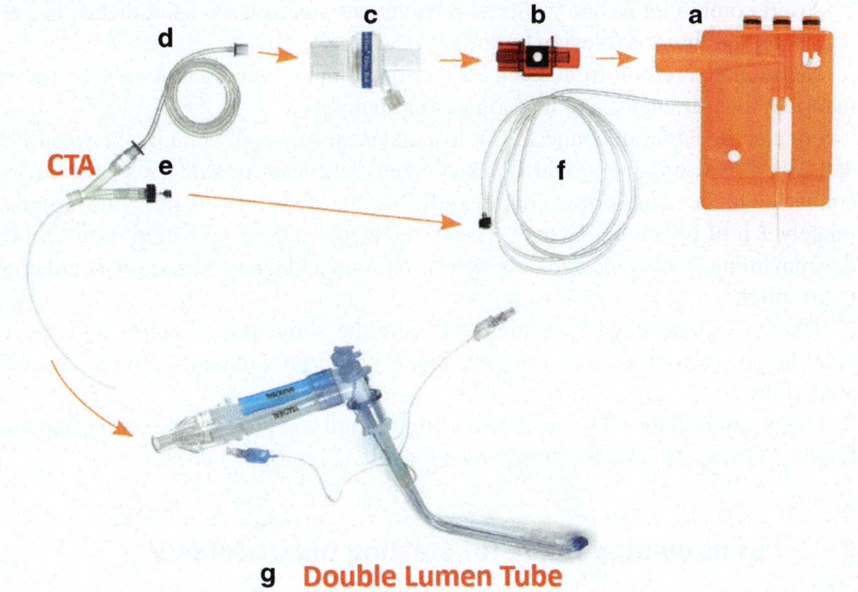

Fig. 7 All parts of the breathing unit for CTA® and double lumen tube connection. (**a**) Cartridge, (**b**) $ETCO_2$ measurement adaptor or airway adapter, (**c**) Humid-vent filter pedi straight, (**d**) Evone breathing tubing, (**e**) Conventional tube adaptor (CTA®), (**f**) Intra-tracheal (IT) tube measurement line, (**g**) Double lumen endobronchial tube (DLT) larger than 35 French (courtesy of Ventinova Medical, Eindhoven, The Netherlands)

6 FCV Device Preparation for the Use

Prior to powering on Evone®, ensure the control unit adjusts to the ambient temperature.

To prepare the device for operation, insert the Evone® Cartridge into the Control Unit.

Upon inserting the FCV Cartridge, assemble the Evone® Breathing System, pairing it either with the Tritube® or a conventional tube adaptor (CTA®) for use with a conventional endotracheal tube.

Ensure the installation of paediatric Heat and Moisture Exchanger (HME) filter between the Evone Airway Adapter and Breathing Tubing/Conventional Tube Adapter (CTA®) to mitigate the risk of contamination in the Control Unit.

Moreover, ensure all parts are securely connected to prevent leakage or disconnection of the breathing system during ventilation. Before employing Evone®, confirm the establishment of the following connections: (1) Medical gases, (2) Electrical power, (3) CO_2 sensor.

For medical gases, FCV features separate connections for medical air and medical oxygen. Before usage, ensure the correct attachment of gas tubing to high-pressure gas supplies within the recommended pressure range of 3.0–6.0 bar.

Avoid combining Evone® with flammable gases or volatile anaesthetics to prevent potential fire or explosion hazards.

Additionally, refrain from using FCV with helium or helium mixtures to prevent incorrect measurements and inadequate ventilation.

For electrical power, connect FCV to a mains power supply ranging between 115 and 230 V AC using the provided power cable. Whenever possible, keep the device connected to the mains power supply as the battery life is limited, providing approximately 1 h of operation. Evone® triggers an alarm and visual battery status when the remaining battery power falls below 30 min, indicating a risk of ventilation interruption.

The device can only be disconnected from the mains power supply by unplugging the power cord, thus ensuring the mains power plug remains easily accessible at all times.

Lastly, connect the CO_2 sensor to the control unit and position the sensor onto the Evone® Airway Adapter for proper functionality (Figs. 5, 6, and 7).

7 Step-by-Step Guide for Starting the Use of FCV

- Switching on and starting up: Switch on FCV using the hard button located on the left-hand side of the control unit. After approximately 10 s, the initial screen will appear. The system initiates various automatic checks for reliable performance. Some startup checks may require user interaction and are optional.
- Self-check: Immediately after powering up, FCV conducts a self-check to verify the basic functioning of valves, sensors, alarm controller signals, and internal communication. This process occurs on-screen.
- Start-up check: Upon successful completion of the self-check, the startup check menu will automatically appear. Users can select tests to perform. It's highly recommended to conduct all tests of the start-up check on a daily basis (every 24 h) before commencing ventilation or before switching between patients' ventilation [1].
- The start-up check necessitates a fully assembled FCV and the connection of Tritube® to an artificial lung. The Evone® Conventional Tube Adapter (CTA®) can be used for this check with adult traditional ETT and lung simulator or artificial lung with certain compliance (TV = 500 ml, PEEP = 0 mbar, Resistance = 20 mbar/l/s, Max TV = 1000 ml).
- The start-up check screen displays actual values for oxygen and air gas supply pressures within the recommended pressure range of 3.0–6.0 bar.
- This process consists of three tests covering various items:
  - Alarm Indication: Generates alarm sounds and light signals. Users confirm low, medium, and high priority alarm signals when prompted (for more details please refer to section "Alarms System").
  - FCV® Mode: Assemble the Evone® Breathing System and Tritube® or CTA® as indicated. Place Tritube® in an artificial lung and inflate the cuff as directed. The following items are tested:

Pressure vessel and sensor
Valve warming-up
Mass flow controllers
Pressure lumen purge pulse
Pressure lumen sensor
Exhaust valve (rotating valve)
Leakage testing

- Following the startup procedure, entering patient characteristics is necessary to establish default ventilation parameters and volume limits.
- Select the patient's gender, which is indicated by a colour change on the screen. Additionally, the patient's length, weight, and age can be adjusted using sliders located on the right-hand side of the screen [1].
- The entered patient's gender and length are utilized to calculate the ideal body weight, which is then employed to determine an inspiratory volume in the initial ventilation cycle. At the bottom of the screen, users can choose to commence with default ventilation settings based on the entered patient data (labelled as 'patient data') or settings from the last use. The default selection is 'patient data' (Fig. 8)
- Clinical workflow during ventilation using Tritube® and conventional tubes:
- Initiation of ventilation with ultra-thin (Tritube®) or CTA Figs. 5, 6, and 7:
  – Initiate total intravenous anaesthesia (TIVA) or target controlled infusion (TCI) because there is no way to use inhalational anaesthetics with FCV.
  – Intubate the patient using Tritube® following the manufacturer's instructions or intubate the patient using the chosen conventional ETT tube or double lumen tube.

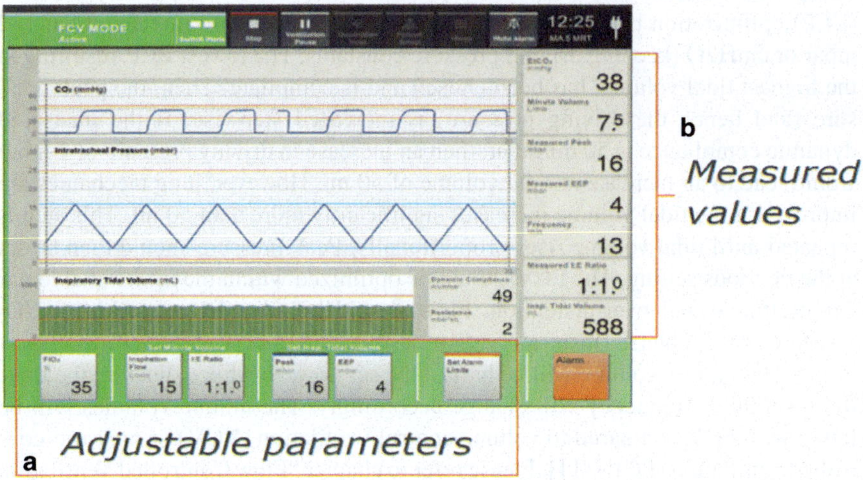

Fig. 8 The Screen of flow controlled ventilator (Evone®): (**a**) Green lower part represents the adjustable parameters and (**b**) Grey part (right vertical) represents measured values (courtesy of Ventinova Medical, Eindhoven, The Netherlands)

- Flush the pressure lumen and ventilation lumen with 10 ml of air to remove any secretions or lubrication gel from inside the lumens.
- Connect Tritube® to Evone®, ensuring connection to both the ventilation lumen and ensure the pressure lumen line as proximal as possible.
- Optionally, commence ventilation with the cuff deflated to facilitate deeper anaesthesia (Jet mode).
- Begin ventilation with the cuff inflated (25–30 mbar) in FCV mode once anaesthesia is deepened. A triangular pressure curve will display on the screen (Fig. 8)
- Adjust ventilation settings if necessary:

  Set FiO_2 per preference.

  Adjust end expiratory pressure (EEP) to preferred levels.

  Modify peak airway pressure to regulate tidal volume.

  Adjust inspiratory flow to manage minute volume and respiratory rate which is more the result of set flow, driving pressure, and patient physics (compliance and resistance).

• It is worth noting that spontaneous breathing is not feasible when the CTA® is connected to the conventional adult endotracheal tube or Ultra-thin ETT (Tritube®) [1].

8 FCV in Special Circumstances

8.1 Special Adjustment of Flow-Controlled Ventilation in ARDS

Ventilation can easily be individualized initially by the end-expiratory pressure (EEP) optimization by changing both EEP and peak pressure increments of 1–2 mbar or cmH2O (keeping driving pressure constant). The lowest EEP, resulting in the highest tidal volume, has been chosen and is compliant. Then, the peak pressure (and hence the driving pressure) is increased stepwise. If the measured dynamic compliance is 50 ml/mbar, then an increase in driving pressure of 1 mbar would lead to an increase in tidal volume of 50 ml. However, lung mechanics are improved if the tidal volume increases significantly more than 50 ml. This step is repeated until tidal volume rises proportionally. Peak pressure should then be set at the previous setting. The FCV should be optimized within the limits of alveolar derecruitment and over-distention. Flow should be adjusted according to CO_2 measurements. The I:E (inspiratory: expiratory) ratio in FCV should always be set at 1:1. The minute volume will be half of the set flow, so while adjusting the flow, the respiratory frequency will change accordingly. The minute volumes will be lower with FCV compared to volume control ventilation (VCV) or pressure-controlled ventilation (PCV) [11]. Please refer to chapter "Flow Controlled Ventilation in ICU Settings" for more details.

8.2 Tritube® and FCV in Airway Canal Stenosis

The application of virtual endoscopy in diagnosing traumatic supra-glottic airway stenosis provides precise anatomical pathology, facilitating the appropriate utilization of the Evone® ventilator in devising effective airway management strategies [12].

Three-dimensional (3D) reconstruction serves as an invaluable tool in improving diagnostic accuracy for airway lesions. Additionally, the ultra-thin endotracheal tube (Tritube®) and the Evone® ventilator offers a safe alternative for airway management in scenarios where standard techniques pose a potential risk of compromising the patient's airway [13, 14].

In tracheobronchial stenosis, virtual bronchoscopy (VB) demonstrates sensitivity ranging from 63% to 100% and specificity from 61% to 99% [15]. This modality permits examination of the post-stenotic segment of the tracheobronchial tree and offers insights into extra-luminal pathology. VB procedures are safe and well-tolerated by critically ill patients, posing no risk of contamination or infection, even in immunocompromised individuals.

Both three-dimensional (3D) reconstruction and virtual bronchoscopy can be conducted by radiologists, anaesthetists, or surgeons using readily available software on appropriate workstations. These techniques generate an internal simulated view of the airway pathology, aiding in the formulation of airway management plans in critical and challenging scenarios.

9 Available Operational Modes of Evone® Ventilator

Flow-controlled ventilator (Evone®) offers two distinct modes of operation:

1. Flow-controlled ventilation (FCV): Suitable for surgical scenarios and ICU settings. This mode is compatible with both the Tritube® or conventional ETT or Double lumen tube.
2. Jet mode: This mode entails traditional high-frequency jet ventilation (HFJV) and can exclusively be utilized with the Tritube® with a deflated cuff, double lumen tubes, jet catheters, or scopes are suitable for jet ventilation.

9.1 Flow-Controlled Ventilation (Fig. 8)

In flow-controlled ventilation, the respiratory cycle's regulation relies on flow for both inspiration and expiration. For this mode, an inflated cuff of the ETT or Tritube® is essential. The adjustable ventilator settings in this mode include:

Inspired FIO_2, inspiration flow rate (L/M), I:E ratio (Inspiratory to Expiratory ratio), peak pressure (cmH_2O), and/or EEP (end expiratory pressure) (cmH_2O).

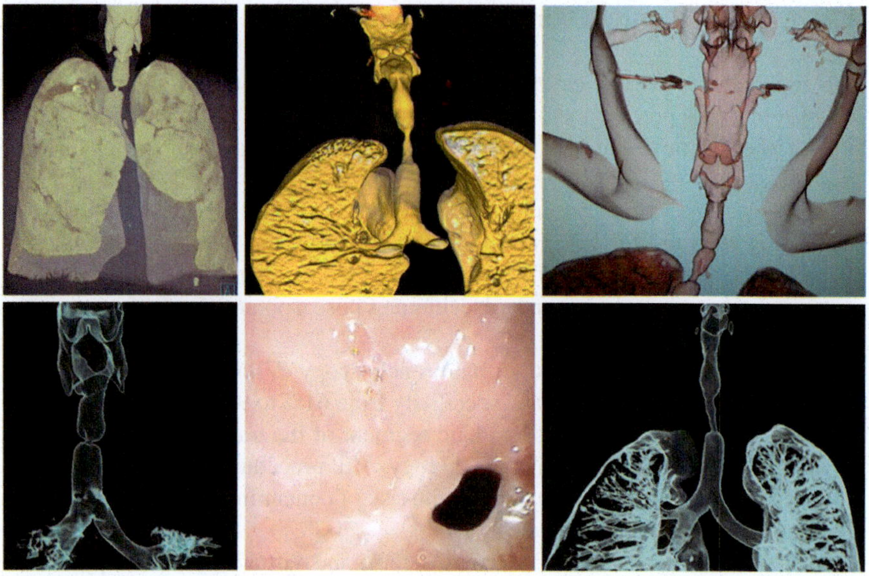

Fig. 9 Different cases of tracheal stenosis diagnosed with CT 3-D reconstruction and virtual endoscopy (VE) were successfully managed using Tritube® and Evone® (Courtesy, Dr. Shallik, Doha, Qatar)

In contrast to conventional ventilation modes such as volume control (VCV) and pressure control (PCV), in FCV, the respiratory rate, tidal volume, and consequently, minute ventilation cannot be directly adjusted or set. Please note that in I:E ratio 1:1, the minute volume (MV) is always half of the set flow (Fig. 9).

9.2 Jet Mode

The Jet Mode can be employed postoperatively to transition the patient from mechanical ventilation to encourage spontaneous breathing. However, the maximum driving pressure is capped at 1.5 Bar. It is important to note that Jet Mode should solely be employed with Tritube® with deflated cuff, jet catheters, devices with single lumen jet or double lumen endotracheal tube but not suitable for the conventional endotracheal tubes [1].

Before initiating jet mode, the cuff must be manually deflated by hand to prevent the risk of barotrauma and allow the unrestricted egress of expiratory gases. However, prior to deflation, it is crucial to inspect the cuff for any accumulated debris to mitigate the risk of infection [1].

To prevent the risk of barotrauma, it's advised not to combine the jet mode with conventional tube adapter (CTA). Additionally, limiting the use of Jet Mode to a maximum of 30 min/patient is recommended to mitigate the risk of dehydration [1].

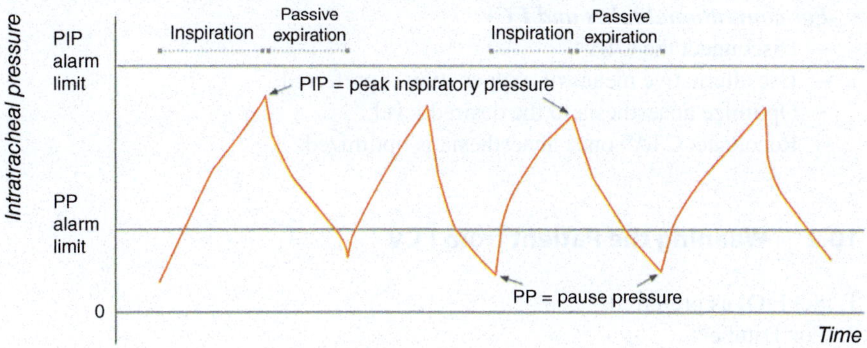

Fig. 10 Jet breathing cycles (courtesy of Ventinova Medical, Eindhoven, The Netherlands)

- The Jet cycle is regulated by three operator settings: (1) FiO_2. Frequency, (2) Inspiration percentage, (3) Driving pressure.

A typical sequence of Jet breathing cycles is illustrated (Fig. 10). Throughout the inspiration phase, the device upholds a consistent driving pressure on the tube, regulated by the set frequency and inspiration percentage. It's anticipated that during inspiration, the peak intratracheal pressure will remain below the predetermined peak inspiratory pressure (PIP) alarm limit. In the subsequent passive expiration phase, the intratracheal pressure should decrease below the operator-configured pause pressure (PP) alarm limit. Failure to do so triggers an alarm, alerting the operator and interrupting the ventilation cycle [1].

10 Trouble Shooting

The patient should be in a deep level of anaesthesia with TIVA, and fully relaxed using muscle relaxant of your choice during Evone® use.

10.1 Management During Light Anaesthesia or Patient Wakefulness

- ***For Tritube® and FCV:***
  - Deflate the cuff of Tritube® to minimize tracheal stimuli.
  - In case of 'early warning' signs (like very small negative pressure drops or weak trigger attempt or increases in pressure curve or weak exhalation attempt) then you have to deepen the sedation.
  - Optimize anaesthesia to attain desired levels.
  - Inflate the cuff when anaesthesia is optimized.
  - Note: Airway remains open, posing a risk of aspiration.

- ***For conventional tubes and FCV:***
  - Disconnect the CTA®.
  - Use alternative means of oxygenation if preferred.
  - Optimize anaesthesia to the desired level.
  - Reconnect CTA® once anaesthesia is optimized.

10.2 Weaning the Patient from FCV

1. Set FiO_2 as preferred.
2. For Tritube®:
   (a) Wake the patient using one of two ventilation options: With an inflated cuff in FCV® mode (e.g., in cases of aspiration risk), please gently wake the patient without much movement, then deflate the cuff and extubate when the patient is awake.
   (b) *Or alternatively,* with a deflated cuff in Jet mode (risk of aspiration). An open airway is required. Adjust settings if necessary (e.g., lower driving pressure with higher frequency may reduce tracheal stimuli).

10.3 Handling Obstructions While Using Evone®

1. Stop ventilation immediately.
2. Vigorously flush the pressure lumen and/or ventilation lumen with 2–5 mL saline, followed by approximately 15 mL of air.
3. If secretions persist in the ventilation lumen, use a suction catheter to remove them. Ensure the airway remains open during the suction from Tritube®. Be sure to do a suction with separate suction catheter above the Tritube® cuff before deflating the cuff.
4. Purge the lumen again with 2 mL of saline followed by air.
5. If using Tritube®: Slightly adjust the Tritube® to prevent contact with the tracheal wall and inflate the cuff. Eventually, oxygenate /ventilate patient with bag/face-mask with Tritube® (empty cuff) in situ, or use Ventrain® as plan B (Fig. 11).
6. Restart ventilation.
7. Prophylactic premedicating with Glycopyrrolate injection and adequate hydration.

For more details, please refer to chapter "Ultra-thin Cuffed Endotracheal Tube (Tritube®)".

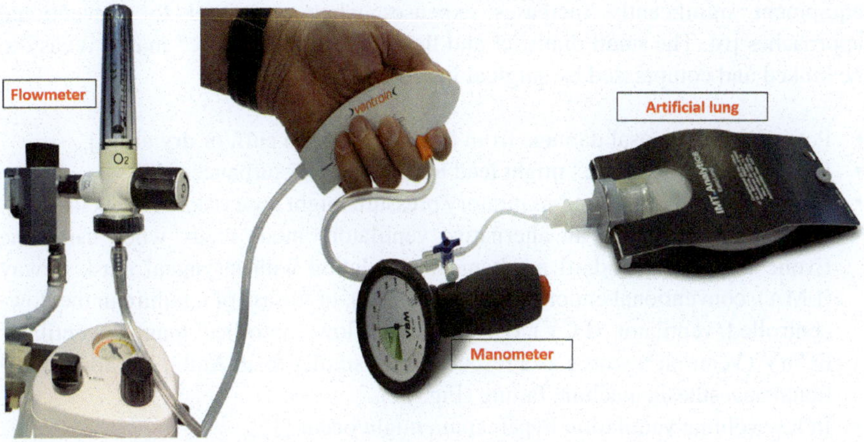

Fig. 11 Anaesthesia machine flowmeter connection with Ventrain®, manometer, and artificial lung. (Courtesy, Dr. Shallik, Doha Airway Equipment Museum, Qatar)

11 Complications and Limitations

A limitation associated with a narrow lumen tube or ultra-lumen is the potential for obstruction due to excessive airway secretions or blood originating from the surgical site. Therefore, it is advisable to use Glycopyrrolate preoperatively to diminish mucus secretion and mitigate potential disturbances in ventilation. When encountering excessive airway secretions, conventional suction catheters may not be viable. Nevertheless, by deflating the cuff, the ventilation lumen can serve as an alternative for suctioning. Deflating the cuff before negative suctioning is necessary to avoid alveoli collapse and atelectasis.

Another drawback associated with Evone® is the potential for displacement of Tritube® from the trachea, which can occur due to factors like coughing, steep surgical positions (Trendelenburg position), increased intra-abdominal pressure (laparoscopic or robotic surgery) or during the emergence from anaesthesia. Moreover, the narrow lumen of the tube increases the likelihood of detachment.

The length and flexible tip of Tritube® could make the Tritube® prone to be placed, just above the carina, too deep, or placed against the tracheal wall. In this case twist and/or withdraw the tube until resistance is removed and / or tube is located in the correct place.

The incompatibility of volatile anaesthetics with flow-controlled ventilation, owing to their physical properties, poses a limitation. Consequently, the necessity for total intravenous anaesthesia (TIVA) or (TCI) and the cost of the specialized equipment significantly increases expenses when compared to conventional approaches [6]. The small diameter and flexibility of the Tritube® makes it easy to be kinked and compressed by surgical instruments.

- Potential for mucosal damage from the tube, balloon cuff, or dry air [1].
- Prolonged use of Evone® might lead to metabolic disturbances [1].
- Negative intrathoracic end-expiratory pressure might pose risks of atelectasis [1].
- It's advisable to have an alternative ventilatory mode ready when using the Evone®, such as standard mechanical ventilation with laryngeal mask airway (LMA), conventional endotracheal tube (ETT), or in case of a failure in the flow-controlled ventilator (FCV) (Evone®), the flow-controlled manual ventilator FCmV (Ventrain®) works as a rescue device similar to an Ambu bag for a traditional anaesthesia machine failure (Fig. 11).
- In low volume ventilation hypercapnia might occur [1].
- Adjust alarm settings individually for each patient to prevent patient harm.
- The exhaust opening of Evone® might get obstructed by any additional device, or the exhaust opening ~~is~~ may get kinked and this will lead to the device malfunctioning. It is recommended that this exhaust is always kept open for proper functioning of the ventilator [1].

12 Alarm System

12.1 Alarm System Overview in FCV Ventilator

- Alarm messages appear as pop-ups in the alarm bar, both audible and visible via the alarm indicator LED on the Evone® Control Unit.
- The alarm sounds can be muted for 120 s by pressing the 'Mute Alarm' button. Subsequent new alarms will also be muted.
- More detailed alarm information can be accessed by clicking the alarm bar during an active alarm, displaying an extended pop-up that can be closed by clicking 'Close'.
- Alarm notifications and history can be viewed by tapping the 'Alarm Notifications' button. The logging of alarms starts from powering on Evone® until powering it off. Note that the alarm history is not stored during power down situations.
- The system can log up to 100 alarm messages. Alarm priority levels and descriptions:
  - Red: High priority alarm indicated by a red blinking light and sound. It signifies an immediate danger situation for the patient. Immediate action is needed to minimize the impact on the patient's well-being.

  - Yellow or orange: Medium priority alarm represented by yellow/orange blinking light and sound. It indicates either a patient-related situation or a device-related error. Investigation and appropriate actions are required.
  - Blue: Low priority alarm indicated by a blue blinking light and sound. It suggests a situation outside normal ranges, signalling an undesired condition. Check and take appropriate actions.
- None: This category signifies obsolete or resolved alarms. There is no current alarm, presenting a list of previous alarms that have been resolved or are no longer valid. Use this list for regular monitoring and take necessary actions if recurring patterns emerge.

12.2 Different Functionalities, Safety Measures, and Alarm Conditions for Evone® [1]

12.2.1 Safety State

- The 'Safety State' activates when Evone® encounters an issue that prevents further device use, potentially posing immediate hazards for the patient.
- It prompts a pop-up screen, allowing the user only one option: to shut down the device.
- During ventilation, if the safety state emerges, switch to alternative ventilation.

12.2.2 Negative End Expiratory Pressure (NEEP)

- NEEP settings (maximally—10 mbar) are strictly limited to use during hypovolemia/severe haemorrhage and concomitant hemodynamic instability [1].
- Lower intrathoracic pressures stimulate blood return.
- Consider NEEP in hypovolemic situations to boost venous blood return, stimulate cardiac output, and maintain peripheral circulation.
- However, NEEP poses risks, including atelectasis. Balancing the risk of metabolic acidosis (during PEEP) against atelectasis (during NEEP) is crucial for hypovolemic patients [1].
- Following NEEP application, consider a recruitment manoeuvre once the patient stabilizes hemodynamically.

12.2.3 Inspiration Hold

- The 'Inspiration Hold' function maintains intratracheal pressure at the peak level for up to 60 s, facilitating clinical recruitment manoeuvres [1].
- After 60 s, ventilation cycles automatically resume to expiratory phase.

12.2.4 Shut Down

- Evone® should be shut down via the shutdown option on the screen, requiring user confirmation before termination. An auditory signal confirms the shutdown.
- Alternatively, pressing the standby button for over 3 s leads to immediate shut down without warning.

12.3 Alarm Text Conditions and Responses

- Various alarm conditions and their corresponding actions and priorities are listed, ranging from fatal alarms (total power loss or internal errors) to gas supply pressures, battery levels, and software malfunctions.
- Device actions include moving to the safety state, ventilation pause, or alarm resets upon resolving the condition.
- User actions involve checking gas supply, switching ventilation methods, contacting the manufacturer, connecting to power sources, and performing self-checks or corrective measures

12.4 FCV Exhaust Filter

It is not advisable to obstruct the exhaust openings on the rear side of the Evone® system. However, utilizing special type of heat and moisture exchanger (HME) filter might offer the advantage of reducing the contamination of the operating theatre air environment (with blood or secretions or infected patient aerosols) and decreasing the noise level during expiration. Further investigation through clinical trial is necessary to assess the efficacy of this adjustment to the exhaust filter. Our centre implemented this method during the COVID-19 era as additional safety to operating room environment as illustrated in (Fig. 12a, b).

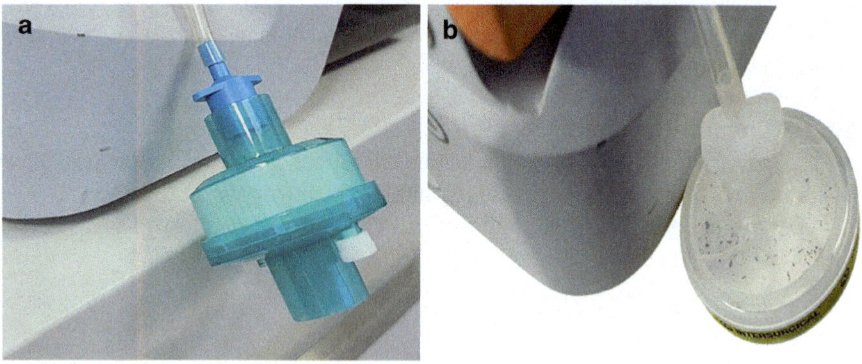

Fig. 12 (**a**) Exhaust Filter attached to FCV, (**b**) Dried blood or rust in the filter

13 Conclusion

In summary, the flow-controlled ventilator (Evone®), employing flow control ventilation concept, represents a novel approach to ventilation. While the evidence supporting its use continues to evolve through clinical trials, it appears to offer safety across various scenarios, particularly in upper airway procedures and certain ICU settings. Compared to standard ventilators such as volume-controlled and pressure-controlled models, the Evone® provides numerous advantages. However, its effective utilization requires expertise and meticulous attention.

Acknowledgments A special thanks is extended to Mr. Abil Luez who artistically captured all images and video clips for this chapter.

Disclaimer Here we introduce the flow-controlled manual ventilator (FCmV), exemplified frequently by the Ventrain®, merely because there is no alternative of its kind on the market and also you may find a particular focus on the only commercially available FCV ventilator, the 'Evone®' ventilator, moreover using of (Tritube®) instead of ultra-thin or straw sized ETT nomenclature due to the lack of other examples and not as commercial endorsement of the products.

The use of the Flow-Controlled Ventilator (Evone®) demands a thorough understanding of the required equipment, the principle and function of the Evone®, technical prerequisites, clinical safety measures, and, most importantly, an appropriate regular training.

References

1. Roggan A. EN instructions for use. 2014. https://ventinovamedical.com/wp-content/uploa6.15_IFUEvone_EN_Final.pdf.
2. Schmidt J, Günther F, Weber J, Wirth S, Brandes I, Barnes T, et al. Flow-controlled ventilation during ear, nose and throat surgery: a prospective observational study. Eur J Anaesthesiol. 2019;36(5):327–34. https://pubmed.ncbi.nlm.nih.gov/30730422/.
3. Shallik N, Elarref M, Khamash O, Abdelaal A, Radi Alkhafaji M, Makki H, Menon A. Management of critical tracheal stenosis with a straw sized tube (Tritube): case report. Qatar Med J. 2020;3:48.
4. Meulemans J, Jans A, Vermeulen K, Vandommele J, Delaere P, Van der Poorten V. Evone® flow-controlled ventilation during upper airway surgery: a clinical feasibility study and safety assessment. Front Surg. 2020;7:6.
5. Filauro M, Mora F, Vallin A, Della Casa P, Arceri C, Gratarola A, et al. Evone® flow controlled ventilation: a new device for laryngotracheal surgery. Acta Otorhinolaryngol. 2022;42(2):189.
6. Weber J, Straka L, Borgmann S, Schmidt J, Wirth S, Schumann S. Flow-controlled ventilation (FCV) improves regional ventilation in obese patients- a randomized controlled crossover trial. BMC Anesthesiol. 2020;20(1):1–10. https://bmcanesthesiol.biomedcentral.com/articles/10.1186/s12871-020-0944-y.
7. Bialka S, Palaczynski P, Szuldrzynski K, Wichary P, Kowalski D, Van Der Hoorn JWA, et al. Flow-controlled ventilation – a new and promising method of ventilation presented with a review of the literature. Anaesthesiol Intensive Ther. 2022;54(1):62.
8. Böttinger L, van der Hoorn JW. Negative pressure ventilation: a special application of expiratory ventilation assistance. Intensive Care Med Exp. 2019;7(1):22.
9. Alhammad MF, Mathias R, Nahid S, Fernando R, Zaki HA, Haidar H, et al. Urinary guidewire and tritube solved the mystery of severe tracheal stenosis management: a case report. Trends Anaesth Crit Care. 2023;50:101257.

10. Grassetto A, Pettenuzzo T, Badii F, Barzaghi F, Carlon R, Dellarole S, et al. A new perspective during laryngo-tracheal surgery: the use of an ultra-thin endotracheal tube (Tritube®) and flow-controlled ventilation-a retrospective case series and a review of the literature. J Anesth Analg Crit Care. 2022;2(1):39.
11. Abram J, Martini J, Spraider P, Putzer G, Ranalter M, Wagner J, Glodny B, Hell T, Barnes T, Enk D. Individualised flow-controlled versus pressure-controlled ventilation in a porcine oleic acid-induced acute respiratory distress syndrome model. Eur J Anaesthesiol. 2023;40(7):511–20.
12. Shallik N, Zaghw A, Dogan Z, Rahman W. The use of virtual endoscopy for diagnosis of traumatic supra-glottic airway stenosis. JCAO. 2017;2(1):103.
13. Kumar N, Dardeer A, Hammad Y, Shallik N, Shaikh N, Ganaw A, Moustafa A. Pushed away: how did 3D reconstruction solve this airway problem? Trends Anaesth Crit Care. 2020;30:e36–7.
14. Mohammed H, Haidar H, Shallik NA, Elhakeem A, Al Abdulla M, Dogan Z. Virtual endoscopy and 3-D reconstruction/prototyping in head and neck surgeries. In: Shallik NA, Moustafa AH, Marcus MAE, editors. Virtual endoscopy and 3D reconstruction in the airways. Cham: Springer; 2019. https://doi.org/10.1007/978-3-030-23253-5_8.
15. Shallik N, Labib A, Ganaw A, Shaikh N, Moustafa A, Hammad Y. Virtual bronchoscopy and 3D reconstruction in the critical care setting. Qatar Med J. 2019;2:81. https://doi.org/10.5339/qmj.2019.qccc.81.

A Narrative Review on the Past, Present, and Future of Small-Bore Ventilation, Expiratory Ventilation Assistance, and Flow-Controlled Ventilation

M. W. P. de Wolf

1 Introduction

Medical knowledge and techniques are constantly evolving and these changes seem to follow a predictable time frame. This has been coined the half-life of facts [1].

Techniques, and therefore possibilities in airway management change over time as well. For instance: most of us will have been taught that ventilation through a small-bore cannula is only possible if the upper airway is open or if expiration is prolonged considerably.

Since the invention of Ventrain®, we know that expiration can easily be facilitated through that small-bore cannula. Subsequently, Ventrain® led to the development of a novel endotracheal tube (the Tritube®), a new approach to ventilation [flow-controlled ventilation (FCV)] and Evone®, a ventilator designed for FCV.

This chapter will describe the development of Ventrain®, Tritube®, and Evone® and the possibilities they bring: Respectively: expiratory ventilation assistance (EVA) to achieve normoventilation through small-bore airways; the possibility of intubating very small diameter airways and facilitating airway surgery; and FCV, a ventilation mode with increased ventilation efficiency and lung protective properties.

M. W. P. de Wolf (✉)
Department of Anaesthesiology and Pain Therapy, Maastricht University Medical Centre, Maastricht, The Netherlands
e-mail: m.de.wolf@mumc.nl

N. A. Shallik (ed.), *Flow Controlled Ventilation Mode Through a Straw Size Tube*, https://doi.org/10.1007/978-3-031-77477-5_8

1.1 Past

The evolution of small-bore ventilation. The development of Ventrain®, Expiratory Ventilation Assistance (EVA), Flow-Controlled Ventilation (FCV), Tritube®, and Evone®.

1.1.1 Front of Neck Access and Ventilation Through a Small Lumen

Surgical tracheostomies were documented millennia before the common era [2]. However, it wasn't until 1956 that continuous oxygen insufflation through a transtracheal 18 G cannula was first described in patients with upper airway malignancies [3]. Already it was well known that a major disadvantage of this technique would be a marked hypercarbia resulting in important respiratory acidosis [4].

To overcome this problem, in 1971, Spoerel and colleagues applied intermittent positive pressure ventilation through a 16 G transtracheal needle in elective patients without upper airway pathology, which even resulted in slight hyperventilation in most patients [5].

Following this, various approaches and devices were developed to ventilate through small-bore transtracheal or endotracheal catheters [6–8]. Self-assembled equipment [9] like tubing from an oxygen source with a side hole cut in it [10] or with a Y connector between the tubing and the cannula are still recommended in the current Acute Traumatic Life Support (ATLS) student course manual and Acute Paediatric Life Support (APLS) guidelines (at the time of writing). The use of a three way stopcock has also been described, where the aperture is occluded during insufflation and released during expiration. However, even with an open aperture, flow will still occur into the patient [11], with a risk for hyperinflation.

These self-assembled setups are not recommended in anaesthetic guidelines.

Licenced appliances for ventilation through a cannula are either pressure regulated (often referred to as jet ventilators) or flow regulated.

Typically, a handheld injector (for instance, Manujet®) or an automated jet ventilator is used for pressure-regulated ventilation. In automated systems, insufflation is automatically cut off when airway pressures become too high [12]. Ventilation with these systems requires an open airway for air to escape during exhalation.

Flow splitters like the Enk Oxygen Flow Modulator® and Rapid O_2® insufflation device rely on a set oxygen flow to insufflate air into the patient by manually occluding several or 1 opening respectively. The flow rate will provide the user with information on how much oxygen is insufflated (e.g., 250 ml/s at a flow of 15 L/min). By releasing the aperture(s) oxygen will be vented into surrounding air, instead of into the patient, and expiratory flow can occur both through the airway catheter/cannula and their own airway if not completely obstructed [13–15].

Resistance to flow increases exponentially with decreasing airway diameter. Therefore, insufflation through narrow-bore catheters/cannulae requires a high-pressure gas source. Oxygen cylinders and oxygen wall outlets can provide sufficient driving pressures but not all anaesthesia machines can, and this should be considered before insufflating through a cannula [16].

Expiration will be a passive process. As a result, as resistance to flow increases exponentially with decreasing airway diameters, so will the time needed to accomplish full expiration. If exhalation is only possible through a 14 G (1.6 mm = 4.8 F) cannula, this can take more than half a minute [17].

Air trapping, even with low minute volumes is a recognised complication of ventilation through a small-bore catheter. Upper airway patency is an important factor but the extent of upper airway obstruction is unknown in most cases and can vary during the course of ventilation. Therefore, one should always monitor outflow of air through the upper airway, and chest movements should be observed meticulously. Most importantly, in emergencies where expiration cannot be controlled, the focus of ventilation through a transtracheal (rescue) cannula should be on oxygenation, not CO_2 removal. Protocols suggest in a critical situation only to insufflate oxygen when a patient desaturates [18].

1.1.2 Aiding Expiration

The first reports on aiding expiration in patients with endotracheal tubes cited Bernoulli's principle or the Venturi effect as their mode of action. Confusingly these terms are often used interchangeably (Fig. 1).

In summary: Bernoulli's (1700–1782) principle states that when speed of a fluid (this includes air and oxygen) increases, this results in a decrease in pressure. (Kinetic energy increases; according to the principle of conservation of mechanical energy, another form of energy must decrease.) The Venturi (1746–1822) effect occurs when a non-compressible fluid flows through a constriction. According to the laws of conservation of mass and of momentum, the fluid has to speed up, so that the same amount of volume can travel through the constriction in the same amount of time. As per Bernoulli's principle, this will lead to a decrease in pressure.

In 1958, in an effort to decrease airway pressures in conventionally intubated and ventilated patients, Eger and Hamilton modified an Ayre's T-piece by incorporating a small bent needle in its side port, with the direction away from the patient's airway. Air and nitrous oxide were driven though the side port of the T piece. Occlusion of the exit port would lead to inspiration. At expiration the exit port was opened, and the jet of air from the needle would entrain air from the patient's airway (Fig. 2a) [19].

In 1963, Keuskamp published his experiences of a similar setup to assist expiration in paediatric patients. He incorporated a small-bore tube inside the Ayre's T piece with a venturi shaped outlet (i.e., with a constriction, gradually widening downstream, resulting in a gradual return of pressure) in the expiratory limb, so that gas flow through it generated a negative pressure during expiration [20] (Fig. 2b).

The first reports of assisting expiration through a transtracheal cannula followed later:

In 1978 Dunlap published his results of a modification with a T piece, which, when open to air, would entrain air out of the trachea with high flow oxygen (800 ml/s or 48 L/min) as driving gas. Expiratory volumes of 185 ml/s could be achieved through a transtracheal cannula [8] (Fig. 2c).

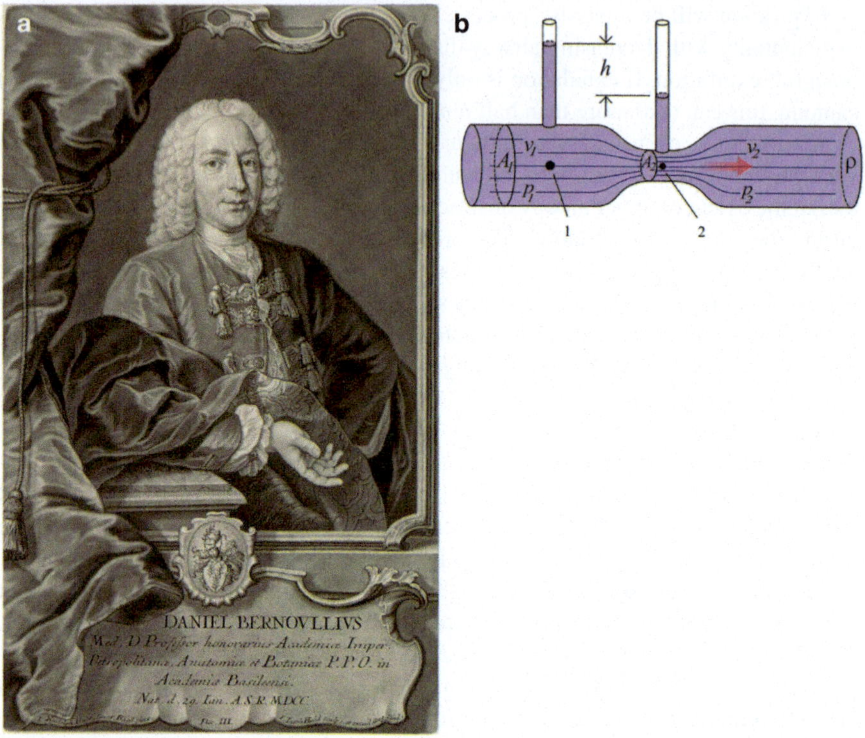

Fig. 1 (**a**) Daniel Bernoulli. (**b**) Venturi effect: at point 2, relative to point 1: speed of fluid increases and pressure decreases. As the tube diverges downstream pressure gradually returns. (**a**, **b**) Public domain image, courtesy of Wikipedia

In the 1990s, several systems were proposed where expiration was assisted by suction [23–25]. These systems required sophisticated equipment or elaborate setups.

In the new millennium, the principle of assisting expiration by using Bernoulli's principle or the Venturi effect formed the basis for further development of devices designed to provide expiratory assistance during ventilation via narrow-bore airways (Fig. 2d–f).

Meissner et al. incorporated the geometry of a conventional Venturi jet pump in a glass T-piece [21] (Fig. 2d). Expiration could be slightly expedited through small-bore cannulas but the overall effect on achievable minute volume was very limited.

1.1.3 The Advent of Ventrain® [26]

Hamaekers et al. introduced expiratory ventilation assistance (EVA) in small-bore ventilation by modification of an industrial injector, designed to pick up parts using suction generated by jetting air through a nozzle [27] (Fig. 2e). In an in vitro model, I:E ratios could be improved, approaching 1:1. However, at low lung-compliances, the device did not work well. In a static situation (where no (expiratory) gas was

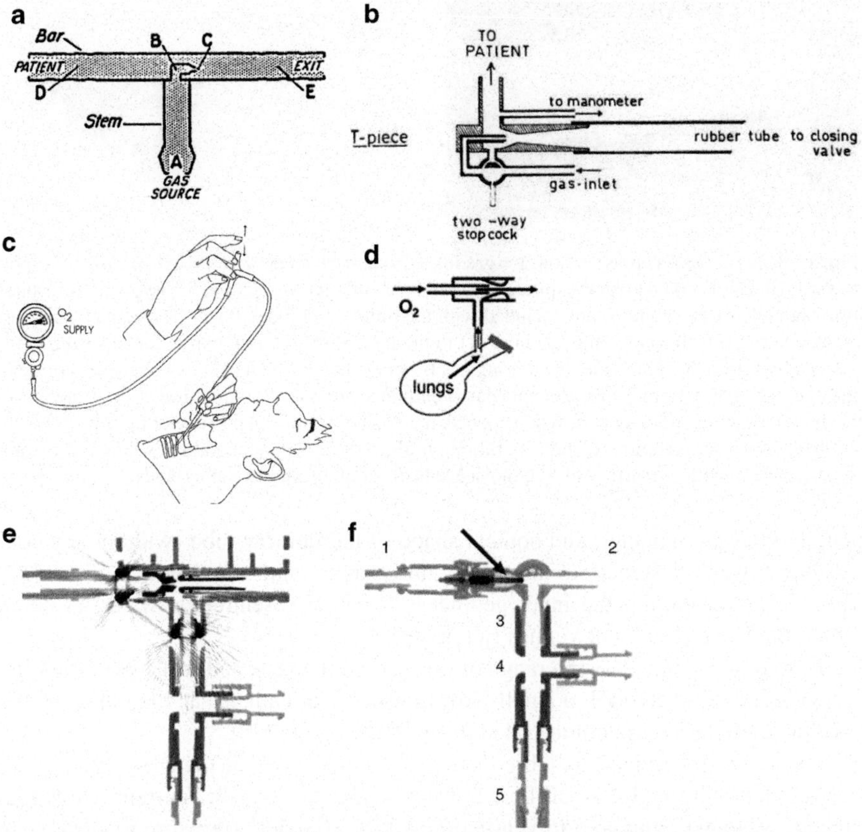

Fig. 2 Different setups to facilitate expiration by the Venturi effect or Bernoulli's principle. (**a**, **b**) A driving gas (typically oxygen) is injected through a small nozzle. The jet of air entrains air during expiration in conventionally intubated patients. Figures (**c**–**f**) illustrate different setups for small-bore ventilation: the patient's small-bore airway is connected to the devices at their side ports (at the bottom of the devices). By closing the outlet (all depicted on the right side of their respective image), insufflated air will flow through the side port into the patient. By opening the outlet, the driving gas will flow forward. Depending on the device's inner architecture expiration is assisted. Figure (**a**) Eger and Hamilton, 1958. From reference 19, with permission. Figure (**b**) Keuskamp. From [20] with permission. Figure (**c**) Dunlap. From [8] with permission. Figure (**d**) Meissner. From [21] with permission. Figures (**e**, **f**) are CT images of prototypes that led to the development of Ventrain. The arrow indicates the 0.7 mm ID nozzle. From [22] with permission

discharged), sufficient sub-atmospheric pressures could be achieved. In contrast, in a dynamic situation (when air was entrained), generated pressures were much less negative. To improve support of expiration by jet-flow generated suction, downstream resistance (i.e., the resistance in the outflow tract of the ejector) had to be diminished. In 2011, the same group published results of a new purpose-made ejector, the DE5 (DE for the inventor Dietmar Enk). To create sub-atmospheric pressures during expiration, oxygen was injected through a 0.7 mm ID jet nozzle with its tip proximal to the side port of the DE5 connected to the small-bore airway. The

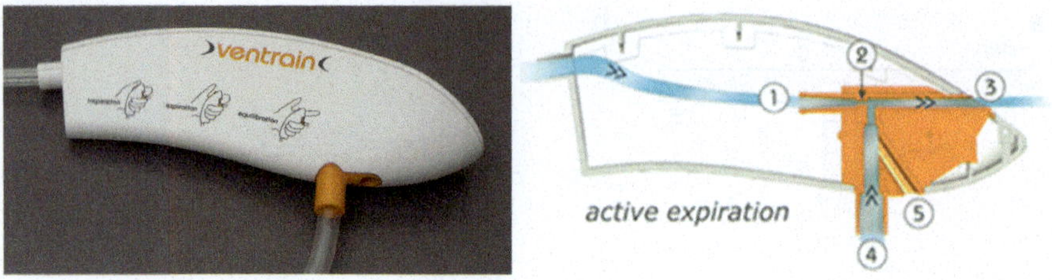

Fig. 3 Ventrain® and a cross section. 1 = gas inlet, 2 = narrow jet nozzle, 3 = exhaust pipe, 4 = port towards (inspiration) and from (expiration) small bore catheter or cannula, 5 = bypass. At inspiration both apertures (3 and 5) are occluded with the thumb and index finger, respectively, and gas (typically oxygen) flows via the gas inlet (1) to the patient (4). During expiration, aperture (3) is opened by lifting the thumb and the driving gas flows via the gas inlet (1) through the jet nozzle to the exhaust (3). By Bernoulli's principle gas is entrained from the patient through (4). The bypass (5) functions as an on/off switch. When opened. there is no significant positive or negative pressure at the catheter tip, resulting in slow equilibration of pressures between patient's lungs and atmosphere. (cross section courtesy of Ventinova Medical, Eindhoven, the Netherlands)

length, internal diameter, and conical shape of the outflow tube (without any constriction) were designed to minimise turbulences and resistance to flow [22] (Fig. 2f). Considering the inner geometry, the DE5 resembles a water jet pump rather than a conventional Venturi (jet pump).

In an in vitro model over a range of flows, compliances, and resistances, ventilation was possible through a small-bore transtracheal catheter at I:E ratios of 1:1. Normoventilation was demonstrated in a porcine model [28].

The Ventrain® device was subsequently developed based on the DE5 [29] (Fig. 3).

Ventilation through a small-bore transtracheal catheter with Ventrain® (flow regulated) was next compared to ventilation with a Manujet® (pressure regulated). In obstructed and partly obstructed airways, airway pressures were lower and oxygenation and ventilation were superior when Ventrain® was used [30, 31]. Contrary to the traditional view that effective and safe ventilation and oxygenation through a transtracheal catheter are only possible if the airway is open, ventilation and oxygenation with Ventrain® were much improved if the airway was obstructed [31] (much like ventilating through endotracheal tubes where cuff inflation improves oxygenation and ventilation).

2 Development of the Tritube® and Evone®

Manual ventilation with Ventrain® through a small-bore catheter has some limitations. When the airway is not completely obstructed, efficiency of oxygenation and ventilation is reduced [31]. Also, and very importantly, airway pressure can only be measured intermittently, leaving chest wall movement to guide ventilation and the risk of unintended high or negative airway pressures.

In response to these issues, a cuffed small-bore ventilation catheter with an integrated manometry channel was developed. Initially, a laserjet catheter (length 40 cm, inner diameter 2.2 mm) with two lumens (one for ventilation and one for intra-tracheal pressure measurements) was modified by attaching a cuff connected to its pilot balloon by a 19 G epidural catheter. Addition of this cuff to seal the airway significantly improved the efficiency of oxygenation and ventilation in pigs and, indeed, enabled normoventilation [32]. Other advantages of a cuff include decreased risk of aspiration or soiling of the trachea during airway surgery, ability to accurately control tidal volumes and to accurately measure end tidal CO_2.

Next, this prototype was further developed and commercially manufactured as the Tritube®, a 40 cm long tube, with an outer diameter of 4.4 mm with three lumens: one for ventilation (inner diameter 2.4 mm), one for cuff inflation/deflation, and one for continuous intratracheal pressure measurement distal to the cuff [33]. In 2020, the length of this tube was increased to 50 cm (Fig. 4).

During early experiments with Ventrain®, ventilation was noted to be much "softer" than conventional pressure-controlled ventilation (PCV) or volume-controlled ventilation (VCV). Bearing this in mind and to automate ventilation via the Tritube®, Evone® was developed (Fig. 5).

Cleary, an automated ventilator adds convenience but also safety: intratracheal pressure, inspiratory and expiratory flow, tidal volumes and capnograph are continuously monitored with alarms to alert to deviation from safe limits.

Expiratory flow, although similar, differs between EVA (in manual ventilation with Ventrain®) and FCV (in automated ventilation with Evone®). With Ventrain®, the flow of the driving gas is constant (typically set at the oxygen driving source) and will generate a consistent negative pressure at the jet nozzle ("2" in Fig. 3). As a result, assisted expiratory flow from the patient will be near-linear but will vary

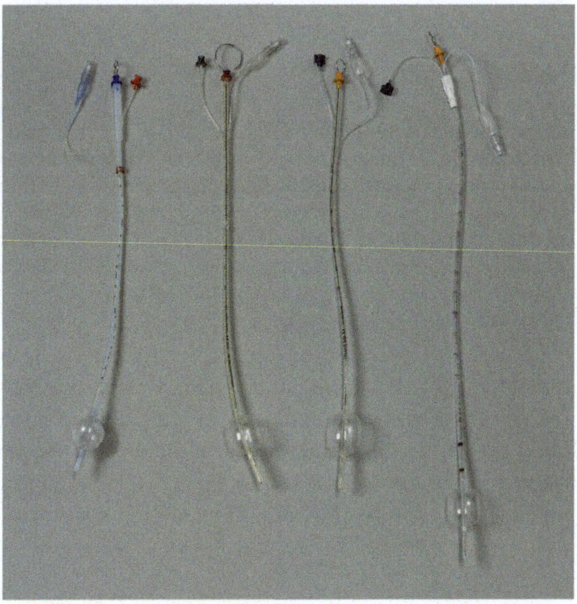

Fig. 4 A prototype made from a laserjet catheter, the cuff of a microlaryngeal tube ID 4 mm, and an epidural catheter, followed by the evolution of Tritube® as manufactured commercially. Intubation is facilitated by a malleable stylet in the ventilation lumen

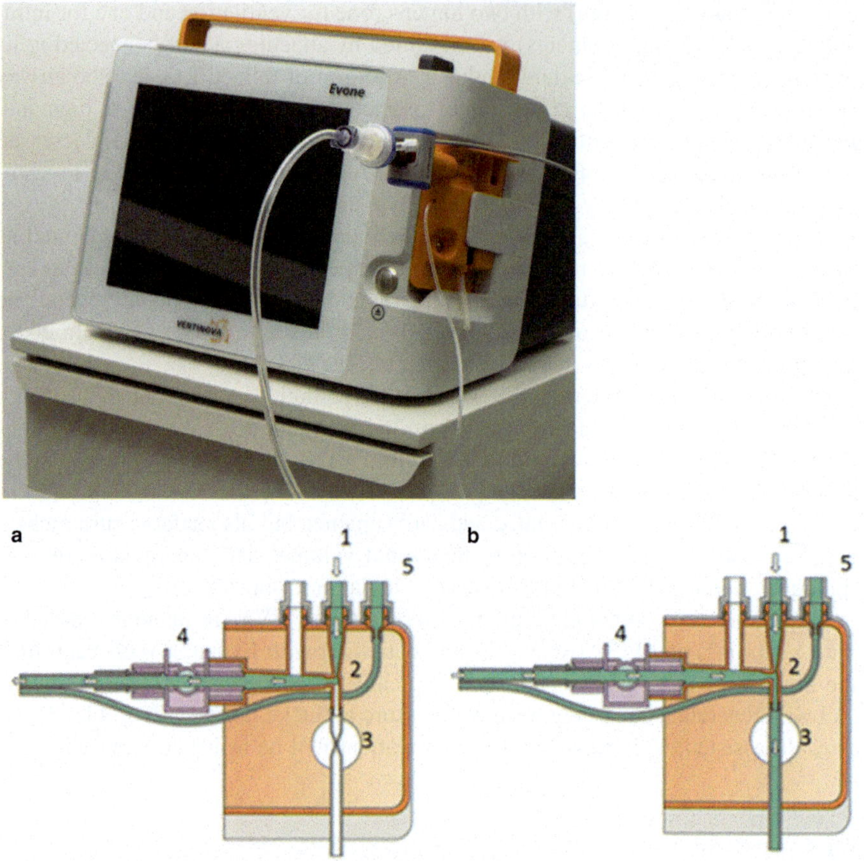

Fig. 5 Evone® and a schematic representation of its cartridge. 1 = gas inlet, 2 = narrow jet nozzle, 3 = exhaust pipe, 4 = port towards (inspiration) and from (expiration) Tritube® and patient. These components are equivalent to those depicted in Fig. 3 (schematic representation of Ventrain®) and represented by the same numbers. 5 = port for continuous intratracheal pressure measurement. (**a**) Closure of the exhaust pipe (3) leads to inspiration (gas flows from 1, via 2 to 4). (**b**) After opening of the exhaust pipe (3), driving gas flows through the jet nozzle (2) and exhaust pipe (3) to the outside. By Bernoulli's principle the flow entrains gas from the patient through port (4). Schematic representation of cartridge courtesy of Ventinova Medical (Eindhoven, the Netherlands)

slightly over the course of expiration. Evone® is designed to maintain a constant expiratory flow from the patient. This is achieved by varying the driving gas flow (and hence negative pressure generated) during expiration. To summarise: with EVA, driving gas flow and therefore the created sub-atmospheric pressure are constant, and expiratory flow is near-linear. In FCV, expiratory flow is constant (mirror image of inspiratory flow, Fig. 6) by slight variation of driving gas flow.

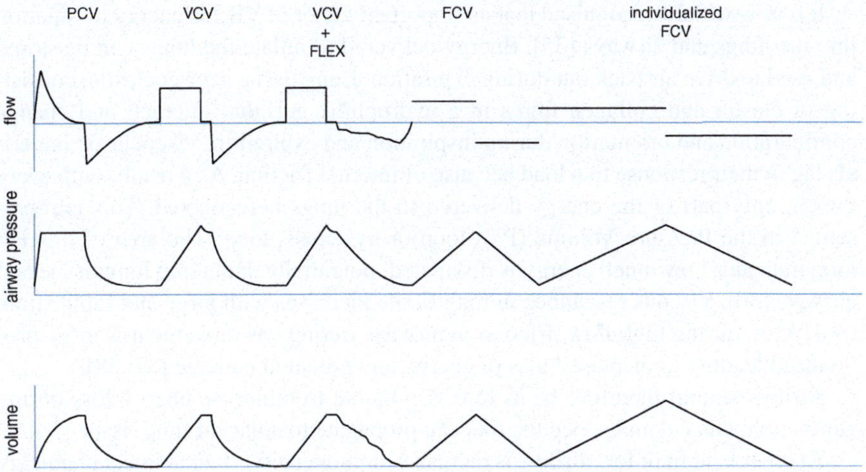

Fig. 6 A schematic representation of flow-, pressure-, and volume curves of different ventilation modes

2.1 Flow-Controlled Ventilation (FCV): A New Mode of Ventilation [34]

The creation of Ventrain® and the ability to normoventilate through narrow-bore catheters clearly marks a major innovation in airway management. However, with the complementary development of flow-controlled ventilation (FCV), the implications are much wider.

In FCV, inspiration is comparable to that in VCV (without a plateau phase): flow is constant and volume is insufflated linearly. Expiration is also controlled: in contrast to conventional ventilation methods where expiration is passive (leading to peak flows at the start and low flows at the end of expiration), in FCV expiratory flow is constant so that intrapulmonary volume decreases linearly (Fig. 6).

This has several significant advantages, including homogeneity of lung aeration, improved ventilation efficiency and lung protective ventilation.

3 Benefits of FCV and Low Continuous Flow

Ventilator-induced lung injury (VILI) is a well-recognised complication of mechanical ventilation. In the search for lung protective ventilation various strategies are recommended, including decreased tidal volumes, low driving pressures, and protocols to optimise PEEP and inspired oxygen fraction. These aim to minimise transpulmonary pressure, strain (ratio of tidal volume to end expiratory lung volume), atelectrauma, and oxygen toxicity.

It is now widely-recognised that an important factor of VILI is energy dissipation into the lungs and airways [35]. Energy delivered to inflate the lungs can be stored and used to drive air back out during expiration. Lung tissue is viscoelastic, consisting of elastin and collagen fibres in a hydrophilic gel, that interact, and change configuration and orientation during inspiration and expiration. Viscoelastic materials lag in their response to a load because of internal friction. As a result, with every breath, only part of the energy delivered to the lungs is recovered. This is represented in the Pressure-Volume (PV) loop or hysteresis loop: The area of this PV loop indicates how much energy is dissipated, potentially damaging lung tissue and airways [36]. Viscous resistance in lung tissue increases with large and rapid strain [36]. Also, during high flow, friction in airways during gas movement is more pronounced leading to increased loss of energy and potential damage [37, 38].

Airflow should therefore be as low as possible to minimise energy loss during ventilation. Once damage occurs, this can propagate to adjacent lung tissue [36].

Another benefit of low airflow is increased homogeneity: If air is injected quickly (high flow), it will preferentially flow to fast lung compartments as only these will be able to inflate quickly enough. At very low flow, the effect of differences in resistances to flow of different lung units becomes much less pronounced [39]. In other words: minimising airflow promotes homogeneous lung aeration [40]. Intuitively, this will improve oxygenation and carbon dioxide clearance and protect fast lung compartments from strain and therefore VILI as insufflated air is spread more evenly. Also, the degree of regional distribution of inspired gas can influence capillary perfusion of alveoli. On the one hand, if air is distributed unevenly over different lung fields, increased oxygen and decreased CO_2 partial pressure will stimulate local capillary blood flow in well-aerated (fast) alveoli. On the other hand, if intra-alveolar pressures are higher in these fast alveoli compared to poorly-aerated (slow) alveoli, (partial) compression of alveolar capillaries could lead to preferential perfusion of the poorly ventilated areas and therefore increase shunting.

In FCV, pendelluft, which is air (with high CO_2 and low oxygen concentrations) passing back and forth between fast and slow lung compartments, will be minimised: Pendelluft occurs due to intra-alveolar pressure differences between fast and slow alveoli, typically when no flow occurs between ventilator and patient (for instance during a plateau pressure phase). At the end of inspiration, this will lead to filling of slow lung compartments with CO_2-rich air from fast lung compartments, leading to a decreased efficiency of CO_2 elimination. At the end of expiration (in conventional ventilation modes), pendelluft may occur the other way round with CO_2-rich/oxygen-depleted gas passing from slow to fast compartments [39]. These effects become more pronounced with increasing flows [40]. In FCV, inspiratory and expiratory flow are low, constant (square flow waveform), and uninterrupted. By minimising a pressure difference between alveoli due to increased homogeneity of lung aeration and by eliminating a plateau pressure phase, pendelluft is largely eliminated and CO_2 elimination is increased.

As expiratory pressure decreases gradually during FCV, intrapulmonary pressure during expiration remains higher than during passive expiration, which will decrease the risk of atelectasis.

Considering these characteristics of continuous, uninterrupted, and low inspiratory and expiratory flow, gas exchange can be expected to improve with FCV. This has been demonstrated in healthy lung, and ARDS porcine models where normocapnia was achieved with lower minute volumes in FCV, compared to VCV and PCV. Oxygenation and lung recruitment were also improved [41–43]. Similar results were found in patients without respiratory disease and in patients living with obesity [44, 45].

4 Reducing Expiratory Flow

In earlier work on lung protective ventilation little focus was put on the expiratory phase. However, as described, reducing expiratory flow and eliminating flow pauses will reduce energy dissipation, atelectasis, and pendelluft.

Rapid expiration can also have cardiovascular consequences, as shown in a rat model, where abrupt deflation of the lungs (from sustained inflation to zero end expiratory pressure) would lead to a surge in pulmonary perfusion, increases in left ventricular pre- and afterload and pulmonary oedema [46].

In the 1990s, peak expiratory flow was reduced by incorporating an expiratory resistance in an attempt to improve ventilation of patients with chronic obstructive pulmonary disease (COPD) (much like pursed lips in spontaneously breathing COPD patients). This counteracted airway collapse during exhalation. However, no clinical benefit in gas exchange was demonstrated. Possible explanations are that hyperinflation occurred [47] or that to prevent hyperinflation, the decrease in peak expiratory flow was less pronounced, and as a result insufficient to improve gas exchange [48].

In 2012, FLEX (Flow-controlled EXpiration) was introduced [49]: a computer regulated variable resistance is incorporated in the expiratory limb of a ventilator and is gradually decreased during exhalation leading to less pronounced fluctuations in expiratory flow. As a result, lung volume and airway pressures decrease more gradually. This led to better lung mechanics and less lung injury in a porcine lung injury model [50]. However, this technique results in variable expiratory flow and suboptimal I:E ratios (1:1.5–1:2) (Fig. 6).

5 Minimising Energy Dissipation

Considering the benefits of low in- and expiratory flow, Barnes et al. calculated that to minimise energy loss to pulmonary parenchyma and airways, flows during inspiration and expiration should remain constant, without inspiratory or expiratory pause, and with an I:E ratio of 1:1.

Firstly: this will result in ventilation with the lowest flow possible both during inspiration and expiration, which will minimise energy dissipation.

Secondly: A continuous and stable flow is energetically most favourable [51].

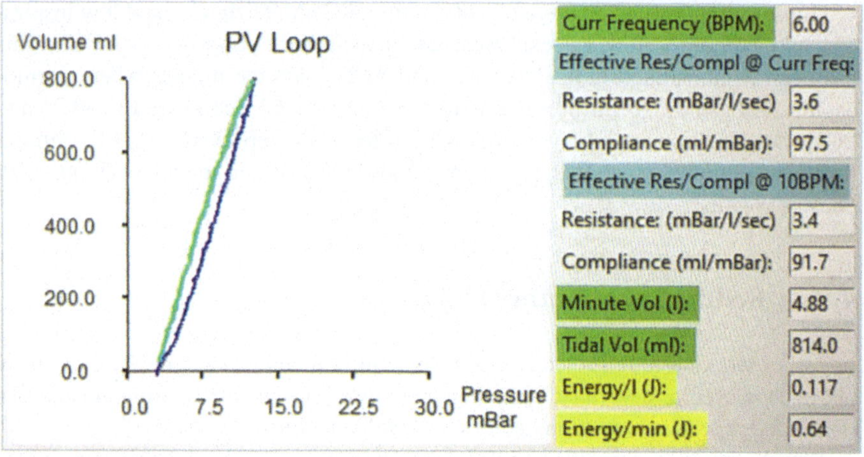

Fig. 7 PV loop of individualised FCV. Values for energy are dissipated energy, which in this case are below that of average work of breathing in a healthy person at rest. Respiratory rate is 6/min and tidal volume 814 ml. The straight inspiratory rise of the PV loop proves that the tidal volume does not exceed the individual range of optimum compliance. (Courtesy of Prof. Dr. Dietmar Enk. Software developed by Prof. Dr. Thomas Barnes)

Using the PV loop on a patient, Barnes and Enk calculated that energy dissipation during FCV, with an I:E ratio of 1:1 was very low, comparable to the lower end of energy dissipation in spontaneous respiration [52].

Typically, individualised FCV (discussed later) leads to lower minute volumes, lower respiratory frequency, and higher tidal volumes compared to current best practice PCV or VCV (Fig. 7). While this might seem to contradict the philosophy of lung protective ventilation which traditionally aims to limit tidal volume, with individualised FCV, inspiratory and expiratory flow can be expected to be (much) lower than with VCV and PCV. Since the respiratory system is viscoelastic, slow changes in pressure and stretch let lung tissue adapt more smoothly to their changes in configuration, and prevent damage from occurring, whereas a quick stretch through high flows will lead to high shear forces [36, 37, 53]. This is nicely illustrated in the following video: https://www.youtube.com/watch?v=E0IRlRcwE3k&t (from minute 15–17).

Indeed, CT scans in patients during individualised FCV showed an increase in normally aerated lungs without an increase in hyperinflation when compared to PCV, despite significantly higher tidal volumes [54].

Further to this, with high tidal volumes, dead space ventilation relative to total minute volume is lower, resulting in an increased ventilation efficiency (on top of previously discussed mechanisms of improved CO_2 clearance), so that minute volume can be further reduced (meaning flow can be set lower).

Minimisation of flow will minimise mechanical power (energy applied to the respiratory system per unit of time) [42, 54–56] (Fig. 7).

Figure 8 summarises the advantages of FCV over conventional ventilation.

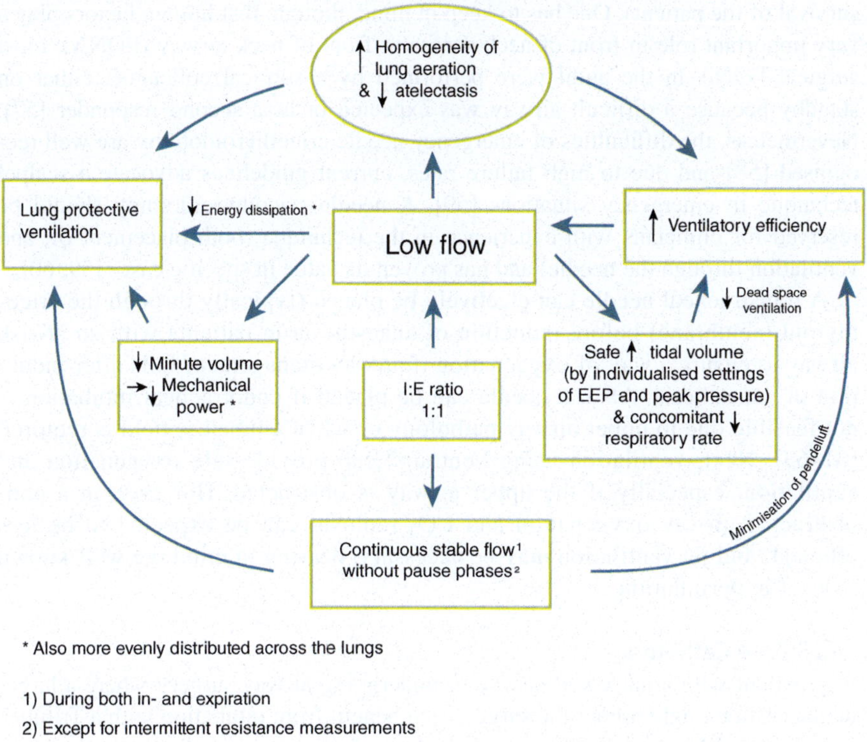

Fig. 8 A summary of lung protective properties of FCV and its increase in ventilatory efficiency

5.1 Present

5.1.1 The Current Use of Ventrain®, Tritube®, and Evone®

Currently, Ventrain®, Tritube®, and Evone® are mainly used for airway management (airway rescue, or more commonly elective advanced airway management), though examples of their use for the benefits of FCV are starting to emerge.

5.1.2 Airway Management

Needle Front of Neck Access

Although a needle cricothyroidotomy can be placed electively in airway management (as will be discussed later) it is more often associated with rescue front of neck acces in a cannot intubate / cannot oxygenate (CICO) situation. NAP 4 (4th National Audit Project) provided insight in the success rates of a surgical technique or placement of a cannula in this situation. 63% of cannula placements by anaesthetists failed (either by wrong placement, use of wrong materials, use of a low-pressure source for oxygenation, or barotrauma) whereas all surgical placements were successful (not necessarily by the first responder and not necessarily resulting in survival of the patient). One has to keep in mind, though, that human factors play a very important role in front of neck access or front of neck airway (FONA): most surgical FONA in the audit were performed by a surgical colleague, either on standby because a difficult airway was expected or as a second responder [57]. Nevertheless, the difficulties of emergency needle cricothyroidotomy are well recognised [58] and due to high failure rates, current guidelines advocate a scalpel technique in emergency situations [59]. A needle cricothyroidotomy should be reserved for clinicians with experience in the technique (both placement of, and ventilation through the needle) and has proven its value in specific cases [59, 60].

A transtracheal needle can electively be placed (typically through the cricothyroid membrane) before induction of anaesthesia in patients with an at-risk airway to ensure a way of oxygenation if airway management fails after induction of anaesthesia. Also, a needle can be placed if endotracheal intubation is not feasible due to upper airway pathology or when a tubeless field is required [61–63]. Next, ventilation using Ventrain® can provide safe oxygenation and ventilation, especially if the upper airway is obstructed. However, in a non-obstructed airway oxygenation and CO_2 removal can be expected to be less efficient, and jet ventilation may be necessary, bearing in mind the well-known risks of hyperinflation.

Small-Bore Catheters

Any patient with a narrowed airway or undergoing airway surgery where a larger diameter tube might hinder the surgeon can benefit from intubation with a Tritube® or other small-bore airway. Typical examples include patients with subglottic stenosis, patients undergoing tracheal surgery and upper airway surgery [64]. Due to its smaller diameter, intubation with Tritube® instead of conventional microlaryngeal tubes will increase surgical exposure of laryngeal structures [33, 64–66].

A Tritube can also be placed as a FONA. By doing so, less steps in acquiring an airway are needed. However, ventilation through the Tritube will require a Ventrain or Evone, and the clinician will need experience in their ventilation modes, before performing them in an emergency situation.

Use of Ventrain® through small-bore catheters has been described in various settings of airway management. Most case reports describe oxygenation and ventilation through endotracheally placed intubating or airway exchange catheters [67–71], but any airway with a Luer lock connection can be used, like bronchoscopes or endobronchial blockers [72, 73]. Disadvantages are that these airways have no cuff and, without a sealed airway, the efficiency of ventilation is greatly reduced. Also, pressure monitoring can only be performed intermittently. However, a Tritube® is not always available for clinicians working with challenging airways.

Low flow Ventrain® ventilation (typically 6 L/min) can also be applied for supplemental oxygenation over the collapsed lung in one lung ventilation. As flow is low, lung inflation and deflation are very gradual and generally won't hinder the surgical field. This can either be done by placing an airway exchange catheter through a double lumen tube [71] or by ventilating through an endobronchial blocker [73].

When ventilating through an endobronchial blocker one has to keep in mind that due to its small inner diameter and its length, the resistance to flow will be higher than that of a transtracheal cannula ("needle FONA") or airway exchange catheter. Therefore, the low flow of the driving gas will not generate enough sub-atmospheric pressure for complete expiration to occur through the endobronchial blocker in the same amount of time as inspiration. (During inspiration as long as the Ventrain® is connected to an oxygen source that can provide enough pressure, driving pressure will increase as necessary, but during expiration suction pressures are a result of set flow of the driving gas [29].) Depending on patient variables and the size of the endobronchial blocker, one can expect that at 6L/min driving gas flow, an I:E ratio of around 1:2.5 will be needed to safely ventilate with Ventrain® [74].

Lung Protective Ventilation

As intratracheal airway pressures are continuously monitored during FCV with Evone®, and flow always occurs either to or from the patient (i.e., dynamic ventilation mode without static phases), dynamic lung mechanics can continuously and accurately be evaluated.

Ventilation can easily be individualised: First, end expiratory pressure (EEP) is optimised by changing both EEP and peak pressure by increments of 1–2 mbar or cmH_2O (keeping driving pressure constant). The lowest EEP resulting in highest tidal volume is chosen. Next, peak pressure (and therefore driving pressure) is increased stepwise while evaluating change in tidal volume. If for instance the measured dynamic compliance is 50 ml/mbar, then an increase in driving pressure of 1 mbar would lead to an increase in tidal volume of 50 ml. If, however, tidal volume increases more than 50 ml, this indicates an improvement of lung mechanics. This step is repeated until tidal volume increases underproportionally. Peak pressure should then be set at the previous setting.

This way ventilation will be optimised, within the limits of alveolar derecruitment and overdistention.

Of note, during FCV pressures are measured in the trachea, but due to its dynamic properties (flow always occurs during inspiration and expiration), pressures in the lungs will be different: During inspiration alveolar pressures will be lower than intratracheal pressures, and vice-versa during expiration. The pressure differential (between alveoli and lungs) is dependant of flow and airway resistance [75]. Therefore, alveolar ΔP is lower than calculated from measured intratracheal peak pressure and EEP, and this should be taken into account when comparing these values between FCV and VCV or PCV.

Flow should be adjusted according to CO_2 measurements. Because the I:E ratio should always be set at 1:1, minute volume will be half of the set flow. While adjusting flow, respiratory frequency will change accordingly. Typically, minute volumes will be lower with FCV when compared to VCV or PCV.

Current literature on FCV in intensive care patients is limited to case reports or small case-series, mainly in COVID-19 patients. FCV, if individualised (compliance guided), was shown to increase ventilator efficiency and decrease mechanical power [76–78].

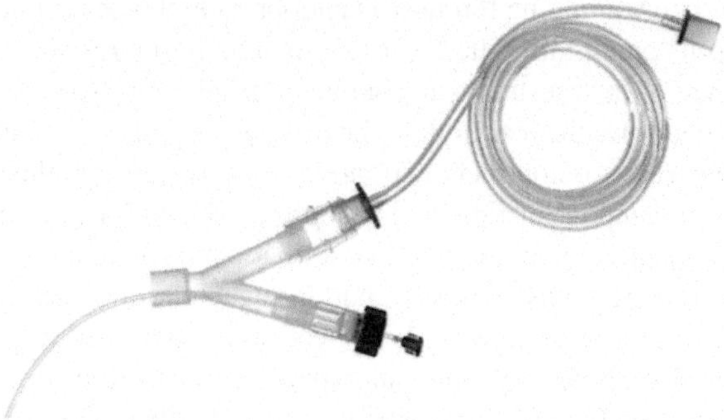

Fig. 9 Conventional Tube Adapter (CTA), consisting of two ports for ventilation with Evone® through conventional endotracheal tubes. One port for continuous intratracheal pressure measurements and one for ventilation (courtesy of Ventinova Medical, Eindhoven, the Netherlands)

FCV by Evone® can only be applied if intratracheal pressures are continuously monitored and the ventilating lumen has a Luer lock connection. Endotracheal tubes cannot be directly connected to Evone®. This can be overcome by placing a Tritube® in the endotracheal tube. However, although this has not been documented, this carries a theoretical risk of avulsion of the cuff during manipulation of the Tritube®. To benefit from FCV in conventionally intubated patients, a conventional tube adapter (CTA) is available for connection of Evone® with endotracheal tubes >5 mm ID (Fig. 9).

Paediatrics

Evone® and Ventrain® are intended for use in patients of 40 kg or more. As a result, paediatric experience with Ventrain® is limited, and mainly used in acute settings. In most of these cases intubation was possible only with the smallest diameter airway available: an 8 Fr intubating or airway exchange catheter. Oxygenation and ventilation can be well established by ventilating with Ventrain® using age or weight appropriate flows [79].

5.2 Future

5.2.1 Prospects of Small-Bore Ventilation and FCV

It seems that most clinicians mainly associate Tritube®, Ventrain®, and Evone® with difficult airway management. Although the introduction of these techniques has dramatically improved management of challenging airways, FCV should also, or mainly, be recognised as a lung protective ventilation mode.

A PV loop (from intratracheal pressure measurement) is currently not displayed on the Evone®, although this would help to monitor dynamic lung mechanics. A near-linear relation between pressure and volume suggests ventilation within safe pressure and volume limits. If the PV loop acquires a sigmoid shape, this would indicate that lung mechanics are not optimal. Representation of the PV loop on

Evone® could further improve clinician decision making in mechanically ventilated patients.

No data are available on FCV in COPD and asthma patients. One can expect that a low, constant expiratory flow will be advantageous in these patients. This will lead to a gradual drop in airway pressure, which will keep the small airways open.

Future research might demonstrate haemodynamic benefits of FCV over conventional forms of ventilation. Intrathoracic pressures influence pre-and afterload of both ventricles in different ways. As intrapulmonary pressures increase and decrease slowly and more smoothly with FCV, pressure swings are minimised, decreasing sudden changes in pre-and afterload. In line with this hypothesis, in a porcine ARDS model FCV resulted in significantly improved haemodynamic stability compared to PCV [80].

Currently, in children, these technologies are only applied in special cases. Future developments of materials might expand the possibilities of EVA and FCV in the paediatric population.

6 Conclusion

Oxygenation and ventilation through a small-bore cannula have evolved from continuous oxygen insufflation without CO_2 clearance (1956)—to intermittent insufflation—to attempts at optimally assisting expiration—to the possibility of complete expiration in the same amount of time as inspiration. In about the same time frame, positive pressure ventilation has become more widespread (from the polio epidemic in Denmark in 1952)—followed by the realisation that this can lead to VILI—and subsequent strategies to prevent this lung injury—to the advent of FCV.

Before the advent of Ventrain®, we were taught that an open upper airway was an absolute prerequisite to normoventilate through a small-bore airway. Now possibilities have changed and an airway seal is even more beneficial with EVA.

Currently, the prevention of VILI in critically ill mechanically ventilated patients remains challenging and typically involves low tidal volumes (relatively) high frequency and (relatively) high flow. These may be the optimal strategies in conventional ventilation but will lead to high mechanical power and risk for lung damage. It is plausible that individualised FCV, typically involving low flows, low respiratory rates and higher tidal volumes, will change this paradigm and, hopefully, decrease the occurrence of VILI.

The half-life of facts doesn't only relate to the realisation that some things we have learned turn out to be wrong or become outdated. Similarly, knowledge, technology, and the publication of these findings grow in a regular way, be it in a linear or exponential function [1]. Use of and research into Ventrain®, EVA and FCV seem to follow this prediction (Fig. 10). It will be interesting to see if current research on

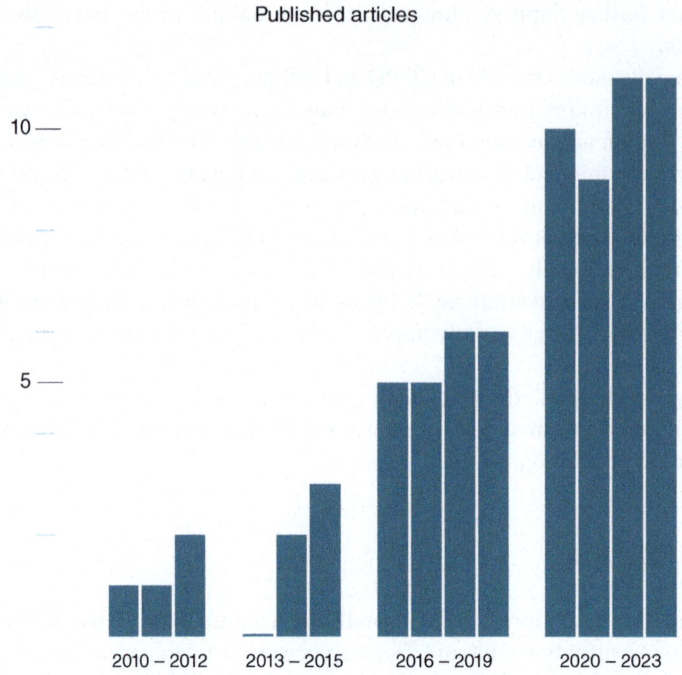

Fig. 10 Graphic representation of increase in published research and reports over the years on small-bore ventilation with EVA and FCV till and including October 2023. Search criteria in PubMed were filtered to title/abstract with search terms "Flow-controlled ventilation OR Ventrain OR Evone OR Tritube OR Expiratory ventilation Assistance". Erratums, responses to and commentaries on articles were excluded

Expiratory Ventilation Assistance and Flow-Controlled Ventilation will continue to follow the current trend and FCV will become more widely adopted.

Acknowledgements I sincerely thank Professor Dietmar Enk, firstly for his inventions and developments which have been described here, and which have revolutionised airway management and ventilation. Secondly for his time and patience while explaining some uncertainties I encountered while preparing this chapter.

Many thanks to Dr John Schutzer-Weissmann for proofreading the text.

References

1. Arbesman S. The half-life of facts: why everything we know has an expiration date. New York: Penguin Publishing Group; 2012.
2. Szmuk P, Ezri T, Evron S, Roth Y, Katz J. A brief history of tracheostomy and tracheal intubation, from the bronze age to the space age. Intensive Care Med. 2008;34:222–8.
3. Flory FA, Hamelberg W, Jacoby JJ, Jones JR, Ziegler CH. Transtracheal resuscitation. JAMA. 1956;162:625–8.

4. Spoerel JP, Kemph JP, Hamelberg W, Hitchcock FA, Jacoby J. Studies with transtracheal artificial respiration. Anesthesiology. 1954;15(1):28–41.
5. Spoerel WE, Narayanan PS, Singh NP. Transtracheal ventilation. Br J Anaesth. 1971;43:932–8.
6. Jacobs HB. Emergency percutaneous transtracheal catheter and ventilator. J Trauma. 1972;12(1):50–5.
7. Klain M, Smith RB. High frequency percutaneous transtracheal jet ventilation. Crit Care Med. 1977;5:280–7.
8. Dunlap LB. A modified, simple device for the emergency administration of percutaneous transtracheal ventilation. JACEP. 1978;7(2):42–6.
9. Scuderi PE, McLeskey CH, Comer PB. Emergency percutaneous transtracheal ventilation during anesthesia using readily available equipment. Anesth Analg. 1982;61(10):867–70.
10. Levinson MM, Scuderi PE, Gibson RL, Comer PB. Emergency percutaneous transtracheal ventilation (PTV). JACEP. 1979;8(10):396–400.
11. Hamaekers A, Borg P, Enk D. The importance of flow and pressure release in emergency jet ventilation devices. Paediatr Anaesth. 2009;19(5):452–7.
12. Ross-Anderson DJ, Ferguson C, Patel A. Transtracheal jet ventilation in 50 patients with severe airway compromise and stridor. Br J Anaesth. 2011;106(1):140–4.
13. Enk D, Busse H, Meissner A, Van Aken H. A new device for oxygenation and drug administration by transtracheal jet ventilation. Anesth Analg. 1998;86(2S):203S.
14. Preussler NP, Schreiber T, Hüter L, et al. Percutaneous transtracheal ventilation: effects of a new oxygen flow modulator on oxygenation and ventilation in pigs compared with a hand triggered emergency jet injector. Resuscitation. 2003;56:329–33.
15. Wexler S, Hall K, Chin RY, Prineas SN. Cannula cricothyroidotomy and rescue oxygenation with the Rapid-O2TM oxygen insufflation device in the management of a can't intubate/can't oxygenate scenario. Anaesth Intensive Care. 2018;46(1):97–101.
16. Fassl J, Jenny U, Nikiforov S, et al. Pressures available for transtracheal jet ventilation from anesthesia machines and wall-mounted oxygen flowmeters. Anesth Analg. 2010;110(1):94–100.
17. Dworkin R, Benumof JL, Benumof R, Karagianes TG. The effective tracheal diameter that causes air trapping during jet ventilation. J Cardiothorac Anesth. 1990;4(6):731–6.
18. Dinsmore J, Lacquiere D, Heard A. Low minute volume rescue oxygenation after cannula cricothyroidotomy in the can't intubate can't oxygenate scenario. Br J Anaesth. 2021;127(2):e54–5.
19. Eger EI, Hamilton WK. Positive-negative pressure ventilation with a modified Ayre's T-piece. Anesthesiology. 1958;19(5):611–8.
20. Keuskamp DH. Automatic ventilation in paediatric anaesthesia using a modified Ayre's T-piece with negative pressure during expiratory phase. Anaesthesia. 1963;18:46–56.
21. Meissner K, Iber T, Roesner JP, et al. Successful transtracheal lung ventilation using a manual respiration valve: an in vitro and in vivo study. Anesthesiology. 2010;109(2):251–9.
22. Hamaekers AEW, Borg PAJ, Götz TAJ, Enk D. Ventilation through a small-bore catheter: optimizing expiratory ventilation assistance. Br J Anaesth. 2011;106(3):403–9.
23. Schapera A, Bainton CR, Kraemer R, Lee K. A pressurized injection/suction system for ventilation in the presence of complete airway obstruction. Crit Care Med. 1994;22(2):326–33.
24. Garry B, Woo P, Perrault DF Jr, et al. Jet ventilation in upper airway obstruction. Description and model lung testing of a new jetting device. Anesth Analg. 1998;87(4):915–20.
25. Kessel G. Transtracheal jet ventilation and the completely obstructed airway: incorporating an active expiratory phase. J Accid Emerg Med. 1999;16(5):390.
26. Enk D. Gasstromumkehr element. Patent application (DE 10 2007 013 385.7). German Patent Office, 16.3.2007.
27. Hamaekers AEW, Götz TAJ, Borg PAJ, Enk D. Achieving an adequate minute volume through a 2 mm transtracheal catheter in simulated upper airway obstruction using a modified industrial ejector. Br J Anaesth. 2010;104(3):382–6.
28. Hamaekers A, Theunissen M, Jansen J, et al. Fast recovery from severe hypoxia through a 2 mm transtracheal catheter in pigs with a completely obstructed upper airway. Eur J Anaesthesiol. 2010;27(47):247.

29. Hamaekers AEW, Borg PAJ, Enk D. Ventrain: an ejector ventilator for emergency use. Br J Anaesth. 2012;108(6):1017–21.
30. Berry M, Tzeng Y, Marsland C. Percutaneous transtracheal ventilation in an obstructed airway model in post-apnoeic sheep. Br J Anaesth. 2014;113(6):1039–45.
31. Paxian M, Preussler NP, Reinz T. Transtracheal ventilation with a novel ejector-based device (ventrain) in open, partly obstructed, or totally closed upper airways in pigs. Br J Anaesth. 2015;115(2):308–16.
32. de Wolf MWP, van der Beek T, Hamaekers AEW, et al. A prototype small-bore ventilation catheter with a cuff: cuff inflation optimizes ventilation with the ventrain. Acta Anaesthesiol Scand. 2018;62:328–35.
33. Kristensen MS, de Wolf MWP, Rasmussen LS. Ventilation via the 2.4 mm internal diameter Tritube® with cuff – new possibilities in airway management. Acta Anaesthesiol Scand. 2017;61:580–9.
34. Enk D. Verfahren und Vorrichtung zur Beatmung eines Patienten. Patent application (DE 10 2016 109 528.1). German Patent Office, 24.5.2016.
35. Gattinoni L, Tonetti T, Cressoni M, et al. Ventilator-related causes of lung injury: the mechanical power. Intensive Care Med. 2016;42:1567–75.
36. Protti A, Votta E. Role of tissue viscoelasticity in the pathogenesis of ventilator-induced lung injury. Annu Update Intens Care Emerg Med. 2018;2018:193–204.
37. Rich PB, Reickert CA, Sawada S, et al. Effect of rate and inspiratory flow on ventilator-induced lung injury. J Trauma. 2000;49(5):903–11.
38. Maeda Y, Fujino Y, Uchiyama A, et al. Effects of peak inspiratory flow on development of ventilator-induced lung injury in rabbits. Anesthesiology. 2004;101(3):722–8.
39. Otis AB, McHerrow CB, Bartlett RA, et al. Mechanical factors in distribution of pulmonary ventilation. J Appl Physiol. 1956;8(4):427–43.
40. Santini A, Mauri T, Dalla CF, et al. Effects of inspiratory flow on lung stress, pendelluft, and ventilation heterogeneity in ARDS: a physiological study. Crit Care. 2019;23(1):369.
41. Schmidt J, Wenzel C, Mahn M, et al. Improved lung recruitment and oxygenation during mandatory ventilation with a new expiratory ventilation assistance device: a controlled interventional trial in healthy pigs. Eur J Anaesthesiol. 2018;35(10):736–44.
42. Spraider P, Martini J, Abram J, et al. Individualized flow-controlled ventilation compared to best clinical practice pressure-controlled ventilation: a prospective randomized porcine study. Crit Care. 2020;24:662.
43. Schmidt J, Wenzel C, Spassov S, et al. Flow-controlled ventilation attenuates lung injury in a porcine model of acute respiratory distress syndrome: a preclinical randomized controlled study. Crit Care Med. 2020;48(3):e241–8.
44. Weber J, Schmidt J, Straka L, et al. Flow-controlled ventilation improves gas exchange in lung-healthy patients – a randomized interventional cross-over study. Acta Anaesthesiol Scand. 2020;64(4):481–8.
45. Weber J, Straka L, Borgmann S, et al. Flow-controlled ventilation (FCV) improves regional ventilation in obese patients – a randomized controlled crossover trial. BMC Anesthesiol. 2020;20(1):24.
46. Katira BH, Engelberts D, Otulakowski G, et al. Abrupt deflation after sustained inflation causes lung injury. Am J Respir Crit Care Med. 2018;198(9):1165–76.
47. Gültuna I, Huygen PE, Ince C, et al. Clinical evaluation of diminished early expiratory flow (DEEF) ventilation in mechanically ventilated COPD patients. Intensive Care Med. 1996;22(6):539–45.
48. Aerts JGJV, van den Berg B, Bogaard JM. Controlled expiration in mechanically-ventilated patients with chronic obstructive pulmonary disease (COPD). Eur Respir J. 1997;10(3):550–6.
49. Schumann S, Vimlati L, Lichtwarck-Aschoff M, et al. Flow-controlled expiration discloses PEEP-dependent dynamic hysteresis of the pressure-volume loop. Crit Care. 2012;16(Suppl 1):105.
50. Goebel U, Haberstroh J, Foerster K, et al. Flow-controlled expiration: a novel ventilation mode to attenuate experimental porcine lung injury. Br J Anaesth. 2014;113(3):474–83.

51. Barnes T, van Asseldonk D, Enk D. Minimisation of dissipated energy in the airways during mechanical ventilation by using constant inspiratory and expiratory flows – flow-controlled ventilation (FCV). Med Hypotheses. 2018;121:167–76.
52. Barnes T, Enk D. Ventilation for low dissipated energy achieved using flow control during both inspiration and expiration. Trends Anaesth Crit Care. 2019;24:5–12.
53. Protti A, Maraffi T, Milesi M, et al. Role of strain rate in the pathogenesis of ventilator-induced lung edema. Crit Care Med. 2016;44(9):e838–45.
54. Spraider P, Abram J, Martini J, et al. Flow-controlled versus pressure-controlled ventilation in cardiac surgery with cardiopulmonary bypass - a single-center, prospective, randomized, controlled trial. J Clin Anesth. 2023;91:111279.
55. Abram J, Spraider P, Wagner J, et al. Short time effects of compliance guided flow-controlled ventilation versus standard of care pressure-controlled ventilation: a prospective porcine trial. Minerva Anestesiol. 2023;89(6):546–52.
56. Spraider P, Martini J, Abram J. Individualised flow-controlled ventilation versus pressure-controlled ventilation in a porcine model of thoracic surgery requiring one-lung ventilation: a laboratory study. Eur J Anaesthesiol. 2022;39(11):885–94.
57. Cook TM, Woodall N, Frerk C. 4th National Audit Project (NAP 4); major complications of airway management in the UK. Report and Findings. 2011.
58. Bick E. Ventrain™ does not make up for needle cricothyroidotomy deficiencies. Br J Anaesth. 2016;116(6):890–1.
59. Frerk C, Mitchell VS, McNarry AF, et al. Difficult Airway Society 2015 guidelines for management of unanticipated difficult intubation in adults. Br J Anaesth. 2015;115:827–48.
60. Heuveling DA, Mahieu HF, Jongsma-van Netten HG, Gerling V. Transtracheal use of the CriCath cannula in combination with the ventrain device for prevention of hypoxic arrest due to severe upper airway obstruction: a case report. A A Pract. 2018;11(12):344–7.
61. Borg PA, Hamaekers AE, Lacko M, et al. Ventrain® for ventilation of the lungs. Br J Anaesth. 2012;109(5):833–4.
62. Fearnley RA, Badiger S, Oakley RJ, Ahmad I. Elective use of the ventrain for upper airway obstruction during high-frequency jet ventilation. J Clin Anesth. 2016;33:233–5.
63. Onwochei DN, El-Boghdadly K, Ahmad I. Two-stage technique used to manage severe upper airway obstruction and avoid surgical tracheostomy: a case report. A A Pract. 2018;10(5):118–20.
64. Grassetto A, Pettenuzzo T, Badii F, et al. A new perspective during laryngo-tracheal surgery: the use of an ultra-thin endotracheal tube (Tritube®) and flow-controlled ventilation—a retrospective case series and a review of the literature. J Anesth Analg Crit Care. 2022;2(1):39.
65. Schmidt J, Günther F, Weber J, et al. Glottic visibility for laryngeal surgery: tritube vs. microlaryngeal tube: a randomised controlled trial. Eur J Anaesthesiol. 2019;36(12):963–71.
66. Meulemans J, Jans A, Vermeulen K, et al. Evone® flow-controlled ventilation during upper airway surgery: a clinical feasibility study and safety assessment. Front Surg. 2020;28(7):6.
67. Wahlen BM, Al-Thani H, El-Menyar A. Ventrain: from theory to practice. Bridging until re-tracheostomy. BMJ Case Rep. 2017;2017:bcr2017220403.
68. Zuercher M, Pythoud-Brügger M, Sandu K, Schoettker P. Combined use of ventrain and S-guide for airway management of severe subglottic stenosis. Turk J Anaesthesiol Reanim. 2019;47(3):238–41.
69. Morrison S, Aerts S, Van Rompaey D, Vanderveken O. Failed awake intubation for critical airway obstruction rescued with the ventrain device and an Arndt exchange catheter: a case report. A A Pract. 2019;13(1):23–6.
70. Willemsen MG, Noppens R, Mulder AL, Enk D. Ventilation with the ventrain through a small lumen catheter in the failed paediatric airway: two case reports. Br J Anaesth. 2014;112(5):946–7.
71. Piccioni F, Caccioppola A, Rosboch GL, et al. Use of the ventrain ventilation device and an airway exchange catheter to manage hypoxemia during thoracic surgery and one-lung ventilation. J Cardiothorac Vasc Anesth. 2021;35(12):3844–5.

72. Escribá Alepuz FJ, García JA, Cuchillo Sastriques JV, et al. Emergency ventilation of infant subglottic stenosis through small-gauge lumen using the ventrain: a case report. A A Pract. 2018;10(6):136–8.
73. Evers VM, Immink RV, van Boven WJP, et al. Intraoperative use of the ventrain for single lung ventilation after iatrogenic trauma to the left main bronchus during thoracoscopy: a case report. Case Rep Dermatol. 2017;9(4):116–8.
74. Instructions for use Ventrain®: http://ventinovamedical.com/wp-content/uploads/2022/05/MSS138.02_IFUVentrain_EN-master_09092021.pdf. Accessed October 2023.
75. Enk D, Spraider P, Abram J, Barnes T. Pressure measurements in flow-controlled ventilation. Crit Care Med. 2020;48(12):e1359–60.
76. Spraider P, Putzer G, Breitkopf RA, et al. A case report of individualized ventilation in a COVID-19 patient - new possibilities and caveats to consider with flow-controlled ventilation. BMC Anesthesiol. 2021;21(1):145.
77. Grassetto A, Pettenuzzo T, Badii F, et al. Flow-controlled ventilation may reduce mechanical power and increase ventilatory efficiency in severe coronavirus disease-19 acute respiratory distress syndrome. Pulmonology. 2023;29(2):154–6.
78. Bergold MN, Otterburg T, Woitzik J, Byhahn C. Flow-controlled ventilation – a novel approach to treating acute respiratory distress syndrome. Trends Anaesth Crit Care. 2020;30:e93.
79. de Wolf MWP, Enk D, Jagannathan N. Ventilation through small-bore airways in children by implementing active expiration. Paediatr Anaesth. 2022;32(2):312–20.
80. Abram J, Martini J, Spraider P, et al. Individualised flow-controlled versus pressure-controlled ventilation in a porcine oleic acid-induced acute respiratory distress syndrome model. Eur J Anaesthesiol. 2023;40(7):511–20.

Ultra-thin Cuffed Endotracheal Tube (Tritube®)

Farah Saleh Hijazi, Hany A. Zaki, and Nabil A. Shallik

1 Introduction

Laryngotracheal surgeries represent a major point of interest amongst the anaesthesiologists and the surgeons involved in performing such complex procedures. The ability to safely perform such surgeries relies on establishing a motionless and visible operative field, maintaining adequate gas exchange, and reducing the risk of complications such as air-trapping and barotrauma. To maximize the visibility of the surgical window, various designs of ETT have been developed. Common among them are the small-diameter tubes such as the microlaryngoscopy tubes (MLTs) and ultra-thin ETTs. Alternatively, a tubeless surgical field could be established either by high-frequency jet ventilation (HFJV) with intermittent periods of apnoea [1, 2] or SponTaneous Respiration using IntraVEnous anaesthesia and Hi-flow nasal oxygen (STRIVE Hi) [3]. In the latter examples, the unsecured airway may be jeopardized by aspiration of gastric contents. Additionally, a subset of patients with an underlying impairment in pulmonary mechanics may not tolerate the high-pressure jet delivered by the HFJV. Furthermore, HFJV may not offer a motionless operative field as the

F. S. Hijazi
Anaesthesia, ICU and Perioperative Medicine Department, Hamad Medical Corporation, Doha, Qatar

H. A. Zaki
Emergency Medicine, Hamad General Hospital, Doha, Qatar

N. A. Shallik (✉)
Anaesthesia, ICU and Perioperative Medicine Department, Hamad Medical Corporation, Doha, Qatar

Clinical Anaesthesiology Department, Weill Cornell Medical College in Qatar, Doha, Qatar

Clinical Anaesthesiology Department, College of Medicine Qatar University, Doha, Qatar

Anaesthesia and SICU Department, Tanta University, Tanta, Egypt
e-mail: nshallik@hamad.qa

N. A. Shallik (ed.), *Flow Controlled Ventilation Mode Through a Straw Size Tube*, https://doi.org/10.1007/978-3-031-77477-5_9

airway structures could be displaced by the jets. Nevertheless, facilitating surgical access is not the only indication for employing a narrow diameter ETT. In many instances, the pre-existing upper airway pathology such as a peri-glottic stenosis or a large intra-oral lesion renders a standard ETT impractical, by virtue of a narrower anatomical lumen, that doesn't accommodate a standard-bore ETT. Therefore, the limitations of the aforementioned airway management techniques inspired the design of ultra-thin cuffed ETT or straw-size cuffed ETT, such as the Tritube® (Ventinova Medical B.V., Eindhoven, The Netherlands). Essentially, a straw-size ETT offers a narrower diameter that preserves the visibility of the operative field and a cuff that seals the airway to protect against aspiration.

The advent of ultra-thin ETT (Tritube®) necessitated manufacturing a novel mechanical ventilation mode called flow-controlled ventilation (FCV) that can accommodate its unique design. A deep understanding of the principles that underlie how these unique equipment functions, as well as the basic principles of FCV, is of utmost importance to ensure patients' safety and troubleshooting throughout the procedures.

This chapter focuses on the ultra-thin cuffed ETT (Tritube®) (Ventinova Medical B.V., Eindhoven, The Netherlands), its specifications, applications in upper airway surgeries, limitations, and a brief discussion on FCV which is covered in detail in the chapter "Specifications of Flow Controlled Ventilator (Evone®)".

2 Ultra-Thin Cuffed Endotracheal Tube: The Conception of the Idea and Prototype Development

The design of ultra-thin ETT was inspired by both, the limitations of the current airway management equipment and the advantages of offered by a narrower diameter ETT. To elaborate, a conventional ETT may obscure the surgical field rendering the surgery technically difficult. Additionally, the pre-existing airway pathology such as stenosis or a mass lesion may not accommodate the relatively larger diameter of the conventional ETT. Moreover, opting for a tubeless operative field runs the risk of aspirating gastric contents and potential displacement of the anatomic structures due to air jets delivered. On the other hand, employing an ETT with a narrower lumen improves the visualization of the surgical field and reduces trauma to the laryngeal mucosa and vocal cords [4].

Hence, combining a narrower-lumen ETT, with a sealing cuff along with a continuous pressure-monitoring port inspired the development of an ultra-thin cuffed ETT, known as Tritube® (Ventinova Medical B.V., Eindhoven, The Netherlands). Initially, a dual-lumen laser-jet catheter (40 cm in length, Inner Diameter (ID) 2.2 mm) was modified by adding a cuff to its distal end, by connecting it to the pilot balloon using a 19 G epidural catheter [4]. The addition of a cuff offers airway protection, establishes normoventilation, and permits accurate measurements of end-tidal Carbon Dioxide (etCO_2). Following that, the Tritube® (Ventinova Medical B.V., Eindhoven, The Netherlands), ID ~2.4 mm, was manufactured with three lumens: a ventilation port, a port to inflate and deflate the cuff, and a port for continuous measurement of intra-tracheal (IT) pressure along with a preloaded stylet. The initial length of the tube was 40 cm, but in 2020, it was redesigned, and the

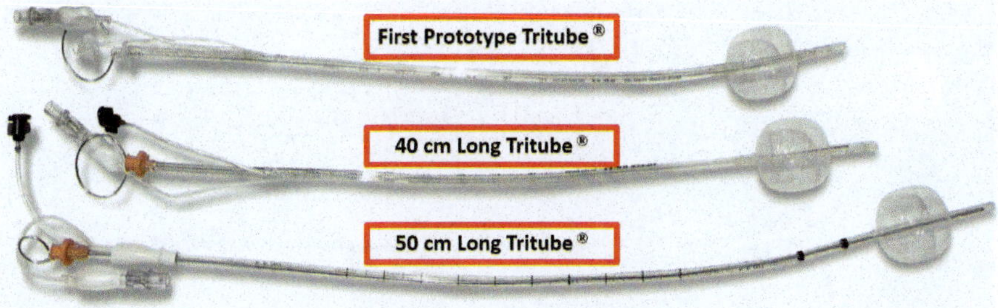

Fig. 1 Three different versions of Tritube® (Ventinova Medical, Eindhoven, the Netherlands). (Courtesy, Dr. Shallik, Doha Airway Equipment Museum, Qatar)

length was increased to 50 cm, and two black marks upstream of the cuff, marking the depth of insertion, were added [2] (Fig. 1).

For more details, please refer to chapter "A Narrative Review of the Past, Present, and Future of Small-Bore Ventilation, Expiratory Ventilation Assistance, and Flow Controlled Ventilation".

3 Ultra-Thin Cuffed Endotracheal Tube: An Overview of the Specifications

One of the most recent advancements in airway management for laryngotracheal surgeries is using an ultra-thin or straw-size cuffed ETT (Tritube® Ventinova Medical, Eindhoven, The Netherlands). The tube is manufactured from polyurethane and could be inserted through the nasotracheal or orotracheal route. The length of the tube is 50 cm and it has three independent ports: a ventilatory lumen that opens at the distal tip of the tube and has a Murphy eye, a pressure-monitoring lumen that continuously measures the intra-tracheal pressure, and a cuff-inflation channel to inflate/deflate the cuff [2]. The ID of the straw-size cuffed ETT is less than 3 mm, and the outer diameter (OD) is 4.4 mm [1] (Fig. 2). The cuff measures 4 cm in length and is elliptical in shape as shown in (Fig. 3). The narrow diameter, hence, the name ultra-thin, yields better visualization of the surgical field. The cylinder-shaped, high-volume low-pressure cuff is located roughly 3 cm from the tip of the tube and seals the trachea, conferring airway protection against aspiration [2]. Another important feature of ultra-thin tubes is the preloaded malleable metal stylet that facilitates intubation.

Given the narrow ID of the ultra-thin tube of 2.4 mm and the presence of an inflated endotracheal cuff, passive expiration through a patent airway may prove impractical [1, 5]. For that reason, the use of ultra-thin tube necessitates utilizing active expiratory techniques, either by using the hand-operated manual ventilator (Ventrain®) or the flow-controlled mechanical ventilator (Evone®) (Ventinova Medical, Eindhoven, The Netherlands). Both airway devices operate using a negative suction, also called expiratory ventilation assistance (EVA), which actively rids the lungs of expired gases. Coupling straw-size cuffed ETT with active expiratory techniques is vital, as a reduction in the expiratory flow relative to inspiratory flow

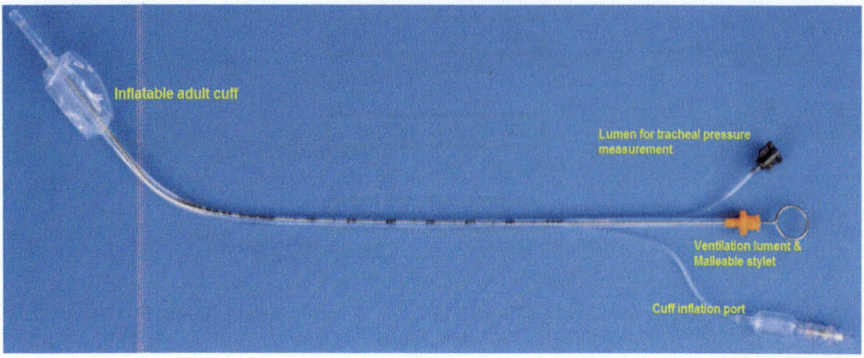

Fig. 2 Ultra-thin or straw-size cuffed endotracheal tube (Tritube® Ventinova Medical, Eindhoven, The Netherlands)

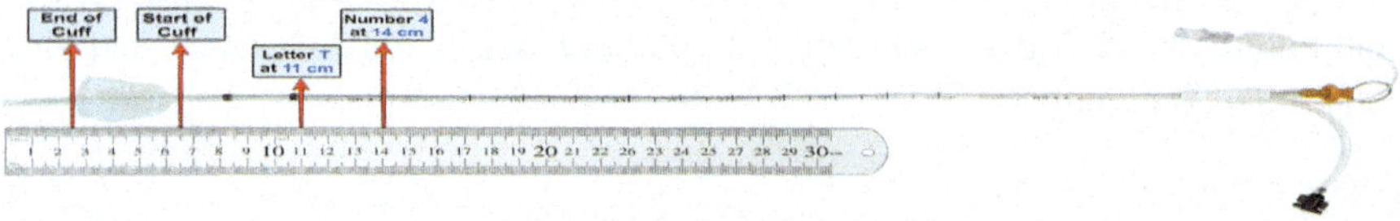

Fig. 3 Estimated cuff length and markings. Note that the cuff is cylindrical in shape and is estimated to measure 4 cm in length and that the letter "T," marking the black line is located at 11 cm. (Courtesy, Dr. Shallik, Doha Airway Equipment Museum, Qatar)

will lead to gas trapping and lung hyperinflation. The pressure-monitoring lumen plays a pivotal role in diagnosing serious lung hyperinflation that may engender hemodynamic instability.

4 Ultra-thin Cuffed Endotracheal Tube: A Window to Greater Possibilities

The narrower OD of the ultra-thin tube ~4.4 mm provides a greater likelihood of securing the airway with less trauma and bleeding; therefore, it confers better preservation of the operative field when a substantial peri-glottic narrowing is anticipated, based on preoperative assessment and diagnostic imaging. Before the advent of ultra-thin tubes, MLT with ID 6.0 mm and OD 8.8 mm would have been considered as an alternative to securing the airway, however, insertion may be difficult or impossible depending on the anticipated peri-glottic narrowing as the OD of MLT is almost double that of an ultra-thin tube (Fig. 4). A randomized clinical trial (RCT) published in 2019, showed that Tritube® (Ventinova Medical, Eindhoven, The Netherlands) was associated with a statistically significant reduction in the concealment of the laryngeal structures compared to MLT [6], ($P < 0.001$). In this RCT, subjects scheduled for elective laryngeal surgery were randomized to be intubated with either a Tritube® (Ventinova Medical, Eindhoven, The Netherlands) or

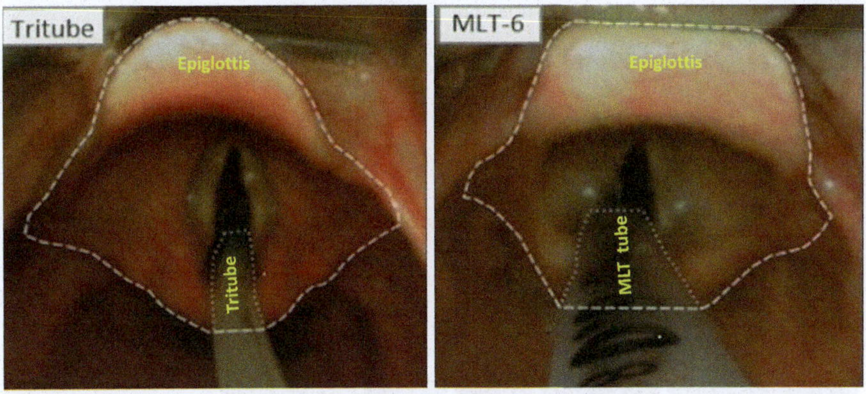

Fig. 4 Glottic visibility using Tritube® vs. microlaryngoscopy tube [6]

MLT. Of note, subjects with a potentially difficult airway were excluded. The concealment of the laryngeal structures was compared using software that compared images obtained during endotracheal intubation using video laryngoscopy. Even if a MLT was inserted successfully, the visibility of the operative window may be compromised by the presence of the tube or due to the trauma and bleeding sustained during intubation. Therefore, the anaesthetist would be left with the option of a tubeless operative field to allow enough debulking of the mass for a tube to be passed through the glottic opening [5]. Inherently, a tubeless airway is at a greater risk of aspiration and post-operative pulmonary complications. Another option would be a pre-laryngectomy tracheostomy. However, the trend is shifting away from a preoperative tracheostomy given the association with suboptimal wound healing and loco-regional recurrence due to tumour seeding [7]. In a case report that was published in 2021, a tubeless debulking of a laryngeal tumour and the need for a pre-procedural tracheostomy were obviated using a Tritube® (Ventinova Medical, Eindhoven, The Netherlands), and the patient was spared the complications associated with tubeless surgeries and a tracheostomy. The authors of the case report stated that inserting MLT 5.0 mm would have been difficult as the airway was too narrow to accommodate it [5]. See Fig. 5 for a comparison of the diameter of conventional ETT and Tritube® (Ventinova Medical, Eindhoven, The Netherlands). At our institution, we encountered a case of marked tracheal stenosis due to impingement of follicular thyroid carcinoma. A preoperative 3D construction and virtual endoscopy estimated the tracheal calibre to be ~4–5 mm. The airway was successfully intubated using Tritube® (Ventinova Medical, Eindhoven, The Netherlands) and it was used throughout the procedure that lasted for more than 6 hours [8].

An important technology that can be combined with ultra-thin ETT is using 3D CT reconstruction and virtual endoscopy (VE) of the upper airway to map out stenotic areas in the airway and deciding on the ETT with the most suitable OD preoperatively. We have encountered various cases at our institution as shown in (Fig. 6)

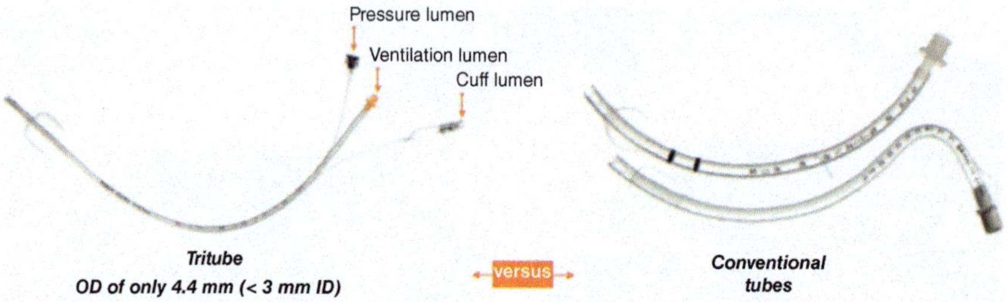

Fig. 5 Comparison between the outer diameter of a Tritube® and conventional tubes. (Ventinova Medical, Eindhoven, The Netherlands)

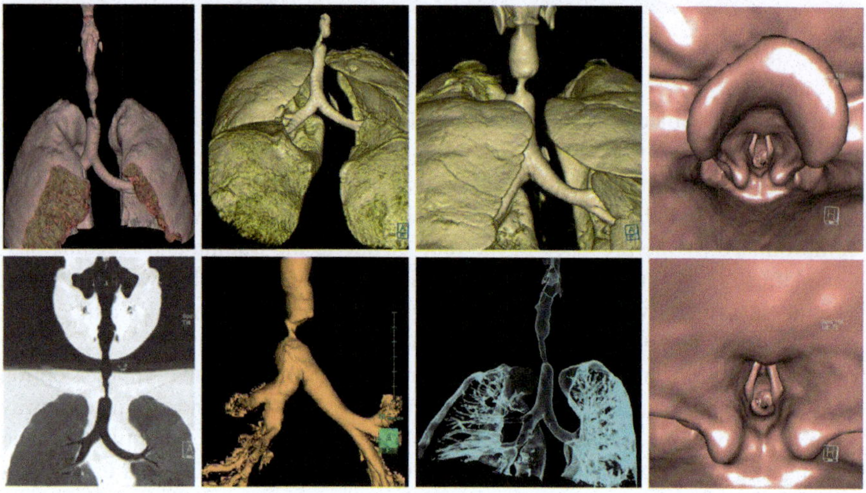

Fig. 6 Different cases of tracheal stenosis diagnosed with CT 3D reconstruction and virtual endoscopy (VE) that were successfully managed using Tritube® and Evone® (Courtesy, Dr. Shallik, Doha, Qatar)

successfully managed using ultra-thin ETT in which the preoperative plan was based on images obtained from VE and 3D CT reconstruction [9, 10].

5 Flow-Controlled Ventilation: The Bernoulli's Principle in Effect

The advent of ultra-thin ETT was accompanied by an innovative mode of mechanical ventilation called FCV, which can accommodate the resistance to airflow caused by the tube's narrow diameter, in addition to, tackling the risk of air-trapping and lung hyperinflation given the presence of an inflated cuff. To fully understand how flow-controlled ventilation operates, it is worth revising

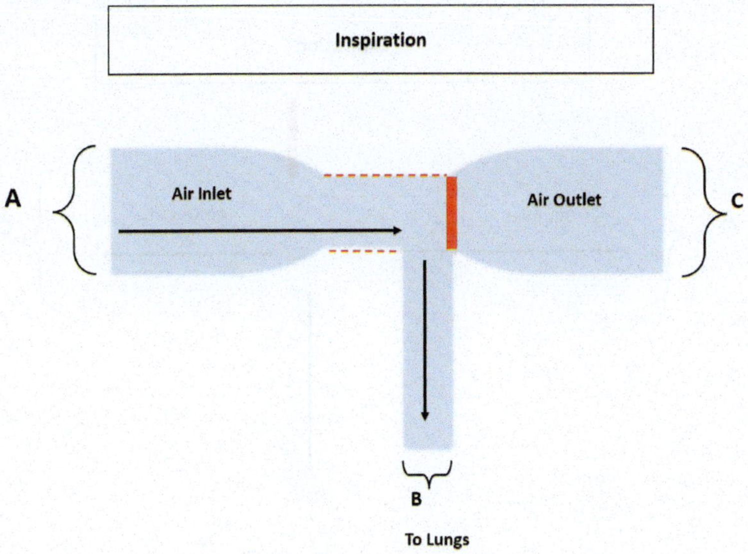

Fig. 7 Bernoulli's principle in the Evone® mechanical ventilator during the inspiratory phase

Bernoulli's principle, the basis of how the hand-operated manual flow-controlled ventilator(Ventrain®) and the automatic flow-controlled mechanical ventilator (Evone®) function.

In essence, Bernoulli's principle describes the relationship between the velocity, pressure, and the flow of a fluid (liquid or gas). It states that, as the speed of a moving fluid increases, the pressure within the fluid decreases [11]. During the inspiratory phase of the respiratory cycle, the air is insufflated from the air inlet of the flow-controlled mechanical ventilator to the patient through the narrow-lumen Tritube® (Ventinova Medical, Eindhoven, The Netherlands) (From point A to Point B, in (Fig. 7) [1, 12]. The air stream has no alternative route as the air outlet is blocked. During the expiratory phase of the respiratory cycle, the blockage at point C is released, giving way to the high-velocity air that is injected through the air inlet to generate negative pressure at point B, with a resultant suctioning force, which actively aspirates gas out of the lungs and into the air outlet (Air flows from Point A to Point C, generating a negative pressure that suctions air from Point B to Point C, as shown in (Fig. 8) [1, 12]). Thus, unlike conventional ventilators that rely on the lung's elastic recoil and passive expiration of gases, FCV actively suctions expired gases out of the lungs to overcome the resistance to airflow imparted by a markedly narrow ETT and the presence of an insufflated cuff.

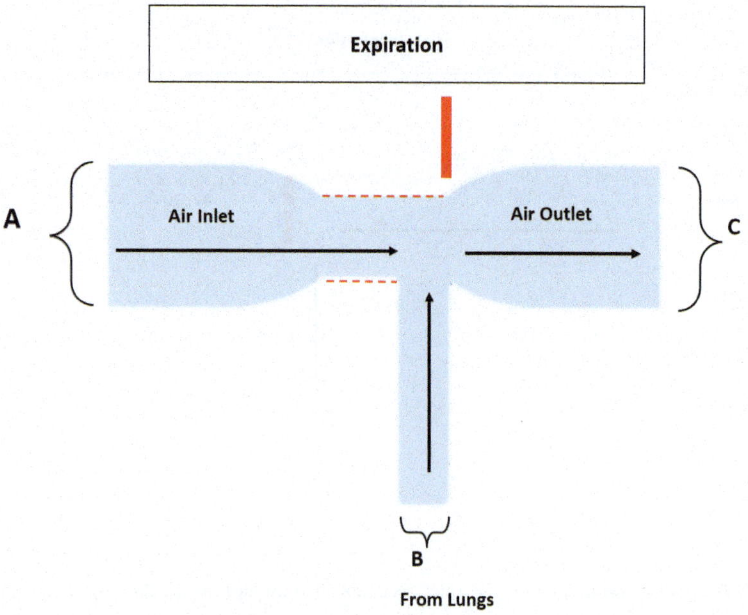

Fig. 8 Bernoulli's principle in the Evone® mechanical ventilator during the expiratory phase

6 A Unique Waveform for a Unique Ventilation Modality!

The uniqueness of the FCV is best depicted using the waveforms of the IT pressure (cmH_2O), volume (ml), and flow (ml s^{-1}) (Fig. 9a, b). During the inspiratory phase, a constant positive flow is provided [13], simultaneously, there is a linear increase in the volume and IT pressure [12]. Once the peak pressure is sensed to have reached the level set by the operator, inspiration ceases, and expiration commences without an inspiratory pause taking place [14]. During expiration, a constant negative flow is provided [13] accompanied by a linear decrease in pressure and volume until it reaches a pre-determined positive end-expiratory pressure [14]. Herein, the air jet is blown through the air inlet, creating a negative pressure that acts as a negative vacuum, actively clearing the lungs from the expired gasses, rather than relying on passive expiration as is the case in conventional modes of mechanical ventilation. Optimal ventilation is ensured by maintaining a continuous inspiratory and expiratory flow.

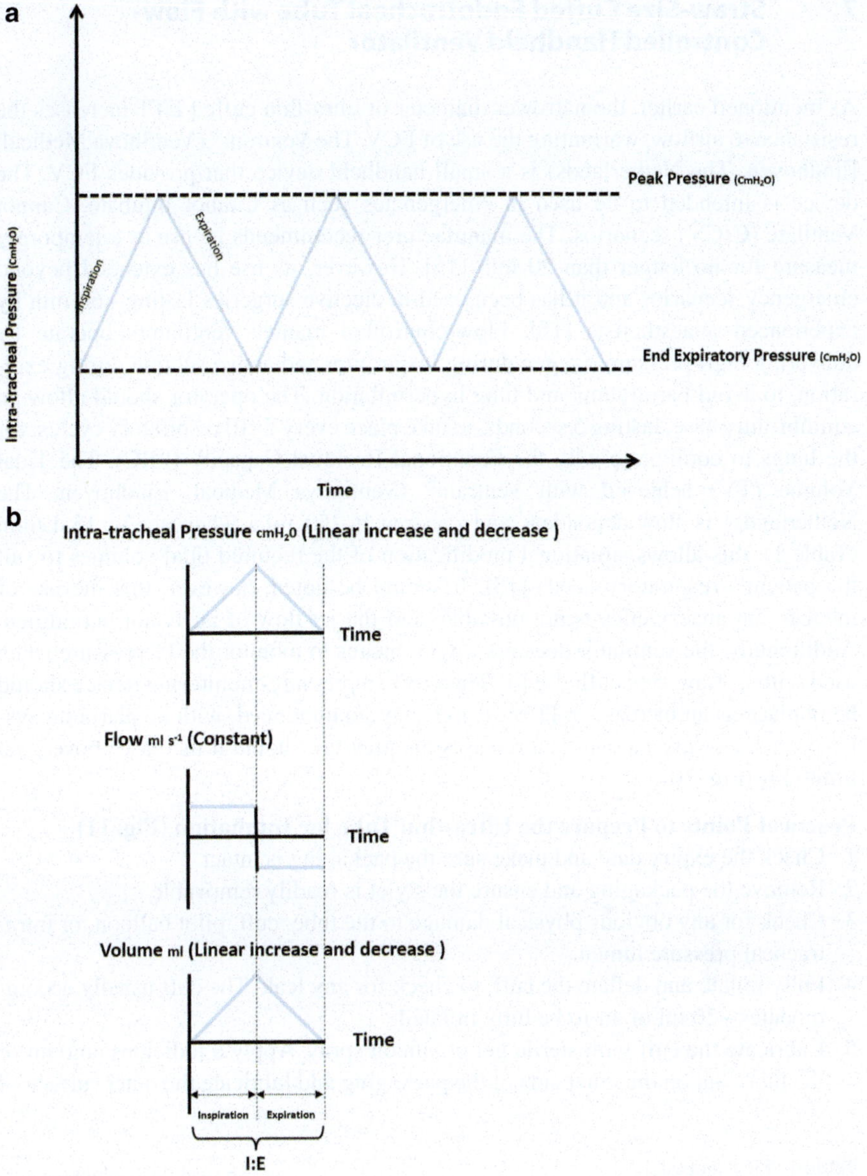

Fig. 9 (**a**) Flow-controlled ventilation pressure waveform. (**b**) Flow-controlled ventilation waveforms

7 Straw-Size Cuffed Endotracheal Tube with Flow-Controlled Handheld Ventilator

As mentioned earlier, the narrower diameter of ultra-thin cuffed ETT increases the resistance to airflow, warranting the use of FCV. The Ventrain® (Ventinova Medical, Eindhoven, The Netherlands) is a small handheld device that provides FCV. The device is intended to be used in emergencies such as Cannot Intubate, Cannot Ventilate (CICV) scenarios. The manufacturer recommends its use as a temporary measure for no longer than 20 min [15]. However, its use has extended beyond emergency scenarios and it has been used in elective surgeries lasting <60 min by experienced anaesthetists [15]. Flow-controlled manual ventilators operate by delivering high-pressure oxygen during inspiration and active suction during expiration, to avoid barotrauma and lung hyperinflation. The operator should allow an equilibrium phase, lasting 5 seconds, to take place every 5–10 respiratory cycles, for the lungs to equilibrate with the Functional Residual Capacity (FRC). The Tidal Volume (TV) achieved with Ventrain® (Ventinova Medical, Eindhoven, The Netherlands) is flow-dependent and can reach 250 ml/s when set to 15 L/min (Table 1), this allows situational modification of the required tidal volumes to suit the patient's respiratory needs [15]. It should be noted, however, that the use of inhalational anaesthetics is not possible, and the jet flow of air is not humidified. Additionally, the ventilator does not offer a means to monitor the IT pressure when used with a straw-size cuffed ETT. Therefore, a pressure-monitoring device should be in place as an increase in IT pressures may go unnoticed, with no alarming system or a safety mechanism that releases the pressure should it increase above a set limit [14] (Fig. 10).

Practical Points to Prepare the Ultra-thin Tube for Intubation (Fig. 11)

1. Check the expiry date and make sure the packaging is intact.
2. Remove the packaging and ensure the stylet is readily removable.
3. Check for any obvious physical damage to the tube, cuff, pilot balloon, or intratracheal pressure lumen.
4. Fully inflate and deflate the cuff, to check for any leak. The cuff usually accommodates ~20 ml of air to be fully inflated.
5. Lubricate the cuff with sterile gel or silicon spray. Apply a judicious amount of the lubricant on the inner side of the packaging and lubricate the outer surface of

Table 1 Flow and tidal volume achieved with the manual flow-controlled ventilator [15]

Flow (L/min)	Expected tidal volume (mL) after manual inspiration lasting 1 s
2	33
4	67
6	100
10	167
12	200
15	250

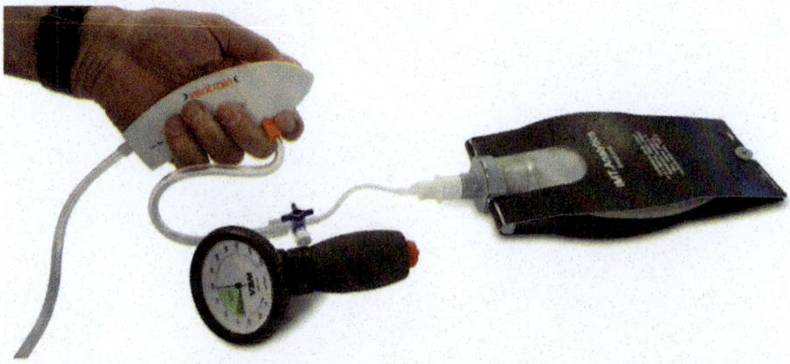

Fig. 10 Pressure-monitoring device attached to an artificial lung and the manual flow-controlled ventilator. (Courtesy, Dr. Shallik, Doha Airway Equipment Museum, Qatar)

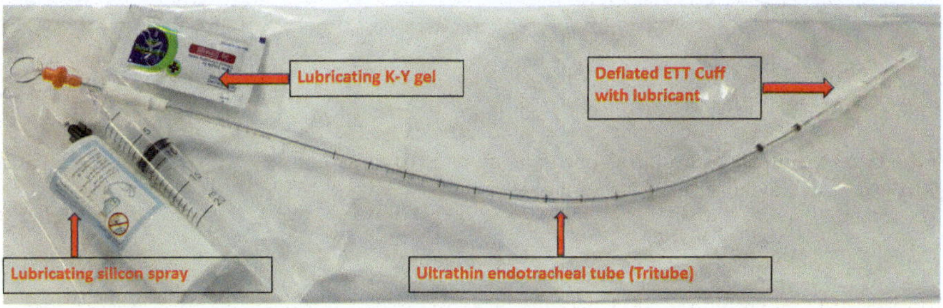

Fig. 11 Preparation of the ultra-thin tube for intubation (Courtesy, Dr. Shallik, Doha, Qatar)

the cuff. Then, deflate the cuff and rotate the tube anti-clockwise while submersing the cuff in the lubricant simultaneously. The idea is to use the lubricant as a "cementing material" to maintain the deflated position of the cuff. This is an important step to ensure smooth insertion as a large cuff can tear easily or obscure the operator's visual field if not fully deflated.

6. The tube is now ready for insertion. Make sure the flow-controlled ventilator, either the manual or the automatic is checked and ready to be used.

8 Tritube® in a Tube to Minimize Aerosol Exposure

Operating on the airway naturally entails exposure of healthcare providers to droplets and aerosols. In a time as critical as that of the COVID-19 pandemic, the need for a novel method to minimize aerosol exposure was of utmost need (Fig. 12). Herein, the combination of conventional ETT with Tritube® (Ventinova Medical, Eindhoven, The Netherlands) and Evone® (Ventinova Medical, Eindhoven, The Netherlands) provides a closed-ventilation system. The novel method was described in an article published in 2021 [16] and utilizes the narrow lumen of the Tritube® (Ventinova Medical, Eindhoven, The Netherlands) as a conduit to be passed through the conventional ETT. After ensuring an adequate plane of anaesthesia is established, ventilation is ceased via the conventional ETT. The latter is cut at its proximal end and a Tritube® (Ventinova Medical, Eindhoven, The Netherlands) is introduced through it. Tritube® (Ventinova Medical, Eindhoven, The Netherlands) is advanced until it emerges at the distal end of the

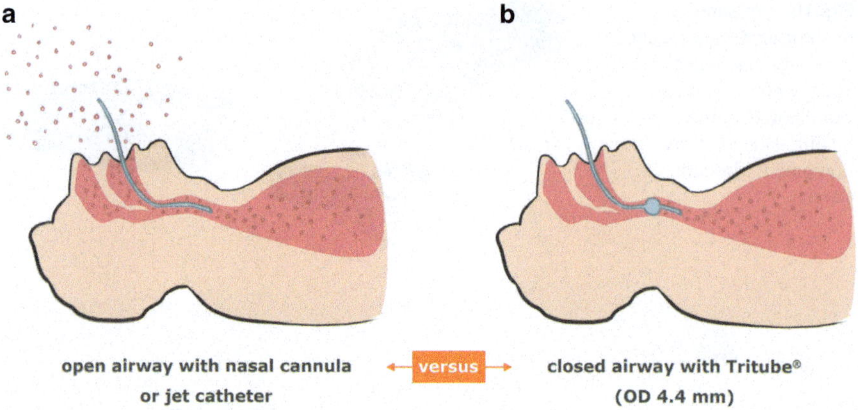

Fig. 12 Aerosol Exposure in (**a**) open airway and (**b**) closed airway with Tritube® (Ventinova Medical B.V., Eindhoven, The Netherlands)

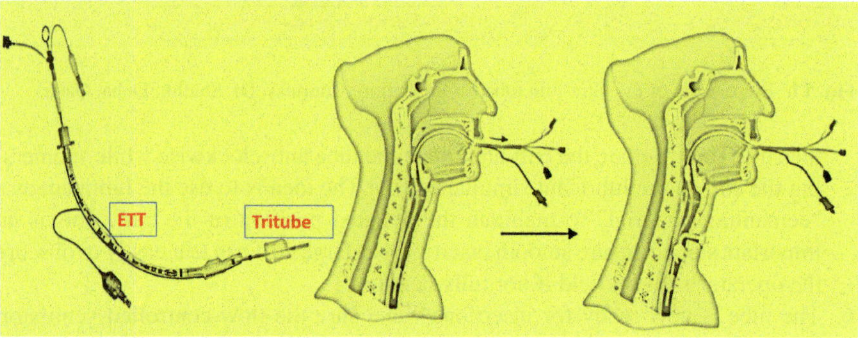

Fig. 13 Tritube® in a tube for tracheostomy in COVID-19 patients to reduce the risk of aerosol exposure (from website of Ventinova Medical B.V., Eindhoven, The Netherlands)[16]

conventional ETT, and the cuff is inflated and connected to Evone® (Ventinova Medical, Eindhoven, The Netherlands) to ventilate the patient. The standard ETT is retracted, to provide optimal working conditions for the surgeons, until the cuff is above the vocal cords. The narrow lumen of Tritube® (Ventinova Medical, Eindhoven, The Netherlands) does not interfere with the working space of the surgical team. Following that, a tracheostomy is created, and ventilation could be attempted through it with a conventional ventilator. Once the functionality of the tracheostomy is confirmed, the cuff of Tritube® (Ventinova Medical, Eindhoven, The Netherlands) can be deflated and removed along with the surrounding conventional ETT. Retracting the Tritube® (Ventinova Medical, Eindhoven, The Netherlands) does not interfere with the tracheostomy given its narrow cross-sectional diameter (Fig. 13). Although the manufacturer does not claim that Tritube® (Ventinova Medical, Eindhoven, The Netherlands) is intended to be used in a conventional ETT, we did use it in our institution and its utility proved useful.

9 Tritube® as a Rescue Measure: Tritube® with Laryngeal Mask Airway (LMA)

So far, we have described the use of ultra-thin ETT in elective settings for pre-selected patients to optimize the visibility of the operative field. But an important question arises, for such a unique tube, are there any applications during emergency scenarios anaesthetists may encounter unexpectedly, particularly those where upper airway stenosis is suspected to be the underlying pathology? A case report that was published in 2023 described a difficult airway scenario, successfully managed with the combination of an LMA, flexible fibre-optic scope, and a Tritube® (Ventinova Medical, Eindhoven, The Netherlands) [17]. The scenario describes a 40-year-old female, posted for an elective gynaecological procedure, who had a childhood history of admission to the paediatric intensive care unit and a need for a tracheostomy. The indication of the tracheostomy is not known as the medical records were not available. After induction, endotracheal intubation was attempted with a standard ETT size of 7.0 mm. However, the tube encountered resistance as it was advanced, and it was subsequently downsized to 6.5 mm, then 6.0 mm, then 5.5 mm, and eventually 5.0 mm to no avail. The primary anaesthetist inserted an LMA as a rescue measure and called for help. Following that, a fibre-optic examination of the airway was carried out, through the LMA, revealing significant tracheal stenosis. To overcome the narrow calibre of the trachea, a urinary guidewire (diameter 0.97 mm and length of 150 cm) (it looks like a central venous catheter guidewire)was inserted through the working channel of the flexible bronchoscope, and a Tritube® (Ventinova Medical, Eindhoven, The Netherlands) was subsequently railroaded, successfully securing the airway [17]. Another rescue combination that we also attempted at our institution is inserting an LMA as a rescue device and then inserting a Tritube® (Ventinova Medical, Eindhoven, The Netherlands) through the LMA to secure the airway as shown in (Fig. 14).

Although more research is required to establish the role of Tritube® (Ventinova Medical, Eindhoven, the Netherlands) in the algorithm for managing difficult

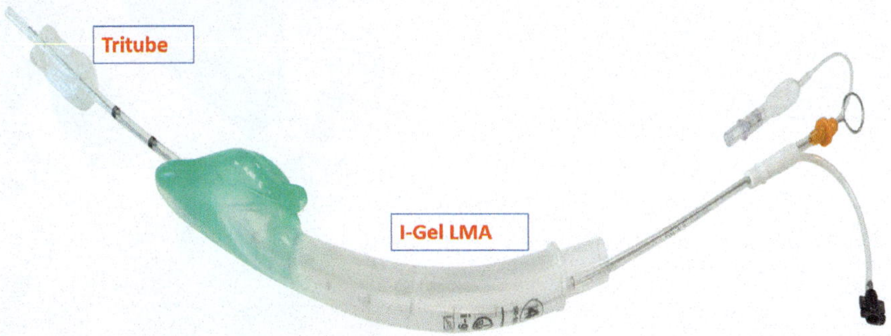

Fig. 14 Tritube® in a laryngeal mask airway (Courtesy, Dr. Shallik, Doha Airway Equipment Museum, Qatar)

airways, its potential should not be neglected, particularly in facilities that carry out Ear, Nose, and Throat (ENT) surgeries. However, it is important to note that in an emergency situations, a manual flow-controlled ventilator (Ventrain® Ventinova Medical B.V., Eindhoven, The Netherlands) should be used by trained personnel as the automatic mechanical ventilator Evone® (Ventinova Medical, Eindhoven, The Netherlands) may not be practical as it needs calibration on an artificial lung, this process takes around 5–10 minutes and time is of essence during emergency scenarios [18].

10 Ultra-Thin Tube in Nasal Intubation

Ultra-thin tubes can be used for nasal intubation for intra-oral or maxillo-facial surgeries, with a few practical points to be considered (Fig. 15).

1. The preloaded stylet should be removed before nasotracheal intubation.
2. In case a Magil's forceps is used to facilitate intubation, care should be taken not to accidentally puncture the cuff, as it would render the ultra-thin tube faulty.
3. Applying a lubricating jelly should be limited to the cuff and not Murphy's eye or the tube's aperture as the jelly might harden forming a crust that occludes either of the lumens, in effect acting like a mucus plug.
4. Consider using a nasopharyngeal airway as a conduit for the passage of the ultra-thin tube to prevent trauma to the nasal cavity.

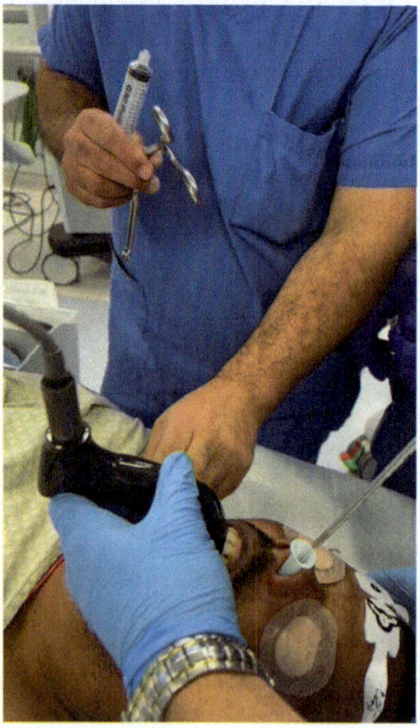

Fig. 15 Nasotracheal intubation using the ultra-thin tube, note the use of a nasopharyngeal airway (Courtesy, Dr. Shallik, Doha, Qatar)

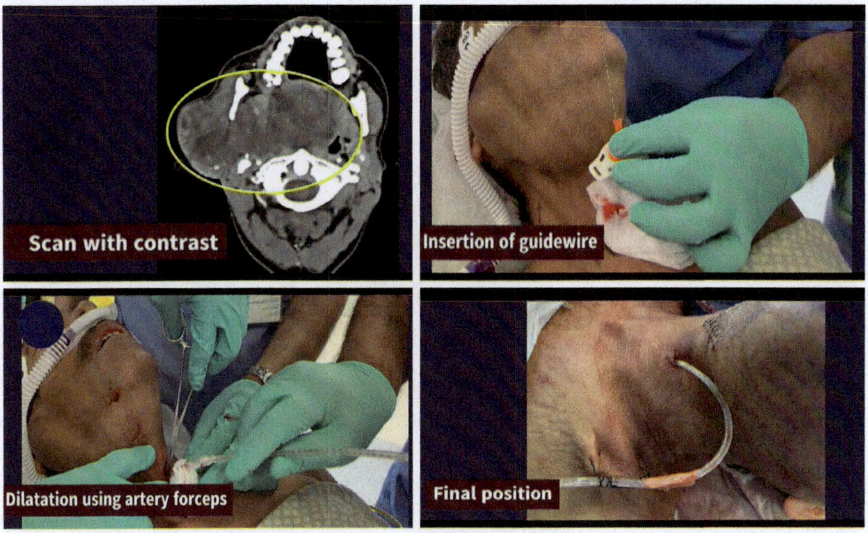

Fig. 16 Plan (A) for airway management is conducting elective front-of-neck access in a patient with a massive parotid gland mass (Courtesy, Dr. Shallik, Doha, Qatar)

11 Ultra-thin Tube in Elective Front-of-Neck Access (FONA)

The use of Tritube® (Ventinova Medical, Eindhoven, The Netherlands) for FONA is not limited to emergency scenarios. The advantages of a narrower lumen may be used in an elective FONA setting, such as that seen in patients who are not amenable to conventional intubation, and a transtracheal route is warranted. For example, patients with extensive head and neck tumours. Securing the airway may prove virtually impossible or risky due to potentially "losing the airway" and failing to restore oxygenation. In this context, it is important to stratify such patients from the outset and plan for a FONA as plan (A) sparing the airway unnecessary trauma with futile attempts. We have used this technique in an elective setting for a patient who presented with a massive parotid mass extending into the oral cavity, we performed a needle Cricothyrotomy using Cricath® (Ventinova Medical, Eindhoven, The Netherlands), following confirming correct placement by observing capnography, we passed a urinary guidewire (it looks like a central venous catheter guidewire) and then the Tritube® (Ventinova Medical, Eindhoven, The Netherlands) was successfully railroaded to the trachea. We conduct such procedures under mild sedation and local anaesthesia at the site of the incision (Fig. 16).

12 Ultra-thin Tube in "Cannot Intubate, Cannot Oxygenate" (CICO) Scenario

Performing an emergent FONA in a difficult airway using a scalpel, then a bougie, and railroading a regular ETT is the recommended approach to obtain surgical access to salvage the airway according to the 2015 Difficult Airway Society (DAS)

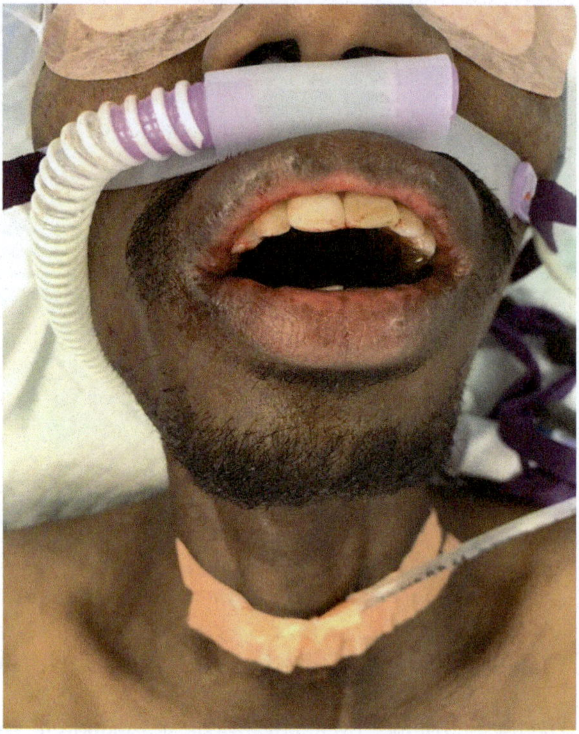

Fig. 17 Emergency front-of-neck access in cannot intubate, cannot oxygenate scenario using ultra-thin tube. (Courtesy, Dr. Shallik, Doha, Qatar)

guidelines [19]. In a CICO scenario, particularly where an upper airway lesion is suspected to be causing the obstruction, a narrower ETT lumen tube may confer the advantage of easier insertion and less trauma (Fig. 17). However, using the ultra-thin tube in such scenarios warrants the presence of either a manual or automatic flow-controlled ventilator. As stated earlier, Evone® (Ventinova Medical, Eindhoven, the Netherlands) needs to be calibrated before usage. Therefore, using Ventrain® (Ventinova Medical B.V., Eindhoven, The Netherlands) is more practical in these circumstances.

13 Tritube® for Difficult Extubation

Much like difficult intubation is expected in patients undergoing laryngotracheal surgery, extubation proves to be more difficult, given the surgical manipulation that took place, the pain, and the agitation at emergence. Therefore, devising a clear plan to safeguard the extubation and to have a conduit in situ, should the need arise, for re-intubation is an approach adopted by many anaesthetists involved in upper airway surgeries. A study published in 2017, demonstrated that Tritube® (Ventinova Medical, Eindhoven, The Netherlands) could be left in situ, after deflating the cuff, while performing face-mask ventilation. This use is rendered practical by virtue of an ultra-thin tube that does not interfere with the mask seal with the face. In that study, the vast majority of the patients tolerated the presence of the tube intratracheally and were able to talk and were transferred to the recovery unit until deemed fit for extubation [20].

From our clinical experience, we found that topicalizing the vocal cords with local anaesthetic drugs using a mucosal atomization device (MAD) and keeping the Tritube® (Ventinova Medical, Eindhoven, The Netherlands) in the retromolar space is well-tolerated by the patients. The tube could be left in situ for less than 24 h for a single tube, as per the manufacturer's leaflet. It is important to note that the cuff must be fully deflated by visualizing a collapsed pilot balloon. A forceful inspiratory attempt by the patient on a fully sealed airway may result in negative pressure pulmonary oedema.

Additionally, Tritube® (Ventinova Medical, Eindhoven, The Netherlands) could be used as an airway exchange catheter in cases where extubation may be deemed risky. The narrow lumen ensures easy passage through the standard tube in a fashion similar to that described in Tritube® (Ventinova Medical, Eindhoven, The Netherlands) in a Tube section.

14 Practical Points for Troubleshooting

With all the advantages offered by a narrower ETT diameter, it renders the tube more susceptible to occlusion by secretions. The occlusive plug interferes with IT pressure monitoring and capnography. The interference is denoted by an irregularity in the pressure curve that also affects the quality of the monitored capnography. Rapid recognition and management in such a scenario are of utmost importance as unrecognized lung hyperinflation can lead to circulatory collapse or halting ventilation altogether.

Below are some strategies to reduce the risk of tube occlusion by secretions (i.e., blood, pus, or mucus).

1. Consider premedicating the patient preoperatively with an anti-cholinergic drug to reduce mucosal secretions such as Glycopyrrolate.
2. Adequate hydration liquifies secretions and renders them less thick and tenacious.
3. Asking the patient to cough to clear the airway.
4. Suctioning the airway before intubating.
5. In case an occlusive plug forms, the operator can use a 10-ml syringe filled with sterile normal saline to flush the lumen(s) of the ultra-thin ETT.
6. Flushing with pressure is required to force any secretions or clotted blood out of the tube.
7. Try connecting a suctioning device to clear any secretions within the lumen(s).
8. Keep in mind that Evone® (Ventinova Medical, Eindhoven, The Netherlands) has a built-in suctioning mechanism that may dislodge an occlusive plug from the ETT to the ventilator upstream causing an occlusion.

Limitations of ultra-thin tube:

1. As is the case for any newly developed device made for anaesthetic practise, there is a learning curve. The previous sections delved into using Tritube®, Ventrain®, or Evone® (Ventinova Medical., Eindhoven, The Netherlands) during elective and emergency scenarios. It is advised against using new techniques or devices in emergencies where the operator lacks the theoretical knowledge and practical skills to use them. We advise providing adequate training and simulation prior to putting the equipment to use. In addition, we recommend using the devices in elective and controlled settings before considering their use in emergencies as a lack of familiarity may aggravate the issue at hand.
2. The ultra-thin tube is not Light Amplification by Stimulated Emission of Radiation (LASER) resistant, and the manufacturer deems using it in LASER surgeries a contraindication, as it is potentially flammable. Nevertheless, there have been some publications whereby Tritube® (Ventinova Medical, Eindhoven, The Netherlands) was used for LASER surgeries, with the standard LASER surgery safety precautions in place [1].
3. As mentioned in the section on troubleshooting, the ultra-thin tube is easily blocked by mucus, blood, or pus.
4. According to the manufacturer's instruction leaflet, the ultra-thin tube is intended to be used in patients weighing >40 kg. Therefore, its use in the paediatrics population is not well-studied.
5. Using an ultra-thin tube with a flexible bronchoscope either for awake or asleep fibre-optic intubation is not feasible, given the presence of a preloaded stylet and a narrow ID. This may impart a limitation for cases in which a flexible bronchoscope is more favourable than direct or indirect laryngoscopy such as cases of cervical spine instability or myelopathy due to cord compression, in which neck movement must be minimized. However, the flexible bronchoscope could be used as a guide for intubation using the working channel of the fibre-optic scope for placing a long guidewire, such as a urinary guidewire (it looks like a central venous catheter guidewire), then retracting the fibre-optic bronchoscope and railroading the ultra-thin tube over the guidewire [17].

15 Conclusion

The clinical utility of straw-size ETT in upper airway surgeries seems promising. The ultra-thin ETT offers stability and better visualization of the surgical field, protection from aspiration of gastric contents, accurate measurement of minute ventilation and airway pressures, and continuous monitoring of $etCO_2$. Additionally, the ultra-thin tube has an important role in securing airways rendered too narrow to accommodate conventional ETT. To be used safely, the operator should have a clear understanding of the physical principles that govern FCV, the novel ventilatory technique that renders adequate ventilation possible while using ultra-thin ETT.

The operator's knowledge and technical skills, coupled with ultra-thin ETT may indeed pave the pathway for a greater possibility in the field of upper airway surgeries.

While more studies are needed, it seems compelling to speculate that straw-size ETT might have a future role in difficult airway management algorithms, particularly in scenarios where FONA is warranted either under elective or emergent circumstances.

Acknowledgments A special thanks is extended to Mr. Abil Luez who artistically captured all images of this chapter.

Disclaimer Here, we introduce the flow-controlled manual ventilator (FCmV), exemplified frequently by the Ventrain®, merely because there is no alternative of its kind on the market. Additionally, you may find a particular focus on "Evone®" as it is the only commercially available FCV. Similarly, using "Tritube®" instead of ultra-thin or straw size ETT terminology is due to the lack of other examples and not as a commercial endorsement of the product(s).

References

1. Grassetto A, Pettenuzzo T, Badii F, Barzaghi F, Carlon R, Dellarole S, et al. A new perspective during laryngo-tracheal surgery: the use of an ultra-thin endotracheal tube (Tritube®) and flow-controlled ventilation-a retrospective case series and a review of the literature. J Anesth Analg Crit Care. 2022;2(1):39.
2. Morrison S, Van Oostende C, Aerts S, Saldien V. The tritube: facilitating upper airway surgery with an ultrathin cuffed airway device. A A Pract. 2023;17(7):e01697.
3. Booth AWG, Vidhani K, Lee PK, Thomsett C-M. SponTaneous Respiration using IntraVEnous anaesthesia and Hi-flow nasal oxygen (STRIVE Hi) maintains oxygenation and airway patency during management of the obstructed airway: an observational study. Br J Anaesth. 2017;118(3):444–51.
4. de Wolf MW, van der Beek T, Hamaekers AE, Theunissen M, Enk D. A prototype small-bore ventilation catheter with a cuff: cuff inflation optimizes ventilation with the Ventrain. Acta Anaesthesiol Scand. 2018;62(3):328–35.
5. Bailey JR, Lee C, Nouraei R, Chapman J, Edmond M, Girgis M, et al. Laryngectomy with a Tritube(®) and flow-controlled ventilation. Anaesth Rep. 2021;9(1):86–9.
6. Schmidt J, Günther F, Weber J, Kehm V, Pfeiffer J, Becker C, et al. Glottic visibility for laryngeal surgery: Tritube vs. microlaryngeal tube: a randomised controlled trial. Eur J Anaesthesiol. 2019;36(12):963–71.
7. Stephens M, Montgomery J, Urquhart CS. Management of elective laryngectomy. BJA Educ. 2017;17(9):306–11.
8. Shallik N, Elarref M, Khamash O, Abdelaal A, Radi Alkhafaji M, Makki H, et al. Management of critical tracheal stenosis with a straw sized tube (Tritube): case report. Qatar Med J. 2020;2020(3):48.
9. Moustafa AH, Shallik NA. Radiological evaluation of the airway: one-stop shop. In: Shallik NA, Moustafa AH, Marcus MAE, editors. Virtual endoscopy and 3D reconstruction in the airways. Cham: Springer; 2019. p. 15–29.
10. Mohammed H, Haidar H, Shallik N, Elhakeem A, Al-Abdulla M, Dogan Z. Virtual endoscopy and 3-D reconstruction/prototyping in head and neck surgeries. Cham: Springer; 2019. p. 85–100.
11. Current JD. Physics related to anesthesia. Mainz: PediaPress; 2010.

12. Filauro M, Mora F, Vallin A, Della Casa P, Arceri C, Gratarola A, et al. Evone(®) flow controlled ventilation: a new device for laryngotracheal surgery. Acta Otorhinolaryngol. 2022;42(2):189–93.
13. Weber J, Straka L, Borgmann S, Schmidt J, Wirth S, Schumann S. Flow-controlled ventilation (FCV) improves regional ventilation in obese patients – a randomized controlled crossover trial. BMC Anesthesiol. 2020;20(1):24.
14. Mallam L, Massingberd-Mundy D, Girgis M, De Zoysa N. Near total intrathoracic airway obstruction managed with a Tritube(®) and flow-controlled ventilation. Anaesth Rep. 2022;10(1):12156.
15. Morrison S, Aerts S, Saldien V. The ventrain device: a future role in difficult airway algorithms? A A Pract. 2019;13(9):362–5.
16. Magasich-Airola NP, Rosal Martins M, Desuter GR, Van Boven MJ. Novel technique for safe tracheostomy during COVID-19 pandemic using Evone® flow-controlled ventilation system. Int J Clin Pract. 2021;75(6):e13863.
17. Alhammad MF, Mathias R, Nahid S, Fernando R, Zaki HA, Haidar H, et al. Urinary guidewire and Tritube solved the mystery of severe tracheal stenosis management: a case report. Trends Anaesth Crit Care. 2023;50:101257.
18. Meulemans J, Jans A, Vermeulen K, Vandommele J, Delaere P, Van der Poorten V. Evone® flow-controlled ventilation during upper airway surgery: a clinical feasibility study and safety assessment. Front Surg. 2020;7:6.
19. Price TM, McCoy EP. Emergency front of neck access in airway management. BJA Educ. 2019;19(8):246–53.
20. Kristensen MS, de Wolf MW, Rasmussen LS. Ventilation via the 2.4 mm internal diameter Tritube® with cuff–new possibilities in airway management. Acta Anaesthesiol Scand. 2017;61(6):580–9.

Use of Tritube for Oropharyngeal and Laryngeal Surgery

Hanne Abildstrøm, Michael Seltz Kristensen, and Jeppe Thue Jensen

1 Introduction

The shared airway between the anaesthesiologist and the ear-nose-throat (ENT) surgeon imposes compromises for both parties. The oral tube being in the middle of the surgical field might create difficulties not allowing the optimal space for the surgical procedure. Therefore, this problem has traditionally been delt with in different ways.

For oral surgery, a small tube size 5.0 or 6.0 mm (outer diameter (OD) 8.8 mm) (Fig. 1), a micro laryngeal tube (MLT), still provides sufficient ventilation for most patients and allows a little extra space for the surgeon with the tube placed in the opposite side of the mouth. Another possibility is the use of a nasopharyngeal preformed tube presenting most of the oral cavity to the surgeon, but the tube still takes up space in the hypopharynx and the larynx.

Subglottic surgery can be performed with the patient in apnoea and intermittently intubated [1]. This approach requires a reasonable degree of apnoea tolerance. However, high frequency jet ventilation (HFJV) is often the choice for tracheal surgery and can also be used for supraglottic procedures, presenting the whole tracheal inlet area to the surgeon. This approach gives no protection of the airway against aspiration of gastric contents in patients at high risk, there is a risk of barotrauma and vibration of laryngeal structures is associated. There is also a risk of viral or bacterial aerosol spread from the patient, this being demonstrated especially with the COVID epidemy. The use of jet ventilation is not well tolerated by all patients and can cause desaturation and insufficient ventilation with a rise in CO_2.

H. Abildstrøm (✉) · M. S. Kristensen · J. T. Jensen
Department of Anaesthesia, Rigshospitalet, Section 6011, Copenhagen, Denmark
e-mail: hanne.harpoeth.abildstroem@regionh.dk; michael.seltz.kristensen@regionh.dk; jeppe.thue.jensen@regionh.dk

N. A. Shallik (ed.), *Flow Controlled Ventilation Mode Through a Straw Size Tube*, https://doi.org/10.1007/978-3-031-77477-5_10

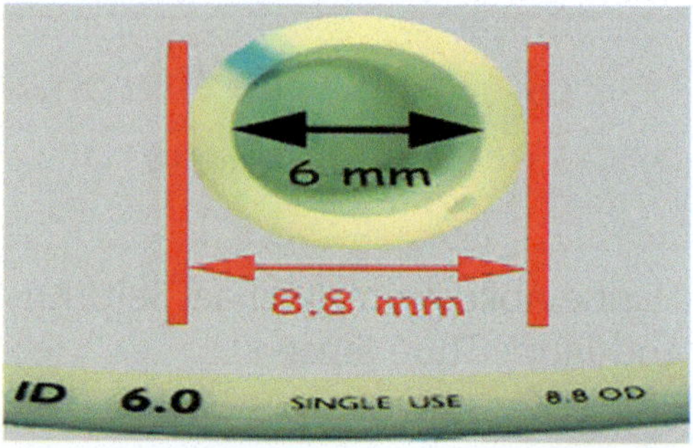

Fig. 1 The relation between inner and outer diameter of a normal sized tube 6.0

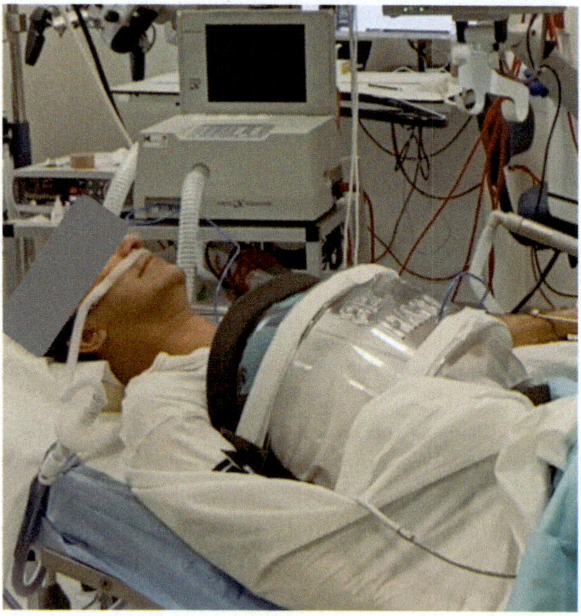

Fig. 2 The Cuirass® ventilator is a modern version of the Iron Lung. It consists of a shell with an airtight seal around the anterior chest and upper abdomen of the patient

Recently, the modern Cuirass® ventilation has been presented for the open airway surgery also with the risk of aspiration of gastric contents with an unsecured airway [2]. The cuirass ventilator consists of a shell with an airtight seal around the anterior chest and upper abdomen of the patient. With the application of negative pressure in the cuirass, the patient is ventilated by sucking air into the patient's lungs. For expiration, there is alternating positive pressure (Fig. 2).

For some major oropharyngeal surgical procedures, a tracheostomy can be performed beforehand in patients needing intensive care for a longer period. The use of a submental tube has been described especially for patients with maxillofacial trauma. In acute cases when there is no other opportunity to get access to the patient's airway Extra Corporal Membrane Oxygenation (ECMO) can be a rescue. This could be the case with a patient that already had a tracheostoma almost occluded by tumour masses or a major blood clot. However, for elective minor surgical procedures, the invasiveness and risk of complications does not justify these extensive methods.

A good choice in many patients presenting for oropharyngeal and laryngeal surgery could be the ultrathin straw sized Tritube®, a small extra-long standardized cuffed tube using flow-controlled ventilation (FVC) with the Evone® ventilator or the manually operated Ventrain®. This method gives sufficient and secure oxygenation and ventilation, and it provides superior surgical exposure for the ENT surgeon [3]. Cuff inflation protects the lower airway and produces a motionless operating field compared to HFJV. Furthermore, this approach provides several advantages or possibilities:

- the Tritube® can be used for the patient with a narrowed trachea
- the extra thin straw sized cuffed tube with FCV gives a better visual field and optimal working conditions for the (ENT) surgeon
- low frequency jet ventilation with an uncuffed tube is an option
- the uncuffed tube can be left in place in the awake patient and is well tolerated as an exchange catheter

2 Tritube® and FCV

The Tritube® has an internal diameter of 2.4 mm and an external diameter of 4.4 mm. The lumen is so small that passive expiration as provided by a standard ventilator is insufficient. The Tritube® requires a flow-controlled ventilation modus either with the manually operated device Ventrain® or via a specially designed ventilator Evone® with the use of both active inspiration and expiration. There is a great difference between the size of the tube and the diameter of the trachea in the adult patient with a normal sized trachea, accordingly the cuff is a high-volume-low-tension cuff. The Tritube® is so thin that it is not possible to breathe spontaneously with the cuff inflated, however spontaneous breathing is possible with the cuff deflated, and it is well tolerated by the patient in the emergence period and to some degree also in the postanaesthetic period [3, 4]. Accordingly, the Tritube® can serve as a tube exchange catheter in patients having or being at risk of developing a difficult airway the first important hours after surgery. This can be crucial in case of postoperative oedema and swelling. The Tritube® left in place can easily be reinflated after sufficient sedation and relaxation of the patient and ventilation with FCV can be applied or the Tritube® can be used as a railroading device for a normal sized tube for standard ventilation.

3 Patient Group, Patient Characteristics

The Tritube® can be used in patients with a weight above 40 kg (ideal body weight). The FCV is a gentle method to ventilate with a minimal amount of stress to the lung tissue with a higher degree of compliance than volume controlled ventilation (VCV) or pressure controlled ventilation (PCV) giving better oxygenation. The Tritube® is an excellent choice in patients known to have narrowing of the trachea caused by different aetiologies needing a sealed airway for non-tracheal surgery.

4 Advantages for the Surgeon

The Tritube® is taking up minimal space in the oro-pharyngeal-laryngeal cavity giving optimal access to the surgical field in the case of oral surgery (Fig. 3). This is a great advantage in many types of ENT procedures, such as biopsies from the oral cavity and tracheal inlet or final surgery for oropharyngeal cancer, tonsillectomy, adenectomy, tracheostomy, and pan endoscopy [3, 5]. Removal of cysts and papilloma in the larynx is also possible with the Tritube® giving excellent space for the surgeon. However, the Tritube® is not laser-resistant and other measures must be taken to minimize the risk of fire in the airway. Wet clothes covering the Tritube® and lowering the FiO_2 below 30% will give a safer procedure [6]. In most cases of maxillofacial surgery, it is necessary with occlusion of the teeth to give optimal surgical result. In case of oral intubation, there is often a little space behind the molars for the Tritube® or it can also be an option to intubate nasally with the ultrathin Tritube® if the space in the nasal cavity is too limited for a standardized nasopharyngeal preformed cuff.

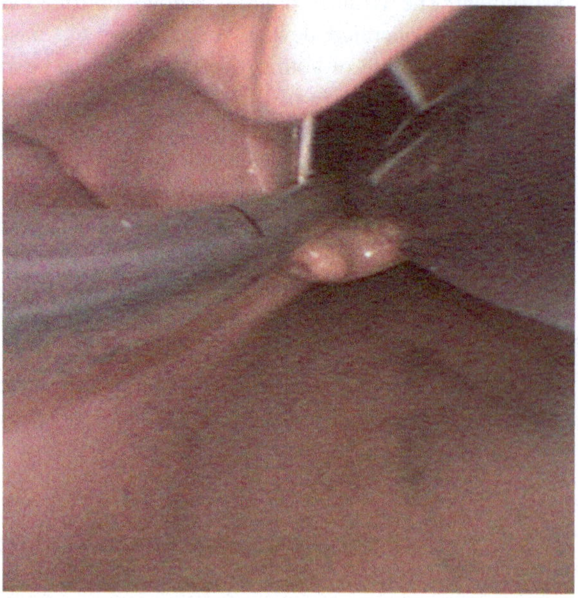

Fig. 3 Comparison of the space taken up in the oral cavity by the Tritube® to the left and a small standard tube size 6.0 to the right

5 Feasibility in Previous Studies

The use of the Tritube® and FCV has been described for ENT surgery. A study group conducted an observational study of 15 ENT patients investigating the potential use of FVC with the Evone® ventilator in this group of patients [4], the outcome measures were minute volume (MV), respiratory rate, intratidal tracheal pressure amplitude (A), and end-tidal CO_2 measured every 5 minutes and the registration of adverse events. FVC proved to give adequate CO_2 levels and MV and A within the normal range. The same study group investigated the use of the Tritube® for glottic surgery compared with a conventional MLT in a dataset of 40 patients [5]. The primary outcome measure was concealment of laryngeal structures evaluated by photos taken by video laryngoscope; better views were obtained with the use of the Tritube®. A secondary outcome was four categorical groups scored by the surgeons ranking surgical conditions, the more experienced surgeons rated the working space in the surgical field with the Tritube® equal to the use of a MLT, however, a subgroup of less experienced surgeons found that the Tritube® gave better working conditions. In this study, the FCV improved lung aeration and respiratory system compliance compared with the group with MLT and VCV.

In one study of seven patients, tracheal intubation was perceived easier with the Tritube® taking up a minimal amount of the visual field with the use of video laryngoscopy [3]. The surgeon rated the field of vision by laryngoscopy and the access to the surgical field excellent with the possibility to move the Tritube around. In patients with an anticipated difficult airway, the authors demonstrated the use of awake intubation in local anaesthesia with two different techniques, oral awake intubation with a video laryngoscope and nasal intubation with the use of a flexible optical scope and a guidewire introduced through the working channel used for railroading the Tritube® into position in the trachea (see video on https://www.airwaymanagement.dk/ressources/2-4mm-tritube). In this study, the Ventrain® device was used to ventilate the patients. The positioning of a guidewire in the trachea during emergence and recovery from anaesthesia can also facilitate fast re-intubation with the Tritube® in a patient with a narrow airway.

6 Step by Step Awake Nasal Flexible Optic Intubation Technique with the Tritube® (Figs. 4, 5, 6, 7, and 8)

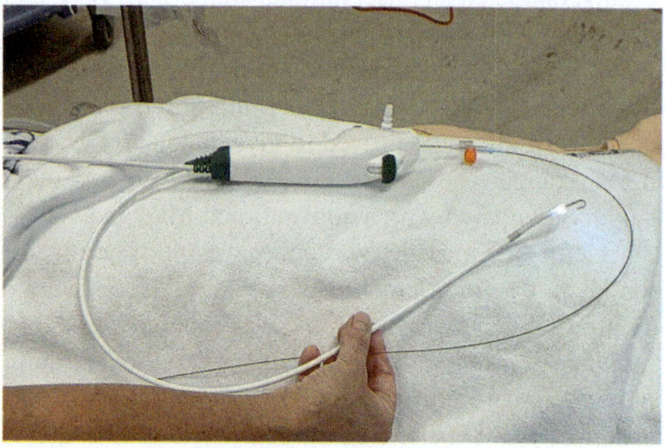

Fig. 4 Use of a long J-tipped guidewire through the working channel on the single use flexible scope

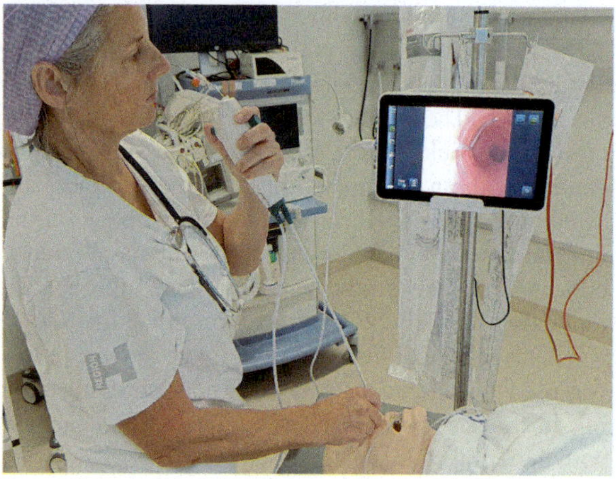

Fig. 5 Nasal flexible optic intubation after appliance of local anaesthesia in the awake patient with advancement of the guidewire into a main bronchus

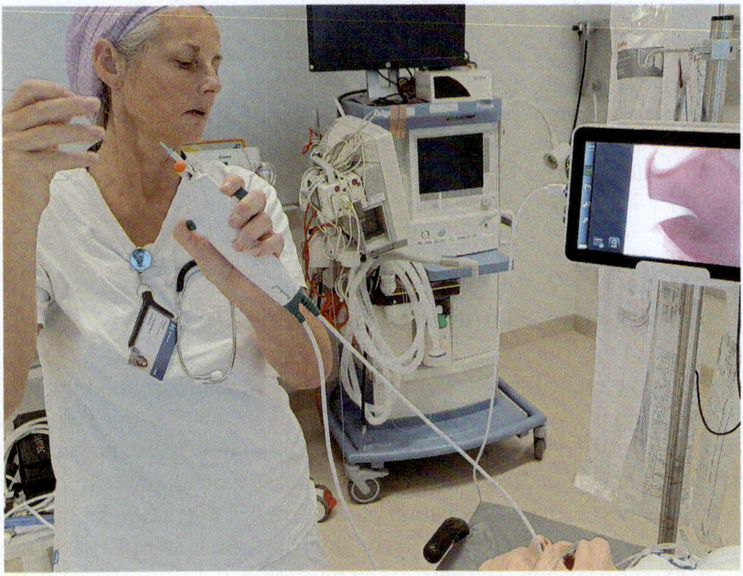

Fig. 6 Retraction of the flexible scope leaving the guidewire in place in the trachea

Fig. 7 The guide wire is used for railroading the Tritube® into the trachea

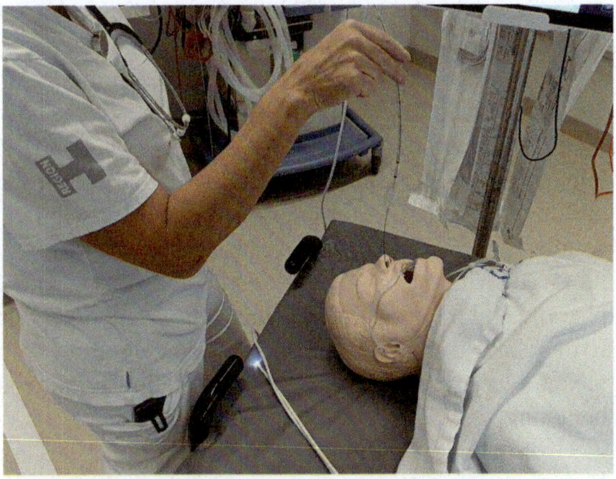

Fig. 8 The nasal uncuffed Tritube® is well tolerated in the awake patient before induction of anesthesia

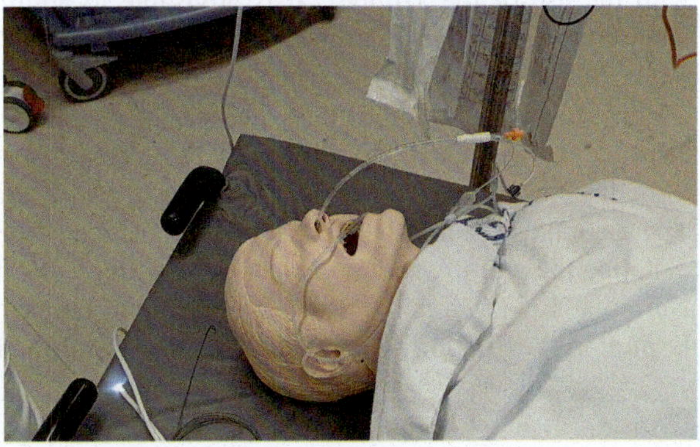

Table 1 Procedure when using FCV and the Tritube® and how to anticipate obstacles

• Thorough election of patients for Tritube® and FCV, avoid heavy secretions
• Give glycopyrrolate ideally 30 min before induction of anaesthesia
• Give muscle relaxants and secure the patient is fully relaxed (TOF = 0) until end of surgery
• Have 10 ml of saline ready to flush the Tritube® in case of obstruction
• Apply suction directly to the Tritube® **AFTER** deflating the cuff in case of obstruction
• Have a MLT ready for back up

7 Adverse Events and How to Handle Them

A typical adverse event is dislocation of the Tritube® and this could happen whatever type of tube is used. However, the risk of dislocation of the Tritube® due to coughing is considered higher, as there is a very high flow resistance in the narrow Tritube® with the cuff inflated [4]. Coughing causes a quick pressure release from the trachea easily causing a dislocation of the Tritube® due to the high rise in flow resistance. ENT surgery predisposes to coughing as there is stimulation of laryngeal reflexes in the surgical area. The patient can be reintubated after increasing the sedation and securing relaxation (Table 1).

It is imperative to have sufficient sedation with remifentanil and/or relaxation of the patient with the use of Tritube® as it is impossible for patients to breathe spontaneously with the cuff inflated. The airway resistance through the ultrathin tube is impossible to overcome in spontaneous respiration. Coping with the issue of getting the patient ready for extubation, there are several possibilities. The jet ventilation modus of the Evone® ventilator can be switched on after deflating the cuff, accordingly spontaneous respiration is a possibility with the Tritube® only taking up a minimum of space in the trachea. Another possibility is to deflate the cuff of the Tritube® after surgery is over and all instrumentation of the patient has been removed. With the patient still sedated, there is no/ little tonus of the muscles in the pharynx and the tongue can act as a tight seal of the airway enabling FCV with the Evone® with a deflated cuff, when the patient is awakening the muscles in the pharynx and larynx become tense creating a lumen in the airway allowing spontaneous breathing.

Obstruction of the tube with secretion is also a common adverse event [4, 6]. First, patients with severe secretions in bronchitis or pneumonia are not compatible with the use of the Tritube®. It is advisable to administer glycopyrrolate before induction of anaesthesia to overcome the problem of secretions beforehand (prophylaxis). In case of a sudden occlusion of the Tritube® despite efforts to avoid it, flushing the tube with saline 0.9% can solve the problem [4, 6]. Accordingly, always have a 10-ml syringe ready at hand. Endotracheal suction is not a possibility as even a small suction catheter cannot enter the narrow ventilation lumen of the Tritube®. The suction can be attached directly to the Tritube® trying to remove secretions after deflating the cuff to avoid severe atelectasis (for more details please see chapter "A Narrative Review on the Past, Present, and Future of Small-Bore Ventilation, Expiratory Ventilation Assistance, and Flow-Controlled Ventilation").

8 Conclusion

The use of the Tritube® and flow-controlled ventilation provides additional advantages in oropharyngeal and laryngeal surgery. This technique gives optimal conditions by offering extra space for the surgeon combined with a sealed airway technique. This technique allows a unique option to handle the airway of a patient with a narrow trachea at high risk of aspiration in a safe way. The use of the Tritube® and flow-controlled ventilation should be an option in major centres for Ear Nose and Throat Surgery.

References

1. Mangahas AM, et al. Anesthesia considerations during management of airway stenosis: a systematic review. Am J Otolaryngol. 2023;44(2):103767. https://doi.org/10.1016/j.amjoto.2022.103767. Epub 2022 Dec 23.
2. Kristensen MS, Hesselfeldt R, Schmidt JF. Modern Cuirass ventilation for airway surgery: unlimited access to the larynx and trachea in anaesthetised patients. Br J Anesth. 2023;131(4):e106–9.
3. Kristensen MS, de Wolf MWP, Rasmussen LS. Ventilation via the 2.4 mm internal diameter Tritube® with cuff – new possibilities in airway management. Acta Anaesthesiol Scand. 2017;61:580–9.
4. Schmidt J, et al. Flow-controlled ventilation during ear, nose and throat surgery: a prospective observational study. Eur J Anaesthesiol. 2019;36:327–34.
5. Schmidt J, et al. Glottic visibility for laryngeal surgery: Tritube vs. microlaryngeal tube. A randomised controlled trial. Eur J Anaesthesiol. 2019;36:963–9714.
6. Grassetto A, et al. A new perspective during laryngo-tracheal surgery: the use of an ultra-thin endotracheal tube (Tritube®) and flow-controlled ventilation—a retrospective case series and a review of the literature. J Anesth Analg Crit Care. 2022;2(1):39. https://doi.org/10.1186/s44158-022-00066-3. PMID: 37386531; PMCID: PMC9411832.

Use of Ultrathin Ventilation Tube in Tracheal Surgery

Jo Mourisse, Marieke Kuut, and Simone Timman

1 Anatomy of the Trachea and Surgical Considerations

The trachea (Fig. 1) is a conduit for air between the outside of the body and the parenchyma of the lungs, connecting the larynx superiorly and the main bronchi inferiorly. The beginning of the trachea is at the lower edge of the cricoid cartilage. The end is at the carina, usually found at the level of the T4 vertebral body. The length of the trachea is 11.8 cm on average with a normal range of 10–13 cm in males. It is comprised of 18–22 D shaped rings with anterior and lateral walls made of C-shaped cartilage and a posterior membranous wall [1]. The trachea tissue has a necessary elastic property and tracheal length vary with neck mobility and respiration. Together with surgical mobilization of the trachea in the laryngeal or hilar region, this elasticity allow resection up to 4 cm or even up to 6 cm in some carefully selected cases [2]. It is important that the result at the end of the operation is a tension-free anastomosis with adequate blood supply. The average external diameter of the trachea is 2.3 and 1.8 cm in the coronal and sagittal dimensions, respectively. The internal diameter of the trachea varies with alterations in intraluminal pressure occurring during respiration, ventilation, and Valsalva maneuvers. Coughing narrows the lumen by causing the trachealis muscle of the posterior wall to pull the cartilaginous C-arms together. With age or obstructive airway disease, the lateral diameter of the lumen narrows, while the anteroposterior diameter

J. Mourisse (✉) · M. Kuut
Department of Anesthesiology, Pain and Palliative Medicine, Radboud University Medical Centre, Nijmegen, The Netherlands
e-mail: jo.mourisse@radboudumc.nl; marieke.kuut@radboudumc.nl

S. Timman
Department of Cardio-thoracic Surgery, Radboud University Medical Centre, Nijmegen, The Netherlands
e-mail: simone.timman@radboudumc.nl

N. A. Shallik (ed.), *Flow Controlled Ventilation Mode Through a Straw Size Tube*, https://doi.org/10.1007/978-3-031-77477-5_11

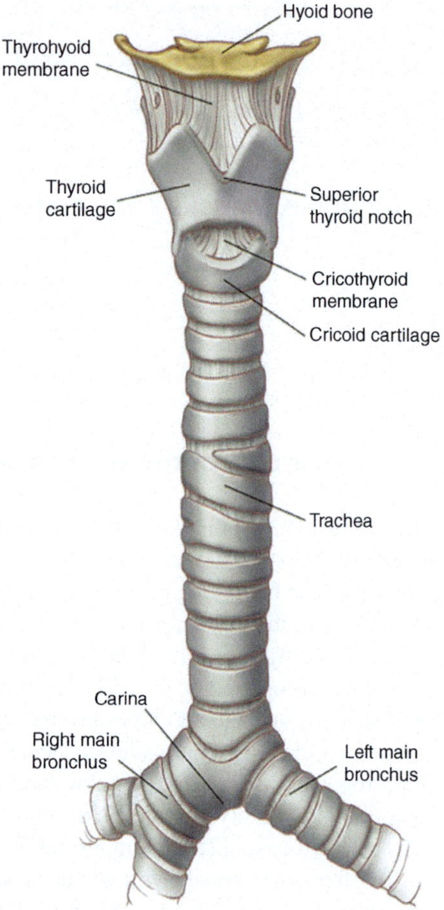

Fig. 1 Structure of the trachea. Anterior view [1]. Picture from Surgical anatomy of the trachea

increases, resulting in the "saber sheath" trachea. In chronic obstructive pulmonary disease ring softening results in AP narrowing of the lumen. This can cause luminal obstruction during expiration or coughing [1]. The cricoid diameter is about 5 mm smaller than the tracheal diameter [3] and after surgery near the cricoid there is more risk for postoperative obstruction due to swelling.

The right and left recurrent laryngeal nerves, branches of the vagus nerves, innervate the true vocal cords. The left recurrent laryngeal nerve arises distal to the aortic arch near the ligamentum arteriosum, at which point it recurs and ascends toward the cricoid cartilage. The right recurrent laryngeal nerve branches off the right vagus nerve just distal to the right subclavian artery. The left recurrent nerve is more susceptible to injury to mobilization of carina and lower trachea. Injury to the recurrent laryngeal nerves can cause vocal cord paresis or paralysis resulting in hoarseness or complete loss of voice or even airway obstruction depending on the extent of injury and the integrity of the contralateral nerve [1].

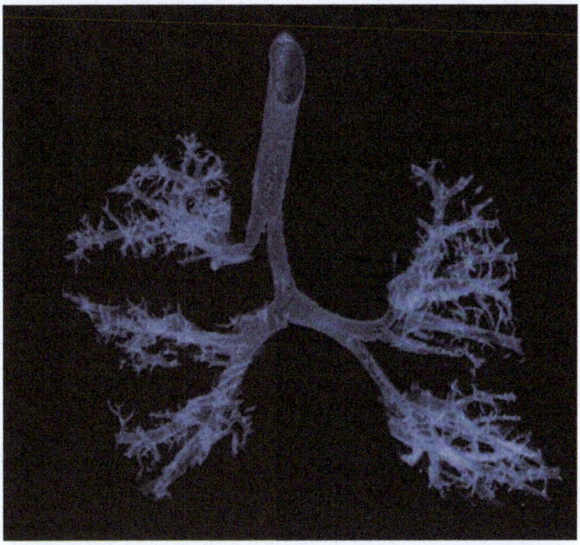

Fig. 2 3D image of a tracheal bronchus arising at the mid-tracheal level. The distal part of the trachea, from the debranching of tracheal bronchus to the main carina, is narrowed. See also Table 1, case 1

The blood supply of trachea consists of interconnected vessels along the lateral tracheal walls and vascularize the trachea in a segmental fashion. These vessels arise from bronchial, intercostal, inferior thyroid, innominate, subclavian, and carotid arteries. Surgical dissection of the trachea should not extend beyond the resected segment because of the risk of ischemia and necrosis [1].

At carinal level, the trachea divides in the left and right main bronchus. The right main bronchus is more vertical, and its length varies from 1.2 to 1.5 cm from the carina to the upper lobe take-off. The diameter is 17.7 [2] and 14 [2] mm (SD) in male and females, respectively. Distal to the upper lobe take-off, it continues as the bronchus intermedius and finally divides into the middle and lower lobe bronchi. The left main bronchus arises at a more oblique angle from the carina and is 1 mm narrower and longer (4–6 cm) than the right main bronchus [3]. It passes under the aortic arch posteriorly to the left hilum and divides into the upper and lower lobe bronchi. Close proximity of the aorta to the airway limits mobilization of the left main bronchus compared with the right side during carinal surgery.

A congenital anomaly in 0.1–3% of the population is a tracheal bronchus that supplies the right upper lobe. In most cases, the tracheal bronchus arises at the level of the carina (trifurcation) and the most severe case the tracheal bronchus arises at mid tracheal level. See Fig. 2. Wheeze or stridor are typical symptoms [4]. Presence of this anomaly is important because of obstruction by an endotracheal tube or problems with one-lung ventilation.

2 Causes of Tracheal Stenosis

Tracheal stenosis can be classified between acquired and congenital tracheal stenosis. Acquired tracheal stenosis can be caused by malignant or benign disease. Primary tracheal tumors are rare. Data from the Netherlands Cancer Registry showed an annual incidence of 0.142 per 100,000 inhabitants [5]. Most were classified as squamous cell carcinoma and adenoid cystic carcinoma. Malignancies are more often located in the mid and distal part of the trachea. Surgical treatment can lead to a significantly better survival, compared to radiotherapy [5]. Metastatic or locally invasive lesions involving the trachea can originate from thyroid, larynx, lung, esophagus, breast or organs. Benign tracheal tumors are also rare and include neurofibroma, chondroma, hemangioma, hamartoma, neurogenic tumors, granular cell tumors, and squamous cell papillomas [6].

Most common reason for partial tracheal resection is iatrogenic postintubation (PITS) or posttracheostomy tracheal stenosis (PTTS) [7]. The initial injury of the tracheal mucosa from the endotracheal tube or tracheotomy cannula is followed by a chronic inflammation with granuloma formation and subsequent stricture formation. Coronavirus Disease 2019 (COVID-19) has been reported to be strictly related to tracheal stenosis. Indeed, longer times of invasive ventilation often with the use of tracheostomy, combined with prone position in patients frequently with obesity, as well as higher rates of iatrogenic intubation injuries, have resulted in significant rise in rate of tracheal stenosis in patients with severe COVID-19 [8, 9].

Acquired tracheal lesion may occur as a result of acute airway injury, inhalation injury or surgical trauma such after lung transplantation, or sleeve resection surgery. Other causes of benign stenosis are autoimmune disease, radiotherapy or classified as idiopathic.

Congenital tracheal stenosis is relatively rare and includes conditions such as vascular rings, tracheal webs, tracheogenic cysts, tracheomalacia, subglottic, and tracheal stenosis.

External tracheal compression can arise from excessive growth of almost every organ nearby the trachea, like thyroid, thymus, lymphoma or aortic aneurysm.

Multiple specialties (e.g., laryngologists, thoracic surgeons, and interventional bronchoscopists) are involved in the management of tracheal stenosis and have resulted in the development of several classification systems with different criteria, the most recently published are Freitag, Ghorbani, and Nouraei [10–12]. Surgery is preferred treatment option for some types of benign stenosis (e.g., in cause of destruction of the cartilage) or after failure after (multiple) mechanical dilatations or laser therapy [13].

3 Airway Management for Tracheal Surgery

The goal of airway management during surgery to the airway is twofold. The anesthesiologists' goal is to have a secured and protected airway with optimal ventilation during surgery. The second goal is to provide the surgeon optimal access with unobstructed view. In these “shared airway” situations close communication between anesthesiologist and surgeon is of utmost importance.

Surgery for tracheal stenosis can be divided into three different phases. The first phase is induction of anesthesia and surgical preparation of the trachea (dissection phase). This phase is followed by incision of the airway, resection of the stenotic part, and anastomosis of the airway (resection phase). The last phase is primary wound closure of the surgical field (closure phase). Different techniques for airway management and ventilation can be used in every phase.

In tracheal and other airway surgery, a number of airway management techniques are being used. All have advantages and disadvantages during the different stages of surgery [14]. In the dissection phase, passing the stenotic airway with a regular or micro laryngeal (MLT) tube can be difficult. Ventilation with a laryngeal mask had also been described in the dissection phase [6]. During the resection phase, a regular of microlaryngeal tube will obstruct access to the posterior tracheal wall. Therefore, cross field intubation (CFI) is the most common used technique during resection of the stenotic part of the airway. During CFI, a controlled exchange of airway devices is required. The surgeon introduces a sterile endotracheal tube in the distal part of the airway. A catheter for high frequency jet ventilation can also be used.

The most recent innovation in upper airway surgery is the use of a very thin cuffed endotracheal tube called Tritube®. It is a polyurethane endotracheal tube with three lumens: a main ventilation lumen, a cuff lumen, and a pressure measurement lumen. It comes in one size, length 44 cm, outer diameter of 4.4 mm (Fig. 3). Because of the small diameter compared to a MLT 5 (internal diameter 5 mm, outer diameter 6.9 mm), it has proven to provide better visibility in laryngeal surgery [15] and it has been used to intubate and ventilate patients with critical airway stenosis [16]. Tritube cannot be used with a conventional anesthesia ventilator but the Evone® ventilator has to be used. It provides flow-controlled ventilation (FCV), by applying constant positive flow during inspiration

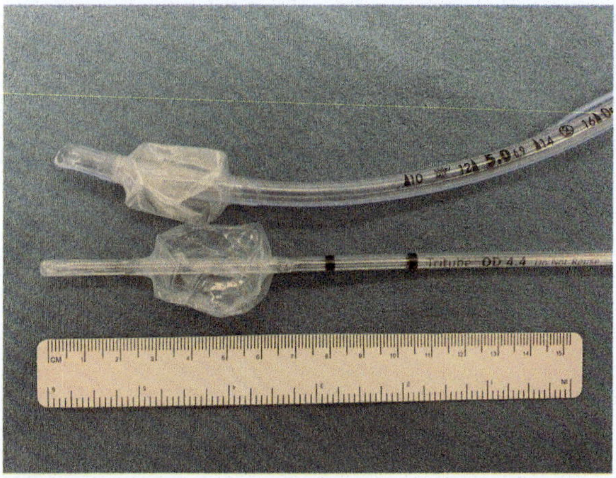

Fig. 3 Distal end of micro larynx tube (MLT) and Tritube®. MLT has an inner diameter (ID) 5.0 mm and an outer diameter (OD) of 6.9 mm. Tritube® has an ID of 2.4 mm and OD of 4.4 mm

and constant negative flow during expiration while measuring tracheal pressure. A comprehensive explanation of FCV can be found in chapter "Conventional Mechanical Ventilation: II—Nomenclature and Basic Modes" of this book. Because of the small outer diameter (4.4 mm), Tritube® can be used in all phases of segmental tracheal resection. An observational study has been published by Kuut [17].

4 Tracheal Intubation Using Tritube®, General Considerations

Before proceeding to surgery, a standard preoperative airway assessment should be performed. Tritube® can be placed after induction of general anesthesia with neuromuscular blocking. Since patients with tracheal stenosis usually suffer from dyspnea and have a reduced functional residual capacity it is important to have a prolonged period of pre oxygenation in upright position using non-invasive positive pressure ventilation if applicable. Tritube® can be placed oral or nasal using a laryngoscope or a videolaryngoscope. For oral intubation the Tritube® can be reinforced with a malleable stylet. Alternatively urinary guidewires which placed through bronchoscope working channel [18, 19] or with the aid of the internal wire of an Arndt blocker® put into the Tritube®, can be used to guide the Tritube® in to the desired place. Nasal intubation can provide more stable fixation. In our first case where the Tritube® was fixed on the upper lip, the tube bended intra-orally and the cuff tended to move upwards into the surgical field. Nasal intubation with Tritube should be performed without malleable stylet. For optimal placement in relation to the stenotic segment, a flexible bronchoscope should be present. After passing the stenosis and cuff inflation, FCV can be started. When excretions are present distal to the stenosis bronchoscopic suctioning can be useful before the start of ventilation. To make repeated flexible bronchoscopy easier, an adjacent nasal or oropharyngeal airway can be placed. The oropharyngeal airway also contributes to a stable fixation of the Tritube®.

In more distal tracheal pathology, Tritube® can be positioned via a regular endotracheal tube that is positioned with the tip above the stenotic airway segment. A schematic presentation of the different levels of the stenosis and the surgical approach is shown in Fig. 4. Also shown is the final position of Tritube® and the eventual position of an endotracheal tube for each situation.

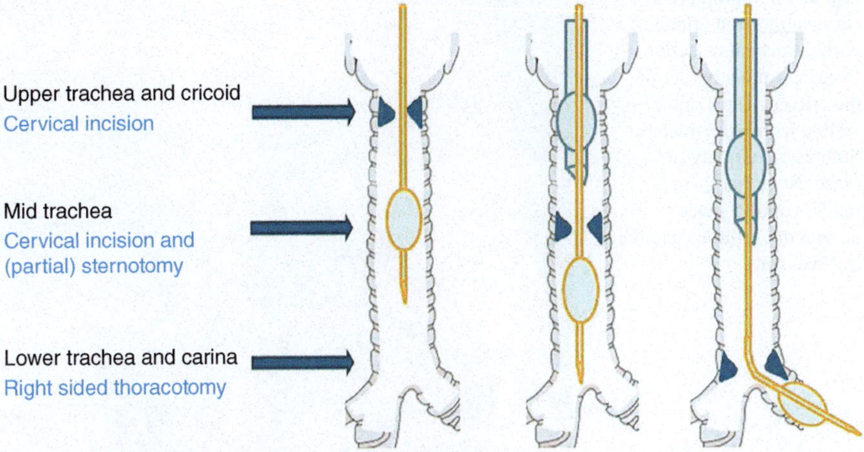

Fig. 4 Schematic representation of tracheal stenosis in proximal, mid, and distal trachea. Indicated on the left side is the surgical approach. The Tritube® is colored in yellow and the endotracheal tube is colored blue

5 Upper and Mid Tracheal Stenosis

Benign stenotic disease of the trachea requiring resection is usually located within the first 3 cm of the trachea. Cricotracheal resection or segmental tracheal resection is performed using a cervical "collar" incision. An observational study [17] showed that Tritube® can be successfully used in most cases of upper and mid tracheal stenosis with good surgical exposure with Tritube® in situ, reducing the need for CFI. After induction of anesthesia, Tritube® can be placed distal to the stenotic airway segment and FCV can be used throughout the dissection, resection and closure phase of surgery. Before incision in the trachea the cuff can be emptied for a very short period, to prevent cuff puncture. If the cuff is emptied or accidentally punctured, Evone® will change automatically to jet modus. Figure 5 shows the surgical exposure after cervical incision and removal of part of cricoid and two tracheal rings. After the anastomosis of the airway is performed flexible bronchoscopy can be performed to check for swelling of the larynx and for the appearance of the (crico-)tracheal anastomosis. In a case of swelling or vocal cord dysfunction, Tritube® can be left in place with the cuff deflated while awakening and with spontaneous ventilation, to evaluate airway patency (Fig. 6).

Surgery for mid tracheal stenosis is performed using a collar incision, partial sternotomy or complete sternotomy. When classifying tracheal stenosis, the distance between the glottis and the stenotic segment is often reported. To evaluate if

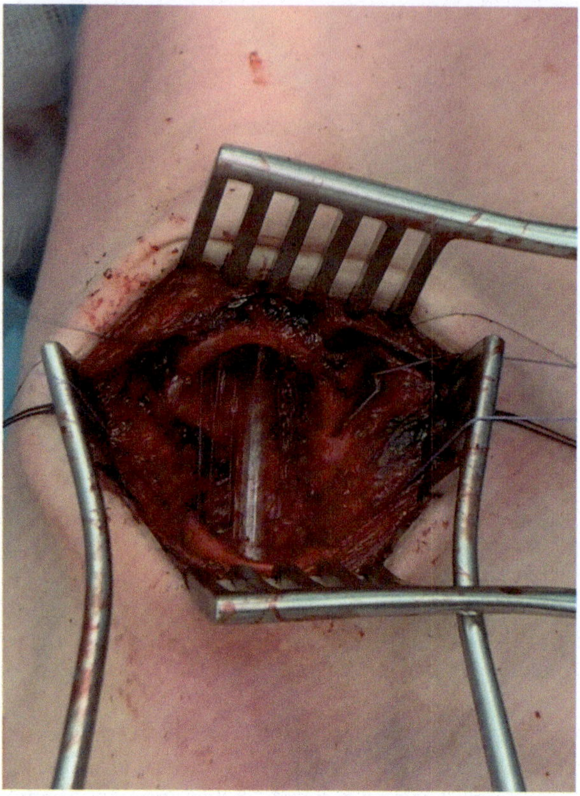

Fig. 5 Photograph of a cervical incision after a partial tracheal resection of two rings and a border of the cricoid. The Tritube® is visible within the trachea. Sutures are already in place. Note that there is much working space around the Tritube® and the tracheal wall

the use of Tritube® is feasible for segmental tracheal resection in mid-tracheal stenosis, it is important to also estimate the distance from stenosis to carina. A preoperative CT scan, 3D reconstruction, and virtual endoscopy (VE) are usually valuable (Fig. 7). The distance from stenosis to carina should be measured. The cuff and tip of Tritube® are about 65 mm long (Fig. 3). So, the distance from stenosis to carina should be at least 65 mm.

In the observational study [17] tube obstruction that needed flushing with air or saline was the most common event during tracheal surgery using Tritube®.

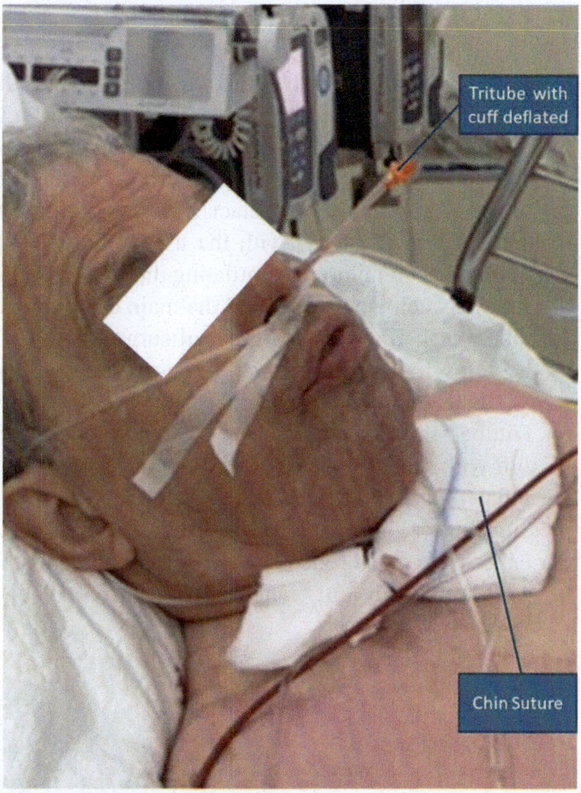

Fig. 6 Nasally placed Tritube® left in situ in a spontaneous ventilating and awaken patient after upper segmental cricoid-tracheal resection. The cuff is deflated. The Tritube will be removed if there is a unobstructed airway

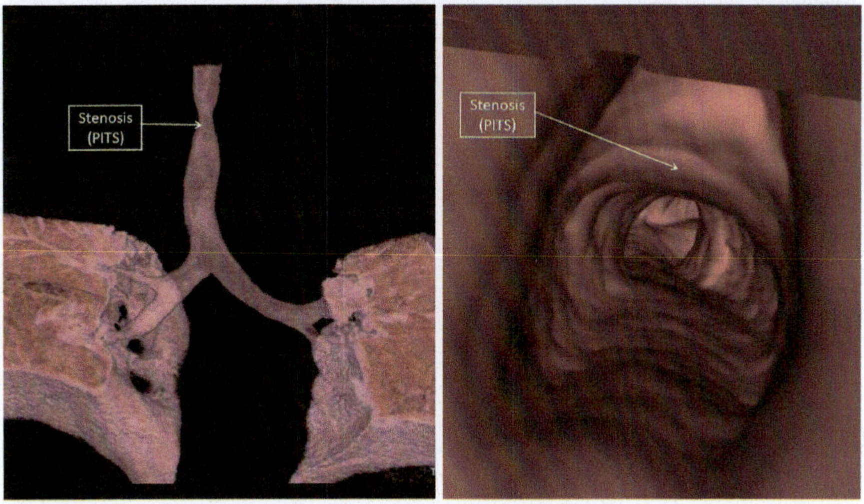

Fig. 7 Still images of 3D (left panel) and virtual endoscopy (right panel) movies of a patient planned for segmental tracheal resection because of post intubation tracheal stenosis (PITS). The relatively mild tracheal stenosis is marked

6 Distal Tracheal Stenosis

Positioning Tritube® behind a stenosis or tumor in the distal trachea can be problematic, because the considerable length of the cuff (35 mm) and the distal end (30 mm). The presence of the cuff impedes resection of the trachea. Also, the Tritube's apertures for the ventilation and pressure measurement channel are at risk for obstruction because of contact with the main carina or bronchial wall. In our published case series [17] with the use of Tritube® for tracheal resections, there were two cases of failure of ventilating through the Tritube® because of shortness of distance between the process and the main carina, which resulted in obstruction of the tube. Furthermore, distal tracheal surgery is often performed by a right sided thoracotomy and therefore one-lung-ventilation (OLV) is required. In our case series, the length of the left main bronchus varied from 4 to 4.5 cm, that is too short for Tritube's tip and cuff. To solve these problems, we reduced the proximal half of the cuff with some surgical knots or taped with Tegaderm® (Fig. 8). The diameter of the inflated cuff is still large enough to fit the left main bronchus. Although low pressure-low volume characteristics of the Tritube® are altered, we believe that with our experience with bronchial blockers, for example the EZ-blocker, we can safely use this modified cuff. The cuff of a bronchial blocker is inflated under

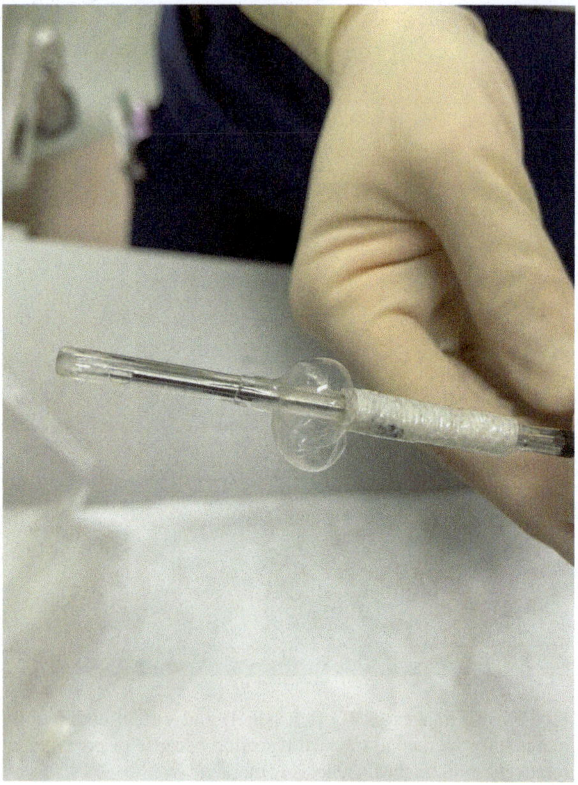

Fig. 8 Example of a modified Tritube®. The proximal end of the cuff is taped with Tegaderm® strips. In this case, the tip was not shorten. Total length of tip and reduced cuff fits the left main bronchus

bronchoscopic view to prevent overinflation. This modified Tritube® is also inflated under bronchoscopic view. In only a few cases, the distal end is shortened to 10 mm, but after cutting the tip of the Tritube®, the lumen for inflation of the cuff is also opened and has to be sealed with glue.

In Table 1, we present ten cases where a modified Tritube® was placed in the left main bronchus. All patients gave informed consent for using a modified Tritube®. One had a congenital tracheal bronchus with distal tracheal stenosis. Nine patients were diagnosed with an acquired tracheal stenosis; 5 of them had a primary malignancy of the trachea (all different tumors) who underwent prior debulking, one had tracheal compression of a surrounding tumor, one had a recurrent fistula after removal of a bronchogenic cyst, one had a benign tumor, and one patient suffered from a saber sheath tracheal stenosis.

In seven cases, surgical access was obtained by right-sided thoracotomy requiring OLV of the left lung (Fig. 9). The other cases were performed via cervical incision and partial or complete sternotomy. Although OLV is then not necessary, we had to put the modified Tritube® in the left main bronchus because lack of space between the stenosis and the main carina.

The modified Tritube® was inserted through an ET tube ID 9 mm in seven cases. The large size was chosen to fit both the Tritube® (OD 4.4 mm) and the bronchoscope (OD 3.5 mm). The ET tube should be placed with the tip above the level of the proximal incision of the airway. After correct placement, the length of the ET tube should be reduced to 25 cm to obtain enough length for Tritube® to reach the left main bronchus. Placement of the endotracheal tube and Tritube® should always be performed using bronchoscopy. The ET provides an easy access for bronchoscopy during the procedure. In three cases, the modified Tritube® was inserted direct orally or nasally.

Mostly, placement of the tip of the Tritube® under bronchoscopic view in to the left main bronchus is easy. If placement is difficult, the aid of the internal wire of an Arnd blocker can be used. This wire can be pulled through the internal lumen of Tritube® and attached to the tip of the bronchoscope and thus guide Tritube® toward the left main bronchus. The External Tracheal Manipulation Maneuver as described by Heir et al. [20] can also help bronchial placement of Tritube®.

In patients who underwent a right thoracotomy, there was good collapse of the right lung and excellent exposure of the surgical field. OLV with FCV provided adequate oxygenation and ventilation with low pressure peak levels. The anastomosis was made with the Tritube® in situ as shown in Fig. 9 (Case 5). There was no need for CFI, which has a drawback of large tubing in the surgical field. In an open airway, Tritube® and Evone® can be used in a jet ventilation mode, comparable to other jet ventilation technique. An important drawback of jet ventilation is the spread of aerosols and an unquiet surgical field. Table 2 gives an overview of quality of surgical exposure and disadvantages of five techniques of airway management for complex segmental tracheal and carinal resections

In these complex distal tracheal surgery cases during the resection phase, the surgical team should always have a back-up plan for airway management present and ready for use. This can be jet ventilation, CFI or ECMO. In case 1, the team

Table 1 First consecutive ten patients who required an adaptation off the Tritube® to make surgery to the distal and or carinal level possible. The reason for surgery (column 2), the type, surgical approach and duration of surgery (column 3), and airway approach (column 4) are given

	Age, sex, weight, length	Reason for surgery	Type, access, and duration surgery	Airway
1	49 years, male, 109 kg, 187 cm	Congenital tracheal bronchus and stenose distal trachea	Sliding tracheoplasty, right thoracotomy, 272 min	ET 9 + modified tritube (reduced cuff and tip) in left bronchus ECMO standby
2	19 years, female, 59 kg, 170 cm	Myofibroelastic tumor 3 cm above carina	Partial tracheal resection (4 rings), right thoracotomy, 221 min	ET 9 + modified tritube (reduced cuff and tip) in left bronchus
3	63 years, male, 76 kg, 175 cm	Adenocarcinoma 4.5 cm above carina	Partial tracheal resection (6 rings), cervical incision and partial sternotomy, 310 min	Modified tritube (reduced cuff and tip) in left bronchus, nasal
4	68 years, male, 76 kg, 177 cm	Adenoid cystic carcinoma 2 cm above carina	Partial tracheal resection (7 rings), sternotomy, 283 min	ET 9 + modified Tritube (reduced cuff) in left bronchus
5	61 years, female, 60 kg, 168 cm	Hamartoma 3 cm above carina	Partial tracheal resection (3 rings), right thoracotomy, 183 min	ET 9 + modified tritube (reduced cuff) in left bronchus
6	72 years, female, 80 kg, 181 cm	Epithelial-myoepithelial carcinoma 2 cm above carina	Carinal resection with end to end anastomosis of right bronchus and end tot side anastomosis of the left bronchus, right thoracotomy, 202 min	ET 9 + modified tritube (reduced cuff) in left bronchus ECMO used for apneic period
7	94 years, male, 95 kg, 176 cm	Saber sheath tracheal stenosis 3 cm above carina	Partial tracheal resection (6 rings), right thoracotomy, 156 min	Modified tritube (reduced cuff) in left bronchus, oral
8	46 years, male, 105 kg, 183 cm	Recurrent fistula at carina after bronchogenic cyst right main bronchus	Sleeve resection of the right main bronchus with end to end anastomosis on the carina via right thoracotomy, 510 min	ET 9 + modified tritube (reduced cuff) in left bronchus
9	35 years, male, 83 kg, 190 cm	Non seminoma germ cell carcinoma with tracheal compression suspected for growth in tracheal wall, 5 cm above carina	Distal tracheal resection, cervical incision and sternotomy, 397 min	Modified tritube (reduced cuff) in left bronchus, oral
10	62 years, female, 76 kg, 164 cm	Carcinoid right main bronchus and main carina	Right upper lobe and sleeve resection with carina resection, right thoracotomy, 275 min	ET 9 + modified tritube (reduced cuff) in left bronchus

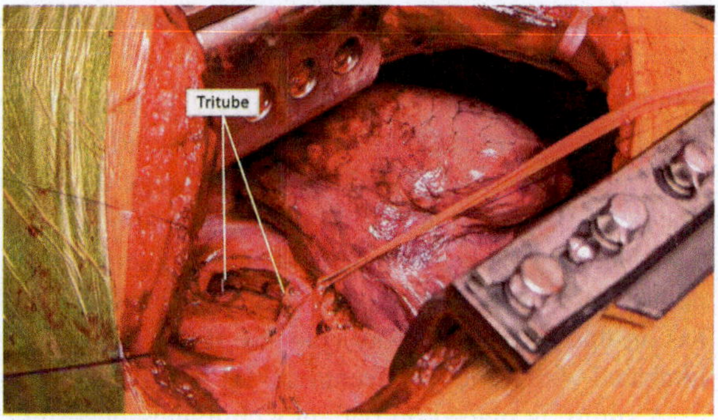

Fig. 9 Photograph of a thoracotomy after removal of three tracheal rings of the distal trachea. The right lung is collapsed. The Tritube® is visible in the trachea and the tip is positioned in the left main bronchus

Table 2 Overview of quality of surgical exposure and disadvantages of five techniques of airway management for complex partial tracheal and carinal resections

Technique	Surgical exposure	Disadvantage
Cross field intubation	Poor	Anesthesia challenging
Jet ventilation	Good	Barotrauma Hypoxia, hypercarbia Aspiration Aerosols (COVID-19) Unquiet surgical field
Tritube	Good	Possible obstruction internal lumen
Spontaneous ventilation	Ideal	Coughing, movement Aspiration
ECMO/CPB	Ideal	Vascular injury Coagulopathy Hemodilution

decided to place the superior cava ECMO cannula in advance, and ready for use when necessary, but it was not needed in the end. In case 6, ECMO was combined with OLV using a modified Tritube®, because an end to side anastomosis for the left main bronchus was made more proximal in the trachea.

Communication and planning are very important during these procedures. Surgical manipulation of the distal airway can cause obstruction alarms or pressure loss in Evone. These alarms have to be solved in close cooperation with the surgical team.

At the end of surgery, final inspection of the sutures by flexible bronchoscopy is easily performed with Tritube® in situ. All patients were extubated in the operating room. There were few complications postoperative. There was an atelectasis (case 3), a period of atrial flutter (case 4), a pneumothorax and dysphagia (case 7). Patients went home on day 6–9 (median 8) except one patient stayed 15 days. Unfortunately, one patient died of massive lung bleeding 1 month after surgery.

We were aware of safety issues around the modification of the Tritube®. We believe that through careful manipulation and meticulous inspection with the bronchoscope we prevented problems.

7 Recovery and Postoperative Management

Extubation immediately postoperatively is the primary goal after partial tracheal resections. Before extubation the glottis, cricoid and anastomoses should be inspected with a bronchoscope or (video-) laryngoscope for edema, bleeding, and dehiscence. The vocal cords should be inspected for dysfunction. If these situations are present, the patient should be left intubated until problems are solved. The Tritube® can be left in the trachea with deflated cuff in an awake patient until it is obvious that the patient has an unobstructed airway (Fig. 6). If the problem persists, the patient should be intubated with a small conventional ETT with the cuff not overlying the anastomosis.

A suture is placed on patient's chin and chest to prevent neck extension and to prevent tension on the fresh anastomosis. Maintaining a free airway in this flexed position of the neck can be challenging directly postoperatively. It is imperative that patient should emerge from anesthesia in a calm, cooperative without vomiting or coughing. Because of swallowing dysfunction, patients will be feeded via nasogastric tube for the first 5 days. Antibiotics will also continue for 5 days.

Postoperative analgesia should be tailored to the surgical approach. For a cervical incision or partial sternotomy systemic multimodal analgesia is sufficient, while for a thoracotomy a thoracic epidural or other neuraxial blockade are recommended. Neuraxial blockades must be placed in accordance with anti-coagulation guidelines.

8 Future Plan

We encourage industry to develop a specifically designed bronchial blocker to ventilate through using FCV, which can be used for distal tracheal surgery and one (left) lung ventilation.

In summary, Tritube® used in combination with the Evone's Flow-controlled ventilation is a novel option for airway management in segmental tracheal resections. It allows an easier intubation and passing of a stenosis, bronchoscopy is possible alongside the Tritube®, and in the meantime providing excellent ventilation. The surgeon can work around the tube without the need for CFI and with less spread of aerosols like in jet ventilation. The use of Tritube® for upper and mid-tracheal surgery has become our primary airway device. Tritube® is not suitable for distal tracheal surgery or it has to be adapted to fit left main bronchus.

References

1. Furlow PW, Mathisen DJ. Surgical anatomy of the trachea. Ann Cardiothorac Surg. 2018;7(2):255–60.
2. Blasberg JD, Wright CD. Surgical considerations in tracheal and carinal resection. Semin Cardiothorac Vasc Anesth. 2012;16(4):190–5.
3. Seymour AH. The relationship between the diameters of the adult cricoid ring and main tracheobronchial tree: a cadaver study to investigate the basis for double-lumen tube selection. J Cardiothorac Vasc Anesth. 2003;17(3):299–301.

4. Conacher ID. Implications of a tracheal bronchus for adult anaesthetic practice. Br J Anaesth. 2000;85(2):317–20.
5. Honings J, van Dijck JA, Verhagen AF, van der Heijden HF, Marres HA. Incidence and treatment of tracheal cancer: a nationwide study in the Netherlands. Ann Surg Oncol. 2007;14(2):968–76.
6. Smeltz AM, Bhatia M, Arora H, Long J, Kumar PA. Anesthesia for resection and reconstruction of the trachea and carina. J Cardiothorac Vasc Anesth. 2020;34(7):1902–13.
7. Gelbard A, Francis DO, Sandulache VC, Simmons JC, Donovan DT, Ongkasuwan J. Causes and consequences of adult laryngotracheal stenosis. Laryngoscope. 2015;125(5):1137–43.
8. Mattioli F, Marchioni A, Andreani A, Cappiello G, Fermi M, Presutti L. Post-intubation tracheal stenosis in COVID-19 patients. Eur Arch Otorrinolaringol. 2021;278(3):847–8.
9. Piazza C, Filauro M, Dikkers FG, Nouraei SAR, Sandu K, Sittel C, et al. Long-term intubation and high rate of tracheostomy in COVID-19 patients might determine an unprecedented increase of airway stenoses: a call to action from the European Laryngological Society. Eur Arch Otorrinolaringol. 2020;278(1):1–7.
10. Freitag L, Ernst A, Unger M, Kovitz K, Marquette CH. A proposed classification system of central airway stenosis. Eur Respir J. 2007;30(1):7–12.
11. Ghorbani A, Dezfouli AA, Shadmehr MB, Pejhan S, Saghebi SR, Ghare-Daghi AS, et al. A proposed grading system for post-intubation tracheal stenosis. Tanaffos. 2012;11(3):10–4.
12. Nouraei SA, Nouraei SM, Upile T, Howard DJ, Sandhu GS. A proposed system for documenting the functional outcome of adult laryngotracheal stenosis. Clin Otolaryngol. 2007;32(5):407–9.
13. Murgu SD, Egressy K, Laxmanan B, Doblare G, Ortiz-Comino R, Hogarth DK. Central airway obstruction: benign strictures, tracheobronchomalacia, and malignancy-related obstruction. Chest. 2016;150(2):426–41.
14. Schieren M, Bohmer A, Dusse F, Koryllos A, Wappler F, Defosse J. New approaches to airway management in tracheal resections-a systematic review and meta-analysis. J Cardiothorac Vasc Anesth. 2017;31(4):1351–8.
15. Schmidt J, Gunther F, Weber J, Kehm V, Pfeiffer J, Becker C, et al. Glottic visibility for laryngeal surgery: tritube vs. microlaryngeal tube: a randomised controlled trial. Eur J Anaesthesiol. 2019;36(12):963–71.
16. Shallik N, Elarref M, Khamash O, Abdelaal A, Radi Alkhafaji M, Makki H, et al. Management of critical tracheal stenosis with a straw sized tube (tritube): case report. Qatar Med J. 2020;2020(3):48.
17. Kuut MH, Honings J, Marres HAM, Mourisse JMJ, Verhagen A. Controlled mechanical ventilation through a narrow bore lumen during tracheal surgery: a prospective observational study. Eur J Anaesthesiol. 2022;39(10):835–7.
18. Meierhans R, Gelpke H, Hetzel J, Madjdpour C. Bronchoscope-assisted Tritube(R) placement for resection of sequential tracheal stenosis. Anaesth Rep. 2022;10(2):e12195.
19. Alhammad MF, Mathias R, Nahid S, Fernando R, Zaki HA, Haidar H, et al. Urinary guidewire and tritube solved the mystery of severe tracheal stenosis management: a case report. Trends Anaesth Crit. 2023;50:101257.
20. Heir JS, Sekhon AK, Thakar DR, Jackson TA, Lasala JD, Purugganan RV. External tracheal manipulation maneuver (ETMM) to facilitate endobronchial blocker placement. J Cardiothorac Vasc Anesth. 2016;30(4):1061–3.

Ventilation Through Small Bore Catheter in Paediatrics

Brahim Boudjenah, Al Moataz Billah Adham, Surendra M. Chinnappa, Rajeev Belludi Babu, Mashael Al-Khelaifi, and Nabil A. Shallik

1 Introduction

Ventilation through smallcalibre tubes poses formidable challenges to the anaesthesiologist, especially in paediatric patients with tiny airways. Clinical scenarios such as emergency transtracheal jet ventilation (TTJV) via a front-of-neck cannula access during "Cannot Intubate, Cannot Ventilate" (CICV) situations, ventilating kids with a stenosed or an oedematous airway, or laryngeal suspension surgeries have always been managed with classical jet ventilation. These consisted of either the traditional three-way stopcock connected to a high-pressure oxygen source or manual jet ventilation (e.g., Manu-Jet). Despite the effectiveness in establishing temporary oxygenation, these techniques carried a high risk of complications such as barotrauma

B. Boudjenah · S. M. Chinnappa · R. B. Babu
Anaesthesia, ICU and Perioperative Medicine Department, Hamad Medical Corporation, Doha, Qatar

A. M. B. Adham
Sidra Medicine and Research, Doha, Qatar

M. Al-Khelaifi
Anaesthesia, ICU and Perioperative Medicine Department, Hamad Medical Corporation, Doha, Qatar

Clinical Anaesthesiology Department, Weill Cornell Medical College in Qatar, Doha, Qatar

N. A. Shallik (✉)
Anaesthesia, ICU and Perioperative Medicine Department, Hamad Medical Corporation, Doha, Qatar

Clinical Anaesthesiology Department, Weill Cornell Medical College in Qatar, Doha, Qatar

Clinical Anaesthesiology Department, College of Medicine Qatar University, Doha, Qatar

Anaesthesia and SICU Department, Tanta University, Tanta, Egypt
e-mail: nshallik@hamad.qa

N. A. Shallik (ed.), *Flow Controlled Ventilation Mode Through a Straw Size Tube*, https://doi.org/10.1007/978-3-031-77477-5_12

or volutrauma (from the uncontrolled pressure), air trapping with hyperinflation (if inappropriate passive expiration), and ineffective CO_2 elimination leading to progressive acidosis, hence limiting the time of their application.

A remarkable evolution in ventilation techniques for children has been attained in the last few years. The concept of manually controlling the inspiratory as well as the expiratory flow has been applied with the purpose of better ventilating the small-calibre airway without causing the problems of the older techniques. Hence, the Flow-Controlled manual Ventilator (FCmV) or Ventrain® (Ventinova Medical B.V., Eindhoven, The Netherlands) has been invented with the aim of "Expiratory Ventilation Assistance" (EVA) working by jet-flow suction to assist in active expiration and to manually control the inspiratory flow, which regulates the volume of inhaled gas per second. Those qualities have proven the Ventrain® to be a safer application as a mode of ventilation for the narrow airways in the paediatric population.

Problems in ventilating children with airway narrowing, Cannot Intubate, Cannot Oxygenate" (CICO) scenarios in children, and shared airway surgeries, are being addressed with ultra-new modalities. This chapter discusses the pathologies of the paediatric airway and the relative application of such innovations.

2 Indications

2.1 Causes of Airway Tract Stenosis in Paediatric Patients

Three main causes can be identified as common pathologies of airway stenosis in children: subglottic stenosis, cysts, or haemangioma.

2.1.1 Subglottic Stenosis (SGS)

Subglottic stenosis (SGS) is defined as a narrowing of the subglottic tracheal lumen ≤4 mm in a full-term neonate and a lumen <3 mm in a preterm infant [1]. It can be congenital but is often acquired, with 95% of the cases mainly resulting from prolonged endotracheal intubations [2]. Gastroesophageal reflux, present in more than 80% of infants with SGS, may exacerbate the pathogenesis of SGS and cause re-stenosis after laryngotracheal reconstruction repair; however, it may be the sole cause of stenosis in infants with no previous history of endotracheal intubation [3]. Patients often present with stridor, commonly biphasic, with signs of respiratory distress, or recurrent infections.

The Myer Cotton staging system described four grades of stenosis based on the degree of reduction in the cross-sectional subglottic area [4]:

- Grade I: Luminal obstruction <50%.
- Grade II: 51–70% luminal obstruction.
- Grade III: 71–99% luminal obstruction.
- Grade IV: Complete stenosis or no detectable lumen.

Management ranges from observation and conservative treatment for the self-limited, less severe stenosis (grade I and asymptomatic grade II) to endoscopic dilation (symptomatic grade II) or laryngotracheal reconstruction using a costal cartilage graft for the high-grade ones (grades III and IV) [1, 4]. Success rates are in the region of 80–90% for this surgery [5].

2.1.2 Subglottic Cysts

A subglottic cyst is a fluid-filled lesion that develops below the vocal cords. It represents a common cause of upper airway obstruction in infants, especially in ex-premature infants with a history of neonatal intubation that has caused mucosal damage resulting in fluid collection [5, 6]. The onset of symptoms occurs after a period of 4–7 months following extubation with a biphasic stridor [6, 7] often necessitating a bronchoscopy and marsupialization of the cyst using micro-laryngeal instrumentation. These cysts may recur, requiring regular follow-up [2].

2.1.3 Subglottic Haemangioma

Subglottic haemangioma is a rare benign vascular tumour due to submucosal endothelial hyperplasia. It is often located on the left side of the subglottic area. It may develop into a circumferential lesion, associated in 50% of cases with cutaneous localization. Asymptomatic at birth, their typical evolution includes two phases. The initial phase is the proliferative phase, with up to 1 year of biphasic symptoms predominantly inspiratory stridor occurring between the ages of 2–6 months and increasing in severity with time [5]. The second phase is the involution phase, between 2 and 5 years of age, and is characterised by the regression of the haemangioma with decreasing symptoms [8].

The management depends on the age of the child, the degree of subglottic narrowing, and the extent of the haemangioma. Medical options include systemic or intralesional steroids or, more recently, the administration of propranolol, which, by its action on the vasoactive endothelial growth facto, encourages involution of the haemangioma. Small unilateral lesions can be treated by CO_2 laser ablation and by an open submucosal excision [8]. Tracheostomy is indicated for bilateral or circumferential haemangiomas with more than 50% loss of the subglottic lumen and is kept in place until the natural regression of the lesion [2].

2.1.4 Other Uncommon Causes

- Laryngeal and laryngotracheal clefts: rare congenital defects with an insufficient division of the respiratory tract and the upper digestive tract.
- Localized tracheomalacia (vascular rings): extrinsic compression of the airway by cardiovascular anomalies (aberrant brachiocephalic artery) or trachea oesophageal fistula.
- Extrinsic compression of the trachea by a mediastinal mass.
- Use of CT-3D reconstruction and virtual endoscopy (VE) of the upper airway is a very crucial step in tracheoa- bronchial stenosis planning and management [9].

2.2 Cannot Intubate Cannot Oxygenate (CICO) Scenario

The incidence of difficult paediatric airways is 0.28% [10]. Thus, “cannot intubate and cannot ventilate” is an extremely uncommon situation, especially in infant patients. However, when encountered, the front of neck access via a needle cricothyrotomy with ventilation through a cannula might be the only life-saving option [11]. An awareness of the anatomical differences between the adult and paediatric airways is vital when performing emergent invasive trans-tracheal airway access. Therefore, cautious attention to the anatomy is mandated during needle cricothyrotomy. In fact, the trachea in infants and neonates is smaller, more mobile, and more easily compressible compared to that of adults [12]. The cricothyroid membrane is narrow and small, to the extent that it is difficult to identify. Compounded by the short neck and cephalad laryngeal position, it renders transtracheal intubation extremely difficult, as well as percutaneous cannula cricothyroidotomy insertion. Hence, the risk of misplacement and posterior tracheal wall perforation is high and adds further challenges to the arduous situation [13, 14]. Small-bore cannulas with an internal diameter <4 mm, such as the kink-resistant Patil (Cook Medical LLC, Bloomington, IN), and Ravussin needle (VBM Medizintechnik, Sulz am Neckar, Germany) (Fig. 1) can be used but requires a high-pressure oxygen source as well as specific ventilation equipment. Intravenous cannulas (16 G = 1.291 mm or 18 G = 1.024 mm) can be a reasonable alternative in case the former items are not available [15]. Efficient oxygenation can be achieved by jet ventilation or the "Ventrain®" ventilation system. Manual jet ventilation exposes the patient to the hazard of serious complications such as barotrauma, air entrapment with auto-PEEP, and inadequate CO_2 washout, along with progressive acidosis. It is contraindicated in cases of upper airway obstruction [16]. On the other hand, the "Ventrain®" system may be easier to perform technically in emergency situations. It also carries a lesser risk of barotrauma and auto-PEEP and provides better gas exhalation due to its active Bernoulli effect [17]. (For more details, please refer to chapter "Flow-Controlled Manual Ventilator (FCmV): A New Horizon in Elective and Emergency Airway Scenarios"). Needle cricothyrotomy is a temporary life-saving measure; hence, the airway operator's priority must escalate to securing a permanent airway as soon as adequate oxygenation is achieved.

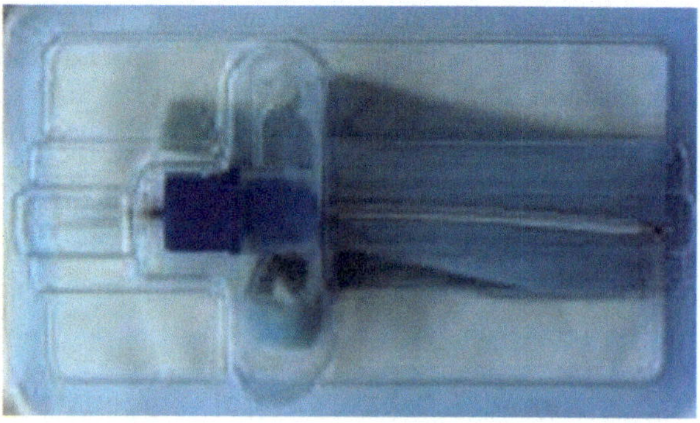

Fig. 1 Ravussin needle ((VBM) Medizintechnik GmbH, Sulz am Neckar, Germany)

3 Ventilation Techniques

3.1 Jet Ventilation

Jet ventilation consists of inserting a small-bore catheter within the airway with a high-pressure air/oxygen mixture aimed to deliver oxygen.

There are two main ways in which the gas pulse can be delivered:

1. At a low or a high frequency jet with distinctly different management concepts for each.
2. A system situated in a supraglottic, trans-glottic, or trans-tracheal position can supply the stream of pulsed gas.

3.1.1 Physiology

In Low-Frequency Jet Ventilation (LFJV), gas exchange is accomplished similarly to spontaneous respiration through bulk flow, also known as convective ventilation, which is the mass movement of gases into and out of the lungs.

Tidal volumes used in High-Frequency Jet Ventilation (HFJV) may be less than those of a series of dead spaces (anatomical plus equipment). Although some gas may enter during HFJV by bulk flow even at volumes below traditional dead space because a few alveoli are close enough to the conducting airways, it is insufficient to sustain efficient gas exchange. Because other modes of gas transport contribute analogously more than other processes, successful gas exchange is obtained in HFJV.

3.1.2 Jet Ventilation Types

Jet ventilation may be high- or low-frequency. Both approaches work on the same general principles: high-pressure sources' jet streams are interrupted by pneumatic or electronically controlled flow interruption devices, creating a tidal volume that is further enhanced by gas entrainment at the jet nozzle. Expiration is dependent on passive lung and chest-wall recoil.

Low-Frequency Jet Ventilation Generally, Low-Frequency Jet Ventilation (LFJV) is supplied by a manually operated apparatus like the Sanders injector (Fig. 2a). The user adjusts the breathing rate, typically between 8 and 10 breaths/min, to provide the lungs and chest wall enough time to passively recoil and exhale [18].

Typically, hand-triggered tools like the Sanders injector or Manujet III (VBM Medizintechnik, Sulz am Neckar, Germany) are used to apply LFJV (Fig. 2b). Its use is typically restricted to brief diagnostic procedures like bronchoscopies or laryngoscopies, but it also plays a significant role in managing a difficult airway or the "can't intubate, can't ventilate" situation when used in conjunction with a cricothyroidotomy cannula. Cannulas or jet-tubes are usually short, narrow-bore, non-compliant, and are frequently already part of instruments like the rigid bronchoscope or laryngoscope. The high-pressure wall-piped oxygen at 4 bar is the

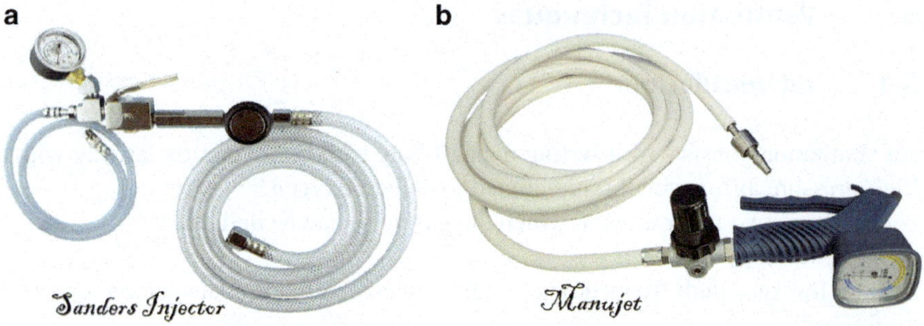

Fig. 2 (**a**) Sanders' injector. (**b**) Manujet III ((VBM) Medizintechnik, Sulz a.N, Germany) (Courtesy, Dr. Shallik, Doha Airway Equipment Museum, Qatar)

oxygen source, also known as the principal gas source. Pressure-reducing valves allow it to pass through, and a regulator located close to the handset allows for additional pressure adjustments up to a level that maintains sufficient gas exchange and oxygenation while resulting in the necessary chest-wall excursion. The handset has a short, stiff piping that needs to be tightly fastened to the cannula, often via a Luer-Lock connection. For the high-pressure jet to function properly, the cannula needs to be tightly attached to avoid dislodgement. If the nozzle or cannula is placed above the glottis, it should be oriented along the axis of the airway in order to be efficient and to prevent gastric distension. The sum of the injected and entrained volumes is known as the tidal volume. A jet frequency of 8–10/min avoids air-trapping and pressure build-up in tiny airways while providing enough time for exhalation through passive recoil of the lung and chest wall. The effective FIO_2 in the trachea is 0.8–0.9 when 100% oxygen is employed as the jet gas due to dilution from ambient air entrainment. If the reduction in oxygen concentration resulting from entrainment is desired, a side-arm attachment to a bronchoscope or a laryngoscope may permit oxygen entrainment instead of ambient air.

High-Frequency Jet Ventilation The equipment needed for High-Frequency Jet Ventilation (HFJV) may deliver a heated, humidified jet at rates of up to 10 Hz [18]. Specialised tools and knowledge about the method are needed for HFJV [19–21] (Fig. 3a, b).

3.1.3 Ventilators (Description and Settings)

There are commercial jet ventilators that operate at 1–10 Hz and provide heated, humidified jets. A high-frequency flow interrupter, which is typically an electrical solenoid valve but can also be a fluidic or spinning cylinder valve, splits continuous flow into square wave pressures. It is possible to modify the driving pressure, frequency, inspiratory time, and jet gas composition. Every ventilator has warnings and automatic shutdown mechanisms to cut off gas delivery when unintentionally excessive airway pressure is detected.

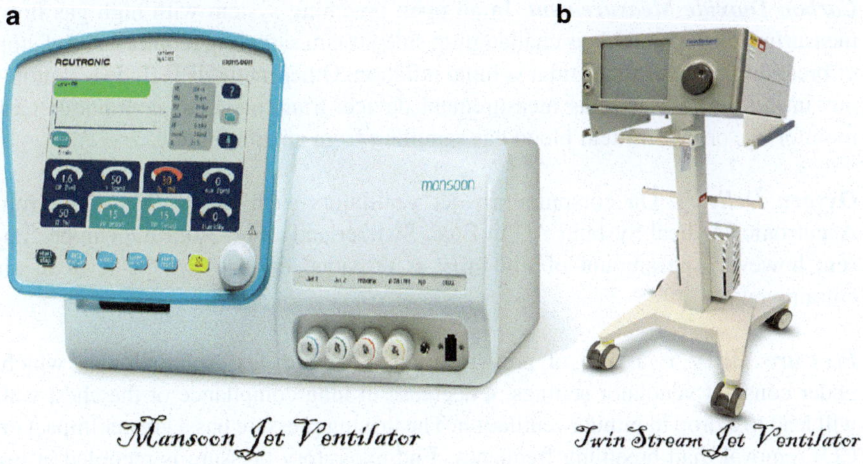

Fig. 3 Automatic jet ventilator; (**a**) Mansoon (Accutronic Medical Systems AG in Baar, Switzerland). (**b**) Superimposed high-frequency jet ventilation (TwinStream, Carl Reiner GMBH, Vienna, Austria). (Courtesy, Dr. Shallik, Doha Airway Equipment Museum, Qatar)

Additionally, the majority features a manual option that permits the administration of high-volume breaths slowly in order to offer the possibility of more precise, albeit sporadic, end-tidal CO_2 monitoring. Due to the drying effects of high gas flows, humidification is crucial in preventing considerable heat loss (Fig. 3a, b).

Disclaimer: Jet ventilators can be used safely in the paediatric age group with caution, and expert anaesthesiologists are always required.

Superimposed High-Frequency Jet Ventilation The Superimposed high-frequency jet ventilator (Twinstream jet ventilator, Carl Reiner GMBH, Vienna, Austria) is a microprocessor-controlled electric jet ventilator that combines simultaneously two different jet streams, one at high-frequency (50–1500/min) and one at low-frequency (1–100/min), resulting in a pulsatile bi-level (p-BLV) mode of ventilation that allows both optimal oxygenation and efficient CO_2 elimination at the same time. Twinstream may also provide HFJV to conventionally intubated patients via ETT or LMA. A Superimposed high-frequency jet ventilator can be used safely in the paediatric age group (Fig. 3b).

Catheters and Delivery Routes Jet catheters can be used independently or through tracheal tubes. The catheter tip can be positioned above or below the vocal cords [2, 22]. Similarly, trans-tracheal jet cannulas may be employed. There are wide variations in a catheter's design. Catheters can have several lumens and are often composed of plastic or metal. Intermittent CO_2 sampling or continuous intratracheal pressure are two uses for the extra lumen. There are tracheal tubes that have been particularly modified and fitted with two tiny apertures that open distally for the administration of jet gas and the monitoring of airway pressure, respectively.

Carbon Dioxide Measurement In an open breathing system with high gas flow, measuring carbon dioxide is challenging; side-stream sampling requires a brief stop of breathing after standard tidal volume inflation. Other methods include a continuous intra-arterial blood-gas measurement device, transcutaneous continuous CO_2 monitoring, or intermittent blood gas sampling from an arterial line.

Oxygen Delivery On contemporary jet ventilators such as the (Mansoon from Accutronic Medical Systems AG in Baar, Switzerland) (Fig. 3a), FIO_2 can be chosen; however, the amount of FIO_2 that is provided depends on the level of air entrainment.

Pressure HFJV is a type of pressure-limited, time-cycled ventilation in which, under constant ventilator settings, a decrease in lung compliance or the chest wall will lead to a drop in minute ventilation. The driving pressure has a greater impact on CO_2 removal than breathing frequency. End-expiratory pressure is recorded at the end of insufflation through the injector; however, because of regional variances that are amplified at high frequencies, it may not accurately reflect intra-thoracic pressures. A second airway measurement line, which continually measures the airway pressure apart from the jet insufflation line, is a feature of modern jet ventilators.

Although a frequency-dependent positive end-expiratory pressure is typically present during HFJV, the mean and peak airway pressures that arise are significantly lower than those that occur during conventional ventilation. This characteristic can be used to lower airway pressures in individuals requiring intensive care or gas leaks through bronchopleural fistulas. If there is insufficient air egress during expiration, HFJV creates a fast build-up of pressure. This breathing modality cannot be used safely without a ventilator with an excessive pressure alert and an automated shutdown feature. Oesophageal or intrapleural pressure monitors may provide more accurate data regarding the measurement of peripheral airway pressures and the incidence of gas trapping in patients undergoing extended HFJV.

Parameters and Settings In clinical practice, rate/frequency (f), driving pressure (DP), inspiratory time (I-time; percentage of ventilation cycle), and inspired oxygen fraction (FIO_2) are critical and interrelated factors.

The driving pressure, cannula resistance, inspiratory time, entrainment volume, and respiratory system impedance all affect the tidal volume, which is not fixed. Reactions to changes may appear illogical at first; for instance, if DP and I-time are held constant, raising the frequency can cause hypercapnia by lowering the tidal volume [5]. A potential danger when using HFJV is the intrinsic PEEP, which rises with frequency and is inversely correlated with expiratory time. The likelihood of it surpassing the desired levels is higher in lung units with extended time constants.

A rise in DP causes a decrease in PCO_2, an increase of TV, and an increase in airway pressure. Large increases in DP, however, can cause CO_2 retention if the frequency is set too high to give the shorter respiratory cycle enough time for adequate expiration. Increasing DP, FIO_2, or I-time can increase oxygenation. However, if I-time is set too high to allow sufficient expiration, CO_2 retention may happen. When using a subglottic catheter for HFJV, the preferred parameter sets are DP at 2 ATM, f at 150/min, FIO_2 of 1.0, and I-time at 50%.

3.1.4 Indications of Jet Ventilation

Emergency in Paediatrics

In the Cannot Ventilate, Cannot Intubate (CVCI) situation, LFJV via a trans-tracheal cannula is a temporary life-saving measure (with an ensured gas egress pathway) [23].

Elective Settings in Paediatrics

Elective jet ventilation involves direct laryngoscopy, vocal cord surgery, and pre-emptive implantation of a transtracheal jet cannula to treat the expectedly difficult airway.

Jet ventilation finds extensive use in thoracic and airway surgery, including major airway procedures like tracheal reconstruction, excision of stenosis, and carinal resections.

There is no requirement for an airtight connection between the breathing system and the airway because HFJV requires an open breathing system.

In comparison to traditional ventilation, HFJV also reduces the extent of bronchial and mediastinal excursion. The surgeon can manage the fine jet catheter while performing the procedure by passing it through the surgical field and bridging the defect or disease. Around the tiny catheter, end-to-end anastomosis and airway resection can be performed.

Applying HFJV to the non-dependent lung during surgery, as opposed to just PEEP, can help eliminate CO_2 and increase oxygenation during one-lung ventilation, which lessens the ventilatory pressures on the dependent lung. Since peak and mean airway pressures are lower with HFJV than with IPPV (Intermittent Positive Pressure Ventilation/VC) or *CMV (Continuous Mandatory Ventilation)*, there is a reduced gas leak through pathological low-resistance channels in the management of broncho-pleural fistula and tracheo-bronchial tree disruption. In chronically ventilated patients, as well as in the acute surgical setting, arterial CO_2 tension can be returned to normal.

3.1.5 Complications of Jet Ventilation

The jet ventilation technique exposes the patient to threats of barotrauma (pneumothorax, pneumomediastinum, and surgical emphysema), oesophageal and stomach rupture, air entrapment with auto-PEEP, inadequate CO_2 washout, and progressive acidosis, which comes from inadequate gas exchange (hypoxaemia, hypercapnia).

3.2 The Ventrain® System

The Flow Controlled Manual Ventilator (FCmV) or Ventrain® is a singleuse, small-lumen, manually operated, flow-controlled ejector device connected to a pressure compensated flowmeter oxygen source, initially designed to provide ventilation through narrow-bore catheters (e.g. 2–3 mm ID) in emergencies. It generates an inspiratory positive pressure as well as an active suction during expiration called "Expiratory Ventilation Assistance" (EVA), facilitating the egress of the respiratory gases [23]. The latter effect is facilitated by a built-in mechanism that operates via a Bernoulli phenomenon.

3.2.1 Description

Ventrain is a compact T-piece with gas inflow on one side and two exhaust ports on the other. Two connections can be described as: an inlet tube (length, 213 ± 20 cm; internal diameter, 3.0–4.5 mm) and a short sidearm (length, 20 ± 1 cm; internal diameter, 5.20 ± 0.15 mm). The inlet tube is attached to a high-pressure oxygen source with a controllable flow through either a standard wall outlet with a pressure-compensated flowmeter or an oxygen cylinder with a flow regulator. The short side-arm is located at the bottom of the FCmV and has a distal T-piece that connects the patient's small-bore airway via a male Luer Lock connector. A side port of the distal T-piece allows intermittent measurement of end-tidal CO_2 concentration. The inlet channel inside the shell narrows to a diameter of 0.75 mm before splitting into a T-shape. The gas is directed either along the inspiratory/expiratory sidearm to the airway or along the exhaust channel toward an opening on the upper surface [24]. FCmV has an internal dead space volume of 5 mL [25] (Fig. 4).

3.2.2 Mode of Action

FCmV is manually operated by intermittently occluding and releasing one or two apertures, resulting in three operational phases: inspiration, expiration, and equilibration [25].

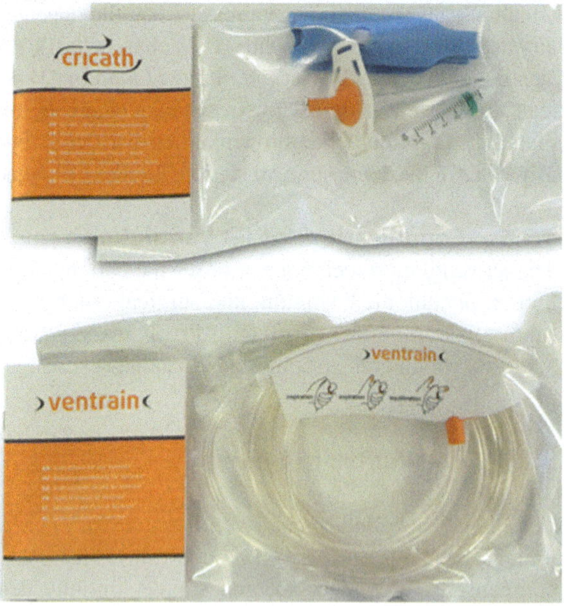

Fig. 4 Flow-controlled manual ventilator (FCmV) or Ventrain® with Criocath. (Courtesy, Dr. Shallik, Doha Airway Equipment Museum, Qatar)

During inspiration, the lower and upper openings are occluded by the index and the thumb. Under high proximal driving pressure, oxygen flow is accelerated across the nozzle and diverted along the inspiratory channel via the sidearm towards the patient's airway.

During expiration, the upper aperture is released by lifting the thumb while maintaining the lower one closed. The oxygen flow, on its way through the ejector, is accelerated by the 0.75 mm ID jet nozzle. This increases the dynamic pressure of the flowing gas and leads to a decrease in the static pressure of the gas surrounding the jet emerging from the nozzle (Bernoulli's principle). The high-speed oxygen flow creates a subatmospheric pressure distal to the nozzle and subsequently exerts a suction effect on the air inflowing from the patient's side (active expiration) due to the Bernoulli effect [26, 27].

During equilibration, both apertures are open, resulting in slow equilibration of intrapulmonary and ambient air pressure and allowing lung volume to stabilise near functional residual capacity, while fresh oxygen escapes via the exhaust. This effect will avoid inadvertent hyperinflation and excessive suctioning on the lungs. An equilibrium pause should always be performed every 5-ventilation cycle for at least 5 s, especially when there is no intratracheal pressure measurement available.

3.2.3 Flow Control

Ventrain is an inspiratory and expiratory flow-controlled device. Inspiratory tidal volume can easily be estimated and controlled over time by setting an appropriate flow and inspiratory time: a flow of 6 L/min (=6000 ml in 60 s) will insufflate 100 ml of tidal volume per second after 1 s of inspiration and 200 ml after 2 s (Table 1) [23]. In clinical practice, the volume delivered will be lower than the one estimated from the set flow due to some air leakage around the small-bore airway and may need to increase the flow and/or inspiratory time. Expiratory tidal volume depends on many factors: set flow, resulting in subatmospheric pressure, resistance to flow, and leakage. Increasing the flow results in more subatmospheric pressure leading to an increase in the suction capacity as well as the expiratory volume per time unit [26]. Respiratory frequency is determined by the duration of the manual inspiratory/expiratory cycle. An I:E ratio of 1:1 is proven to be safe in most paediatric patients during ventilation with FCmV and results in similar inspiratory and expiratory tidal volumes, especially with the proper length and ID diameter of paediatric airway catheters used.

Table 1 Flow set, and volume administered per time [23]

Flow (L/min)	Insufflated volume (ml) after 1 s inspiration	Insufflated volume (ml) after 2 s inspiration
2	33	66
3	50	100
6	100	200
9	150	300
12	200	400
15	250	500

For more details, please refer to chapter "Flow-Controlled manual Ventilator (FCmV): A New Horizon in Elective and Emergency Airway Scenarios—A New Horizon in Elective and Emergency Airway Scenarios".

3.2.4 Advantages of the Ventrain® System

In comparison to jet ventilation, the Ventrain® system offers many advantages. It provides sufficient oxygenation and effective ventilation at lower airway pressures. Thus, it may be able to limit any unintentional hyperinflation and high intrapulmonary pressures when ventilating through long, small-bore catheters. Therefore, it may significantly minimise the risks of barotrauma and air trapping and their consequent deleterious haemodynamic effects [27, 28]. Expiratory ventilation assistance is another main advantage. It exerts a suction effect and actively supports the egress of airflow from the patient due to the Venturi effect. Finally, FCmV allows the possibility of capnography monitoring when ventilating through small lumen tubes, making it inherently safer than jet ventilation. Lastly, it can measure the pressure by connecting the FCmV with the manometer through a Luer lock alternating with the $ETCO_2$ line (Fig. 5).

3.2.5 Disadvantage of the Ventrain® System

Although a very proficient device, the Ventrain® system presents some disadvantages. It requires manual operation, which is challenging to handle whenever dealing with stressful, life-threatening CICO situations. Another disadvantage is the lack of continuous pressure monitoring; hence, the need to observe chest movements is crucial in order to minimise the risk of lung injury [29]. The auxiliary oxygen outlet of some anaesthesia machines should not be used for ventilation without a pressure compensation flowmeter attached to the anaesthesia machine because it cannot generate the required pressure and runs the risk of delivering lower flows than desired [30]. Also, caution must be exercised when high oxygen concentrations are used in flammable environments like LASER surgery. Lastly, during the expiratory phase, debris is ejected out of the thumb hole, including blood or organisms, so it should either be pointed away from bystanders or covered without occluding the holes.

Disclaimer: The use of the Ventrain® demands a thorough understanding of the required equipment, the principle, and function of the Ventrain®, technical prerequisites, clinical safety measures, and, most importantly, appropriate regular training.

3.2.6 Use of Flow-Controlled Manual Ventilator (FCmV) in Paediatric Patients

Setting the Correct Flow and I:E Ratio in Paediatric Patients [24]

Several steps need to be followed to set up the FCmV system for paediatric applications:

- First, attach the long inlet of the FCmV to a high-pressure oxygen source. Then, connect the short tubing to the patient's small-bore airway (catheter or cannula) via the Luer lock connector.

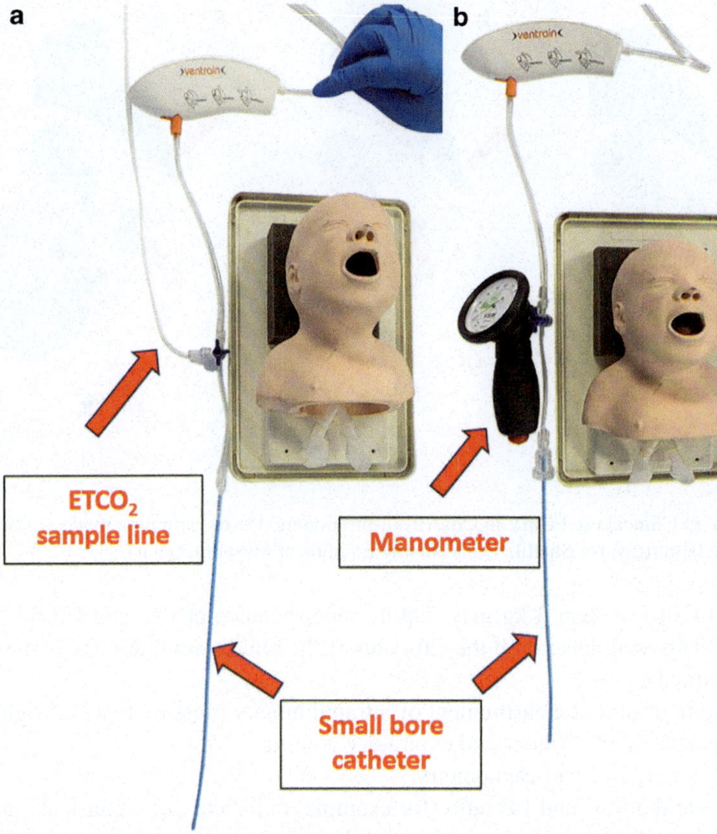

Fig. 5 Flow-controlled manual ventilator (FCmV) (Ventrain®) connection with manometer or $ETCO_2$ sample line and small-bore catheter in kids (courtesy, Dr. Shallik, Doha Airway Equipment Museum, Qatar)

- Set the initial flow at 1 L/min per year of age, with a normal range from 2 L/min to 15 L/min. Estimate the desired tidal volume based on the flow set and aim for a tidal volume of 6–10 ml/kg of the child's weight (Table 1).
- Start ventilation by occluding both lower and upper apertures with an inspiratory time of 1 s (0.5 s if the child weighs less than 3 kg) (Fig. 6a).
- Release the upper opening to start expiration (Fig. 6b).
- Continue with an inspiratory: expiratory ratio of 1:1.
- Closely monitor the chest wall movements, as this may help to adjust the I:E ratio appropriately.
- Release both apertures at the end of expiration every 5 cycles (equilibration mode) for at least 5 s while carefully observing the chest wall excursion. A visible rebound of the chest and/or upper abdomen during this phase indicates an intrapulmonary pressure build-up. To prevent this, expiratory ventilation assistance should be prolonged when resuming ventilation (Fig. 6c).

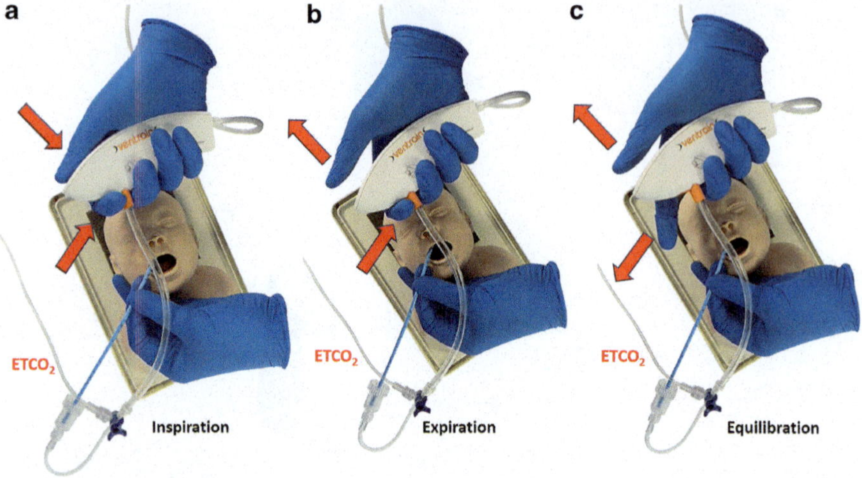

Fig. 6 (**a**–**c**) Clinical use FCmV in kids. (**a**) Inspiration mode, (**b**) expiration mode, (**c**) equilibration mode (Courtesy, Dr. Shallik, Doha Airway Equipment Museum, Qatar)

- A baby of less than 3 kg may require more balance phases and a different I:E ratio. This will depend on the situation of the child's ventilation and chest wall movements.
- Set up intermittent measurement of intrapulmonary pressure to avoid significant imbalances in inspiratory and expiratory volumes.
- Consider intermittent capnometry.
- Evaluate the flow and I:E ratio (for example, in the case of an air leak, increase the flow or lengthen the inspiration to obtain an adequate tidal volume). In case of complete upper airway obstruction, a longer expiration time might be necessary, and more balance phases might be necessary).
- Once sufficient oxygenation and ventilation are re-established, proceed to plan the next step in managing the airway.

Disclaimer: Flow-Controlled manual Ventilator (FCmV) or Ventrain® in the paediatric patients can be used safely in paediatric age group with caution, and expert anaesthesiologists are always required.

Clinical Use in Paediatric Patients

Although Ventrain® can be used for "all patients," the experience with paediatric patients is still limited, and its use should only be granted to expert hands. To our knowledge, there has been no elective use of the Ventrain® in paediatric anaesthesia to date. Only a few animal studies and clinical emergency cases have been reported in the literature so far.

Willemsen et al. reported 2 cases of failed intubation in two small infants rescued by the Ventrain® Ventilation trough small bore catheter (8 Fr intubating catheters (ICs) or airway exchange catheters (AECs)) [31]. The first case was a 2.1 kg ex-preterm baby scheduled for eye cryo-coagulation therapy. After multiple unsuccessful attempts at tracheal intubation in the NICU, a size 1 LMA was inserted before transfer to the operating theatre (OT), and then another trial of direct laryngoscopy was decided due to ventilation difficulty through the supraglottic device. Despite a Cormack-Lehane view grade 1, a 2.5 mm ETT failed to be advanced into the trachea because of a glottic oedema. The infant then experienced an abrupt episode of significant desaturation (SpO_2 <40%) with bradycardia (40 bpm), requiring an urgent airway intervention. A 35 cm long Frova intubating catheter (FIC) [8 Fr = 2.66 mm outer diameter (OD), 5 Fr = 1.66 mm inner diameter (ID); Cook Medical, Bloomington, IN] was pushed with some resistance into the trachea and connected to the Ventrain®. The latter was initially set and started at 2 L flow increased to 4 L and then to 6 L/min, a frequency of 100/min, and a 1:1 I/E ratio while continually monitoring the chest wall movements. Adequate oxygenation with an SpO_2 above 90% could be restored in less than a minute. To secure the airway, a soft tip guide wire was threaded through the FIC and used as a guide to insert a 2.0 mm ID and then a 2.5 mm ID ETT. Postoperatively, a chestXray confirmed the absence of pneumothorax or atelectasis. The second case involved a 4.3 kg infant posted for abdominal surgery. After induction of general anaesthesia, a video laryngoscope offered an appropriate laryngeal view (Cormack-Lehane grade 1), but two attempts at tracheal intubation failed, first with a 3.0 mm ID ETT tube and then with a 2.5 mm ID tube due to laryngeal oedema. Because of difficult mask ventilation, a size 1 LMA was placed, and a subsequent flexible fiberoptic intubation through it was unsuccessful. The airway was finally managed by inserting against slight resistance a Cook tracheal airway exchange catheter (AEC), Cook Medical, Bloomington, IN) (45 cm length, ID 1.66 mm) connected to the Ventrain® with an initial flow rate of 6 L/min. Ventilation with active expiration started at a frequency of 40/min and an I/E ratio of 1:2 with close observation of the chest movements. Reoxygenation was quickly re-established with an SpO_2 of 96%. Then a 3.0 mm ID uncuffed tube was gently advanced over the catheter into the trachea with the help of video laryngoscopy (Fig. 7). The baby was extubated 24 h later, without any complications.

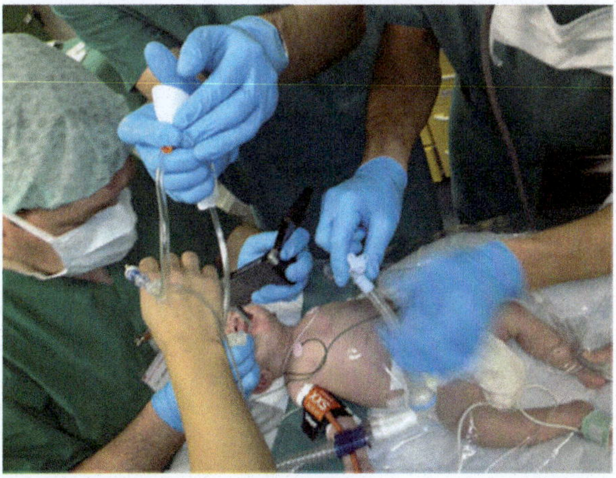

Fig. 7 Ventilation through a 45 cm long, 1.66 mm ID tube exchange catheter using the Ventrain® while advancing a tracheal tube in a difficult airway situation [32]. Published with copyright https://s100.copyright.com/CustomerAdmin/PLF.jsp?ref=d292cef8-67b4-4e74-890b-286b0f53feb8

The third scenario: Escribá Alepuz et al. described how the Ventrain® device rescued a 7-monthsold, 3.7 kg, ex-preterm (25 gestational weeks) infant with a neonatal history of prolonged intubation who was admitted in PICU for a deteriorating respiratory distress with tachypnoea, wheezing, aphonia, and frequent episodes of desaturation despite regular nebulization requiring a high level of oxygen [32]. An urgent flexible bronchoscopy revealed the presence of two posterior subglottic cysts that occupied 50% of the subglottic space. In the operating room, after a smooth tracheal intubation, a microsurgical incision of both cysts was conducted, and the infant was moved back to the PICU after an uneventful extubation. One day later, she developed acute respiratory failure. A rigid bronchoscopy revealed significant subglottic oedema, whereas a Ventrain® device connected to its working channel ensured efficient ventilation. The trachea was then intubated with a size 2 mm ID ETT with some difficulty, then connected to the conventional PICU ventilator, resulting in high peak pressure (above 50 cmH_2O), limited chest rise, significant hypercapnia (above 120 mmHg), and desaturation with an SpO_2 of 85%, which required the help of the Ventrain® device at a flow of 2 L/min for a short while. After sedation, the baby was reconnected to the PICU ventilator before uneventful extubation 24 h later.

Fayoux et al. described a wide use of airway exchange catheters (AECs) to manage the airway of neonates and infants with laryngeal stenosis posted for surgery where an ETT could not be placed due to its size [33] whereas De Wolf et al. have successfully combined Ventrain® with ICs/AECs for ETT exchange in many paediatric patients with a high risk of desaturation or with a previous history of difficult intubation [23].

In brief, the Ventrain® was developed with the goal of providing "Expiratory Ventilation Assistance" (EVA) by jet-flow suction to aid in active expiration, as well as manually controlling the inspiratory flow, which regulates the volume of inhaled gas per second. These characteristics have demonstrated that the Ventrain® is a safer means of breathing for young patients with restricted airways [34].

3.3 Flow-Controlled Ventilator (FCV) (Evone®)

Another advancement in the ventilation of the narrow calibre airway has been established with the invention of "Flow-Controlled Ventilators (FCV)," such as the Evone®, which applies the same principle of action as FCmV but with a constant flow of gas with an inspiratory to expiratory I:E ratio of 1:1. This constant flow and ratio allows for a decrease in energy dissipation (which is a main factor in barotrauma), and ventilation through extremely narrow calibre tubes such as the Tritube® (<3mm ID), which also has the advantage of securing the airway with its cuff, hence allowing the asset of prolonging the ventilation time through the small-bore space [35–37]. However, this new modality is still of limited use in children below 40 kg, pending validation in smaller age groups [38–40].

4 Conclusion

Ventilation through a small calibre tube may be indicated to manage some specific challenging airway situations in the paediatric population, such as the "cannot intubate, cannot ventilate" scenario and narrowed airways, but it exposes the patient to serious complications when the traditional manual jet ventilation is used. The recent introduction of Flow Controlled manual Ventilator (FCmV) may overcome all these risks and turn ventilation via a "straw in the airway" into an efficient mean of oxygenation and ventilation. Another advancement in the ventilation of the narrow calibre airway has been established with the invention of the "Flow-Controlled Ventilators (FCV)" (Evone®), which applies the same principle of action of the Ventrain® but still not approved to be used in age below 40 kg.

Acknowledgments A special thanks is extended to Mr. Abil Luez who artistically captured all images and video clips of this chapter.

Disclaimer Here we introduce the flow-controlled manual ventilator (FCmV), exemplified frequently by the Ventrain®, merely because there is no alternative of its kind on the market, and also because you may find a particular focus on the only commercially available FCV ventilator, the "Evone®" ventilator, due to the lack of other examples and not as a commercial endorsement of the products.

References

1. Jefferson ND, Cohen AP, Rutter MJ. Subglottic stenosis. Semin Pediatr Surg. 2016;25:138–43.
2. Bradley J, Lee GS, Peyton J. Anesthesia for shared airway surgery in children. Pediatr Anesth. 2020;30:288–95.
3. Eid EA. Anesthesia for subglottic stenosis in pediatrics. Saudi J Anaesth. 2009;3(2):77–82.
4. Redondo-Sedano J, Anton-Pacheco JL, Valverde RM, et al. Laryngeal stenosis in children: types, grades and treatment strategies. J Pediatr Surg. 2019;54:1933–7.
5. Oshan V, Walker RW. Anaesthesia for complex airway surgery in children. Contin Educ Anaesth Crit Care Pain. 2013;13:47–50.
6. Lim J, Hellier W, Harcourt J, Leighton S, Albert D. Subglottic cysts: the great Ormond Street experience. Int J Pediatr Otorhinolaryngol. 2003;67:461–5.
7. Watson GJ, Malik TH, Khan NA, Sheehan PZ, Rothera MP. Acquired paediatric subglottic cysts: a series from Manchester. Int J Pediatr Otorhinolaryngol. 2007;71:533–8.
8. Rahbar R, Nicollas R, Roger G, et al. The biology and management of subglottic hemangioma: past, present, future. Laryngoscope. 2004;114:1880–91.
9. Chinnadurai S, Sathe NA, Surawicz T. Laser treatment of infantile hemangioma: a systematic review. Lasers Surg Med. 2016; 48:221-233.
10. Engelhardt T, Virag K, Veyckemans F, Habre W, APRICOT Group of the European Society of Anaesthesiology Clinical Trial Network. Airway management in paediatric anaesthesia in Europe—insights from APRICOT (Anaesthesia Practice in Children Observational Trial): a prospective multicentre observational study in 261 hospitals in Europe. Br J Anaesth. 2018;121:66–75.
11. Berger-Estilita J, Wenzel V, Luedi MM, Riva T. A primer for pediatric emergency front-of-the-neck access. A A Pract. 2021;15(4):e01444.

12. Navsa N, Tossel G, Boon JM. Dimensions of the neonatal cricothyroid membrane - how feasible is a surgical cricothyroidotomy? Pediatr Anesth. 2005;15:402–6.
13. Sabato SC, Long E. An institutional approach to the management of the "can't intubate, can't oxygenate" emergency in children. Paediatr Anaesth. 2016;26:784–93.
14. Johansen K, Holm-Knudsen RJ, Charabi B, Kristensen MS, Rasmussen LS. Cannot ventilate-cannot intubate an infant: surgical tracheotomy or transtracheal cannula? Paediatr Anaesth. 2010;20(11):987–93.
15. Black AE, Flyn PE, Smith HL, Thomas ML, Wilkinson KA. Development of a guideline for the management of the unanticipated difficult airway in pediatric practice. Paediatr Anaesth. 2015;25:346–62.
16. Mahfouz AK, Al Hadifi T, Rashid M. Cannot intubate and cannot ventilate scenario in an infant for airway assessment. Saudi J Anaesth. 2019;13:83–4.
17. Berry M, Tzeng Y, Marsland C. Percutaneous transtracheal ventilation in an obstructed airway model in post-apnoeic sheep. Br J Anaesth. 2014;113(6):1039–45.
18. Evans EBP, Bedforth N. Jet ventilation. Contin Educ Anaesth Crit Care Pain. 2007;7:2–5.
19. Rezaie-Majd A, Bigenzahn W, Denk DM, et al. Superimposed high-frequency jet ventilation (SHFJV) for endoscopic laryngotracheal. surgery in more than 1500 patients. Br J Anaesth. 2006;96:650–9.
20. Ihra G, Hieber C, Adel S, Kashanipour A, Aloy A. Tubeless combined high-frequency jet ventilation for laryngotracheal laser surgery in paediatric anaesthesia. Acta Anaesthesiol Scand. 2000;44:475–9.
21. Tang MM, Xu Z, Ren J, Zou J, Chen G. Superimposed high-frequency jet ventilation used for endolaryngotracheal surgery in a child with congenital subglottic stenosis: a case report. Transl Pediatr. 2022;11(12):2057–62.
22. Rosal Martins M, Van Boven M, Schmitz S, Hamoir M, Veyckemans F. Technical description of a modified jet ventilation injector for airway laser surgery in neonates and infants: retrospective analysis of 20 cases. J Clin Anesth. 2016;32:142–7.
23. Bolton P. Emergency jet ventilation in children. Paediatr Anaesth. 2009;19(5):425–7.
24. de Wolf M, Enk D, Jagannathan N. Ventilation through small-bore airways in children by implementing active expiration. Pediatr Anaesth. 2022;32:312–20.
25. Dos Santos Rocha A, Habre W, Albu G. Novel ventilation techniques in children. Pediatr Anesth. 2022;32:286–94.
26. Morrison S, Aerts S, Saldien V. The ventrain device: a future role in difficult airway algorithms? A A Pract. 2019;13(9):362–5.
27. Hamaekers AE, Borg PA, Enk D. Ventrain: an ejector ventilator for emergency use. Br J Anaesth. 2012;108:1017–21.
28. Doyle DJ. Ventilation via narrow-bore catheters: clinical and technical perspectives on the ventrain ventilation system. Open Anesth J. 2018;12:49–60.
29. de Wolf MWP, Gottschall R, Preussler NP, et al. Emergency ventilation with the Ventrain® through an airway exchange catheter in a porcine model of complete upper airway obstruction. Can J Anesth. 2017;64:37–44.
30. de Wolf MW, Gottschall R, Enk D. Monitoring during ventilation with Ventrain. Anaesthesist. 2017;66:207–8.
31. de Wolf M, Schutzer-Weissmann JM. Response to "Impact of oxygen sources on performance of the Ventrain ventilation device". Acta Anaesthesiol Scand. 2016;60:1477–8.
32. Willemsen MG, Noppens R, Mulder AL, Enk D. Ventilation with the ventrain through a small lumen catheter in the failed paediatric airway: two case reports. Br J Anaesth. 2014;112(5):946–7.
33. Escribá Alepuz FJ, Alonso García J, Cuchillo Sastriques JV, Alcalá E, Argente NP. Emergency ventilation of infant subglottic stenosis through small-gauge lumen using the Ventrain: a case report. A A Pract. 2018;10(6):136–8.
34. Mann CM, Baker PA, Sainsbury DM, Taylor R. A comparison of cannula insufflation device performance for emergency front of neck airway. Paediatr Anaesth. 2021;31(4):482–90. https://doi.org/10.1111/pan.14128.

35. Fayoux P, Marciniak B, Engelhardt T. Airway exchange catheters use in the airway management of neonates and infants undergoing surgical treatment of laryngeal stenosis. Pediatr Crit Care Med. 2009;10:558–61.
36. Meulemans J, Jans A, Vermeulen K, Vandommele J, Delaere P, Van der Poorten V. Evone® flow-controlled ventilation during upper airway surgery: a clinical feasibility study and safety assessment. Front Surg. 2020;7:6.
37. Schmidt J, Günther F, Weber J, Wirth S, Brandes I, Barnes T, Zarbock A, Schumann S, Enk D. Flow-controlled ventilation during ear, nose and throat surgery: a prospective observational study. Eur J Anaesthesiol. 2019;36(5):327–34.
38. Schranc Á, Balogh ÁL, Diaper J, Südy R, Peták F, Habre W, Albu G. Flow-controlled ventilation maintains gas exchange and lung aeration in a pediatric model of healthy and injured lungs: a randomized cross-over experimental study. Front Pediatr. 2022;10:1005135.
39. Enk D, Spraider P, Abram J, Barnes T. Commentary: Flow-controlled ventilation maintains gas exchange and lung aeration in a paediatric model of healthy and injured lungs: a randomized cross-over experimental study. Front Pediatr. 2023;11:1122434.
40. Shallik N, Elarref M, Khamash O, Abdelaal A, Radi Alkhafaji M, Makki H, Menon A. Management of critical tracheal stenosis with a straw sized tube (Tritube): case report. Qatar Med J. 2020;3:48.

Utility of Flow Controlled Ventilation in Laparoscopic and Robotic Abdominal Surgery

Arunabha Karmakar, Anas N. Shallik, and Nabil A. Shallik

1 Introduction

Laparoscopic surgery is performed by qualified surgeons for the management of abdominal organ pathologies in a minimally invasive manner. In contrast to open surgery, laparoscopic surgery has benefits of minimal tissue damage, less pain, reduced post operative analgesic requirements and early post operative ambulation and recovery. It has thus become the standard of care in most hospitals.

The steps of laparoscopic surgery are shown below (Figs. 1 and 2):

A. Karmakar
Anaesthesia, ICU and Perioperative Medicine Department, Hamad Medical Corporation, Doha, Qatar

A. N. Shallik
Royal College of Surgeons in Ireland Medical University of Bahrain, Manamah, Bahrain

N. A. Shallik (✉)
Anaesthesia, ICU and Perioperative Medicine Department, Hamad Medical Corporation, Doha, Qatar

Clinical Anaesthesiology Department, Weill Cornell Medical College in Qatar, Doha, Qatar

Clinical Anaesthesiology Department, College of Medicine Qatar University, Doha, Qatar

Anaesthesia and SICU Department, Tanta University, Tanta, Egypt
e-mail: nshallik@hamad.qa

N. A. Shallik (ed.), *Flow Controlled Ventilation Mode Through a Straw Size Tube*, https://doi.org/10.1007/978-3-031-77477-5_13

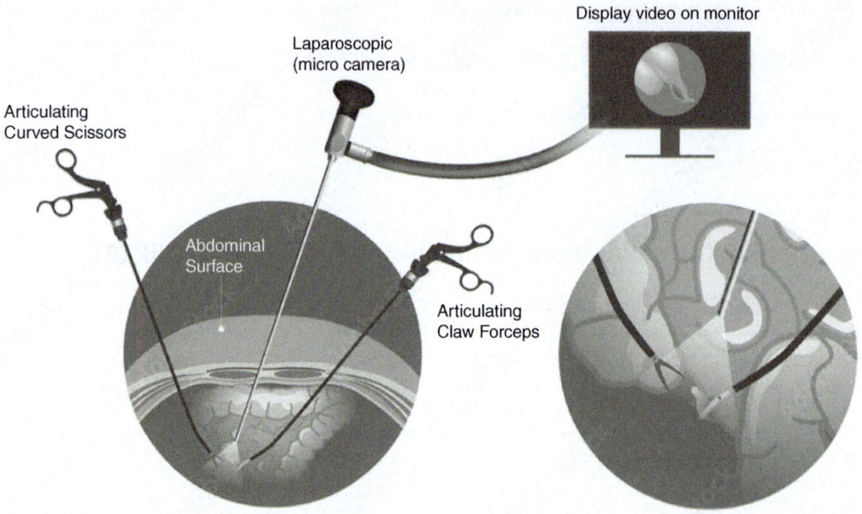

Fig. 1 Graphical description of laparoscopic surgery (free download from https://stock.adobe.com/qa/search?k=&token_type=bearer&expires_in=86399&asset_id=175646829)

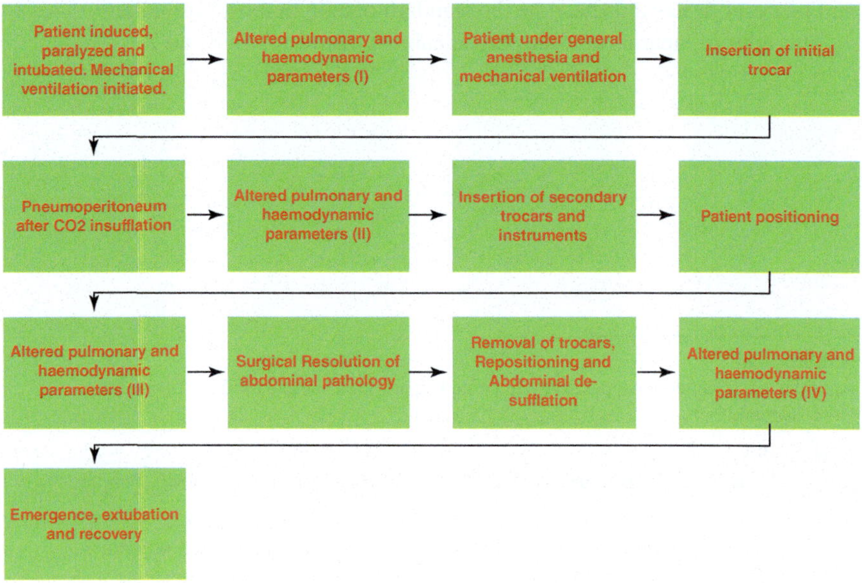

Fig. 2 Critical steps in patient management during laparoscopic surgery. The surgical patient can undergo significant pulmonary and haemodynamic changes on at least four separate instances during a laparoscopic surgery

2 Physiological Changes

Laparoscopy is associated with significant physiological changes in the patient due to pneumoperitoneum and extreme positioning. These changes are described below:

1. Change in lung mechanics: Abdominal distension due to insufflation of carbon-dioxide (CO_2) gas, limits diaphragmatic excursion, increases intra-thoracic pressure, reduces pulmonary compliance and functional residual capacity (FRC), and increases pulmonary atelectasis [1, 2]. Chest walls become stiffer at low volumes [2]. Cephalad diaphragm displacement along with increased minute ventilation, increases airway pressures. There is increased peak and plateau pressures [3].
2. Ventilation-perfusion mismatch (V–Q mismatch): Splinting of diaphragm, reduced lung volumes and atelectasis causes V–Q mismatch leading to increased partial pressure of CO_2 (PCO_2) and reduced partial pressure of O_2 (PO_2). As CO_2 is highly blood soluble, it is absorbed across the large peritoneal surface into the circulation and later expired by the lungs causing increases in end-tidal CO_2 [3, 4].
3. Increase in intra-abdominal Pressure (IAP) and changes in haemodynamics: As Intra-abdominal volume increases, compensatory mechanisms minimize initial change in IAP. There-after IAP increases, causing compression of inferior vena cava and major arteries. There is thus reduced cardiac preload, reduced cardiac output, and increased systemic vascular resistance [3, 4].
4. Effects of position: Most physiological changes in laparoscopic surgeries due to pneumoperitoneum are increased due to position changes. Trendelenburg position (as adopted in laparoscopic appendectomy) increases reduction in lung volumes and atelectasis but preserves venous return and cardiac output. Reverse-Trendelenburg position (as adopted in laparoscopic cholecystectomy) reduces the changes in lung volumes and atelectasis but reduces venous return and cardiac output [3, 4].
5. Changes in arterial blood gas (ABG): CO_2 insufflation into the abdomen along with V–Q mismatch causes increased CO_2 in the patient's system, which if not excreted by adequate minute ventilation will lead to hypercapnia and respiratory acidosis. There can also be reduced PO_2 [4].
6. Alveolar recruitment maneuver: Alveolar collapse especially in basal lung segments occur because increased intra-abdominal pressure in addition to effects of positioning, contribute to reduced functional residual capacity, intra-pulmonary shunt and V–Q mismatch [5]. Alveolar recruitment maneuver is performed to re-open collapsed alveoli thereby improving oxygenation. Studies have also shown improved respiratory mechanics after recruitment. This is especially useful before peritoneal insufflation has taken place, as improved oxygenation (increased PO_2 and reduced Alveolar-arterial gradient) due to the alveolar recruitment maneuver, is sustained even post peritoneal insufflation (if there is otherwise no PEEP by the ventilator) [5, 6]. Another study looked at the combined effects of recruitment maneuver and PEEP in obese and non-obese patients undergoing laparoscopic surgery, after pneumoperitoneum was established [7].

Both obese and non-obese patients experienced improved end-expiratory lung volumes after administration of PEEP, post pneumo-peritoneum. However, PEEP alone, did not significantly change oxygenation. It was found that alveolar recruitment maneuver in addition to PEEP further improved end-expiratory lung volumes and was found to be superior to PEEP alone, in improving end-expiratory lung volume, lung mechanics, and arterial oxygenation [5, 7]. Another study in morbidly obese patients (BMI >40 kg/m^2) found a combination of alveolar recruitment and PEEP is more effective at reducing atelectasis and improving PO_2:FiO_2 ratio than either alone [8]. Because of these reasons, use of alveolar recruitment maneuvers and PEEP in maintaining improved oxygenation is essential in patients undergoing laparoscopic surgeries and its effect has been found to be sustained even after peritoneal insufflation.

3 Airway and Ventilation

Most anaesthetists will choose to intubate patients with a cuffed endotracheal tube (ETT). Because of increased intra-abdominal pressure, there is a theoretically increased risk of gastric regurgitation [9–12]. This combined with the patient's pre-existing abdominal pathology may lead to increased risk of pulmonary aspiration. Use of a cuffed endotracheal tube provides protection against aspiration. An alternative is the use of a laryngeal mask airway (LMA) with adequate seal incorporated into the design (e.g. LMA Pro-seal™ or LMA Supreme™) [12–15].

Additionally, it is important for the airway device to tolerate the driving pressure from the ventilator to maintain adequate gas flow during ventilation of the patient with a pneumo-peritoneum. Use of an ETT will reduce chances of gas leaking in the system during positive pressure ventilation allowing sufficient tidal volumes and positive end-expiratory pressure (PEEP) to be maintained. This contrasts with a LMA which in response to high driving pressures may increase gas leak due to inadequate seal.

Because of these reasons, *the de-facto technique of airway and ventilation for laparoscopic patients remains intubation with a cuffed ETT, with intermittent positive pressure ventilation and a PEEP of at least 5 cmH$_2$O and adequate minute ventilation to maintain normocapnia* [1, 3, 4].

4 Volume Control Mode, Pressure Control Mode and Flow Dynamics (Fig. 3)

Both volumes controlled (VC) and pressure controlled (PC) ventilatory modes have been extensively used in laparoscopic surgeries. VC maintains pre-set tidal volume with variable airway pressures depending on lung compliance and airway resistance i.e. dynamic pulmonary compliance. Physicians must adjust for I:E ratio and respiratory rate. PC maintains constant airway pressures with varying tidal volumes depending on dynamic pulmonary compliance.

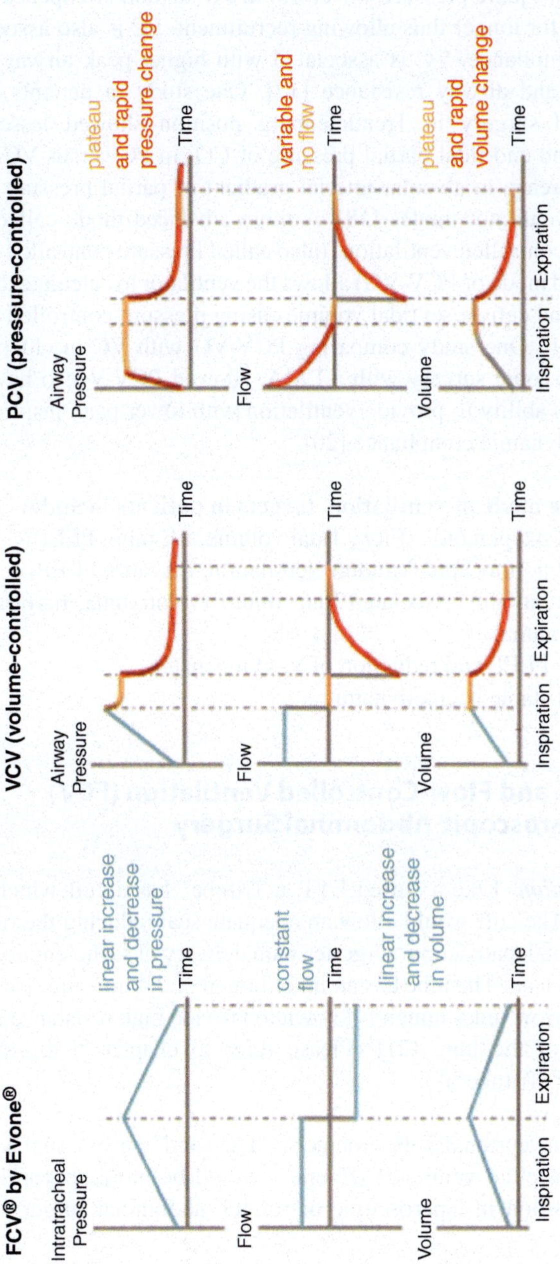

Fig. 3 In volume-controlled ventilation (centre): Square flow waveform and descending airway pressures. In pressure-controlled ventilation (right): descending flow waveform and square pressure waveform. In flow controlled ventilation (left): constant positive and negative flow and linear increase and decrease in pressure. (Ventinova Medical (Eindhoven, the Netherlands))

Compared to VC, PC maintains lower peak airway pressures and higher mean airway pressures during surgery. This may translate to improved oxygenation [16]. Additionally with a square pressure waveform in PC, alveoli are opened much earlier and stay open for longer thus allowing recruitment. PC is also associated with improved lung compliance. VC is associated with higher peak airway pressures, plateau pressures and airway resistance [17]. One study in patients posted for robotic abdominal surgery in Trendelenburg position showed lesser gradient between arterial and end-tidal partial pressure of CO_2 in PC versus VC. However, there was no difference in alveolar-arterial gradient of partial pressure of oxygen between the two ventilator modes [18]. A more advanced mode called 'pressure regulated volume-controlled ventilation' (also called Pressure controlled ventilation volume-guaranteed mode or PCV-VG) allows the ventilator to calculate the patient's lung compliance and deliver set tidal volumes using pressure-controlled ventilation flow dynamics [19]. One study comparing PCV-VG with VC in elderly patients undergoing laparoscopic surgery with a LMA, showed PCV-VG to have superior results to VC in its ability to provide ventilation with lower peak inspiratory pressures and greater dynamic compliance [20].

Irrespective of the mode of ventilation, targets in patients include:

1. Maintenance of oxygenation (FiO_2, Tidal volume, I:E ratio, PEEP)
2. Maintenance of normocapnia (minute ventilation, I:E ratio, PEEP)
3. Avoidance of ventilator associated lung injury (volutrauma, barotrauma, biotrauma, atelectrauma)
4. Maintenance of PEEP and reduction of V–Q mismatch
5. Maintenance of stable haemodynamic

5 Tritube® and Flow-Controlled Ventilation (FCV) for Laparoscopic Abdominal Surgery

Airway Consideration Like a cuffed ETT, a Tritube® has a cuff which is placed below the glottis. The cuff would allow an adequate seal reducing the risk for pulmonary aspiration in laparoscopic surgeries with delivery of sufficient tidal volumes without significant leak. The tube has an inner lumen of 2.4 mm and outer diameter of 4.4 mm. The narrow inner lumen is known to provide high resistance and reduce passive deflation of the lung [21] (Please refer to chapter "Ultra-thin Cuffed Endotracheal Tube (Tritube®)").

The use of a Conventional Tube Adapter (CTA®) and conventional adult cuffed ETT and flow-controlled ventilator (Evone®) would be more appropriate during Trendelenburg position in laparoscopic or robotic abdominal surgery with FCV (Figs. 4, 5, and 6).

Ventilator Consideration Flow controlled ventilation (FCV) in the Tritube® allows for linear increase and decrease in intra-tracheal pressures, which is measured

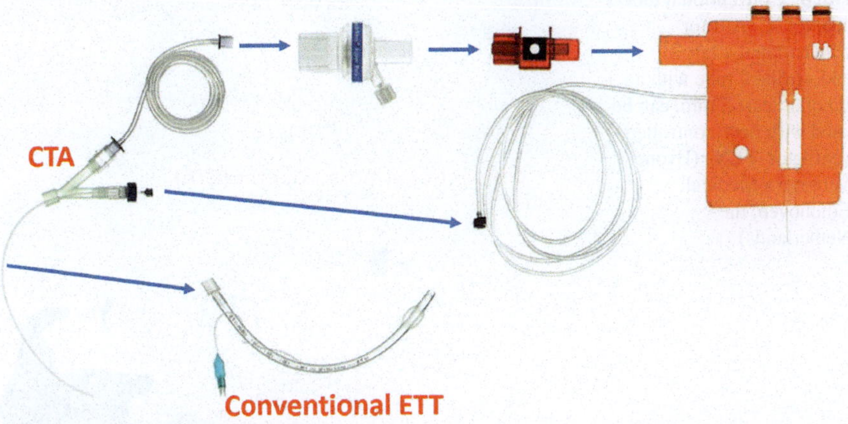

Fig. 4 Conventional tube adaptor (CTA®) and conventional adult endotracheal tube, can be used with flow-controlled ventilator (FCV) (Evone®) in laparoscopic or robotic abdominal surgery (Ventinova Medical, Eindhoven, the Netherlands)

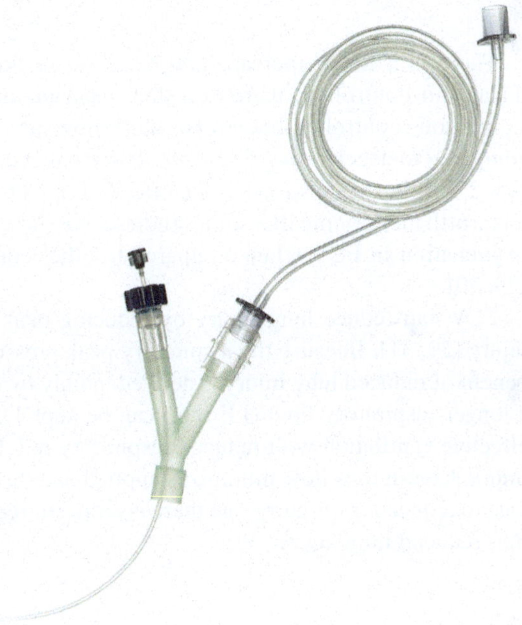

Fig. 5 Conventional tube adaptor (CTA®) (Ventinova Medical, Eindhoven, the Netherlands)

through one of the three lumens [21]. The difference in tracheal pressures accounts for the flow. The physician can set the inspiratory flow rate, I:E ratio, peak inspiratory pressure, FiO_2 and end-expiratory pressure (EEP). Inspiratory and expiratory flows are kept constant and low (<20 l/min) [22].

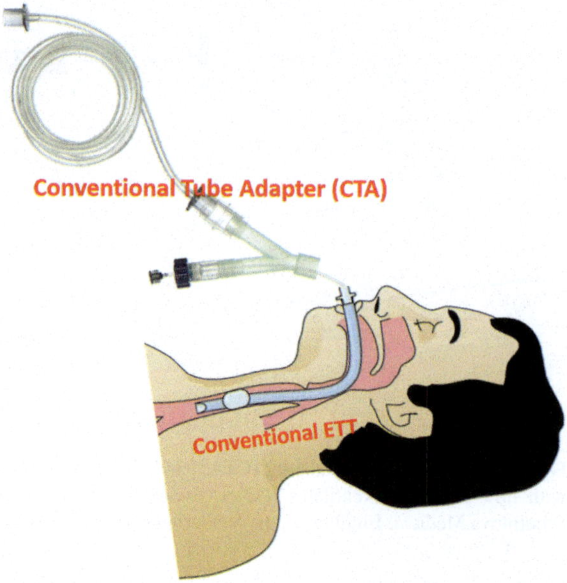

Fig. 6 Conventional tube adaptor (CTA®) for conventional adult endotracheal tube with an ID of at least 5 mm, can be used with flow-controlled ventilator (FCV) (Evone®) Ventinova Medical, Eindhoven, the Netherlands)

There is a linear increase and decrease in tidal volume. Since expiration is linear and controlled, there is a decreased incidence of alveolar collapse [23]. Continuous controlled linear expiratory flow also improves ventilatory efficiency compared to decelerating flow [24]. These enhance gas exchange and oxygenation [25–27]. It has been shown to be effective in CO_2 elimination [27, 28]. However, it is worth mentioning that some studies have shown similar (rather than increased) oxygenation in FCV when compared to other conventional modes of ventilation [29, 30].

FCV can reduce lung injury by reducing peak inspiratory flow induced shear injury [29, 31]. Because the inspiratory peak pressure pattern is same as in VC, the benefit of reduced lung injury is derived mainly by reduced flow with no pauses and a longer inspiratory time (I:E ratio can be kept 1:1). Additionally, it can maintain effective ventilation with reduced respiratory rate further reducing the risk of lung injury. Continuous flow minimizes applied and dissipated mechanical energy [27]. Due to reduced respiratory rate there is reduced frequency of energy dissipation and thus reduced lung injury [32].

In FCV since flow is controlled in both the inspiratory and expiratory phases of ventilation, it is possible to attain the lowest possible flow to attain a given minute ventilation provided both inspiratory and expiratory flows are made equal. With lowest overall flow there is least amount of energy dissipation to the lung parenchyma and airways [32].

A study by Weber et al compared FCV and VC in obese patients undergoing elective bariatric surgery. FCV was associated with lesser decrease in end-expiratory lung volumes and mean lung volumes when compared to VC. 'Mean tracheal pressures' (for the whole ventilatory cycle) and 'Mean tracheal pressures during expiration' were higher in FCV [21]. Just as it can effectively prevent atelectasis in obese patients, it has been postulated to be able to prevent compression atelectasis in other high-risk patients such as laparoscopy and those in the Trendelenburg position [28].

FCV has been described to improve aeration without overinflation in animal studies by calculating and incorporating individualized patient lung compliance values [27]. This is possibly advantageous in patients undergoing laparoscopy as pneumo-peritoneum could lead to reduced and variable compliance for the duration of surgery.

Emergence, post-surgery, and pre-extubation can be facilitated by use of jet ventilation feature of the tri-tube [28, 33].

Haemodynamic Considerations Most studies have shown stable and comparable haemodynamics between FCV and other ventilation modes in otherwise healthy patients [21, 34]. It has been theorized that increased intra-thoracic pressures due to increased PEEP, mean airway pressures and lung volumes may decrease venous return and pre-load thereby affecting cardiac output. However, since the EEP in FCV is not significantly different from PEEP in other modes of ventilation, it would not translate into significant changes in pre-load. Additionally increased mean airway pressures in FCV may not translate to different haemodynamics in patients as the difference in mean airway pressures between FCV and other modes of ventilation may be small [26]. A study in a porcine model showed increased venous return, cardiac output and mean arterial pressure in FCV compared to other conventional ventilatory modes, because of the slow and stable mean increase/release intrathoracic pressure [35].

A summary of possible benefits is shown in Table 1.

Table 1 A summary of possible benefits of FCV and ultra-thin cuffed endotracheal tube

Potential benefits of Tritube® and FCV in laparoscopic surgery	Scientific rationale
1. Reduced aspiration risk	Cuffed Tritube® below the glottic opening
2. Improved CO_2 clearance	Active continuous expiration, low flow with stable inspiratory and expiratory flow pattern and advantages of 1:1 I:E ratio
3. Reduced alveolar collapse	Controlled expiratory flow and maintenance of higher mean airway pressure and end-expiratory pressure (EEP)
4. Maintained tidal volume	It is possible to individualize each patient's compliance and set ventilator settings to achieve the target tidal volume and minute ventilation
5. Reduced incidence of ventilator induced lung injury	Better and homogenous aeration of lungs due to continuous and controlled flow during inspiration and expiration. Reduced application and dissipation of mechanical injury. Reduced respiratory rate for the same amount of ventilation thus reducing the number of respiratory cycles and frequency of energy dissipation
6. Stable haemodynamics	The increase in mean airway pressure, end-expiratory pressure and lung volumes is not significant enough to reduce pre-load to the heart
7. Upper airway stenosis situations	Ultrathin endotracheal tube (Tritube®) is very useful in intubating the trachea of patients during laparoscopic abdominal surgery, if they have critical airway stenosis or partial upper airway obstruction [36]. Use of 3D CT reconstruction and Virtual Endoscopy (VE) of the upper airway are also valuable in trachea- bronchial stenosis planning and management [37]
Potential practical concerns for Tritube®	Scientific rationale and management
1. Easy dislodgement	Since it is a narrow tube with high resistance, there is an increased risk of dislodgement especially if a patient coughs or if there are steep surgical positions. It is advisable to pay extra caution to securing the tube well It may be advisable to use CTA® and traditional ETT to overcome this problem
2. Blockage of inner lumen	This has been reported as the most common complication due to secretions and kinking. Once an obstruction is detected, there will be an alarm (see below) and the anaesthetist will have to clear the obstruction. If the obstruction is due to secretions, it is possible to clear its by using the jet ventilation mode of the ventilator. Additionally, one may try to decrease secretions by anti-sialagogue treatment. Good hydration also liquifies secretions and renders them less thick and sticky (in the event of blockage by secretion, flow controlled ventilator wouldn't be able to deliver the intended flow, and therefore the tidal volume). Alarm of unattained tidal volume will start, and possibly also the alarm of increased airway pressure. In that case one should disconnect and use a 10-ml syringe filled with normal sterile saline and flush the lumen(s) of the Tritube®. Flushing with pressure is required to force any secretions or clotted blood out of the tube. Connect suction to clear any secretions within the lumen(s). Better to use CTA® and traditional ID diameter of ETT to overcome this problem (Figs. 4, 5, and 6)

6 Practical Considerations

The Tritube® is very small and can easily dislodge, especially in steep positions. Since dislodgement is one of the most common complications associated with its use, it is essential to gain practice in securing it well [33]. For the same reason, it is also essential to keep the patient deeply anaesthetized and always paralyzed since coughing can easily dislodge the tube [22]. Another common complaint with use of Tritube® is that its lumen can get blocked with secretions or get kinked [22].

During laparoscopic abdominal surgery using the Da Vinci® Robotic System, the differences in abdominal pressure, thoracic compliance, and tidal volume fluctuation can potentially make ventilatory management exceedingly complex by a conventional anaesthetist, when using FCV. Potential adjustments of the flow-controlled ventilator (FCV) can be required and can lead to serious unexpected events.

The use of CTA® with the flow-controlled ventilator would be more practical in laparoscopic surgery because of high abdominal pressures and use of Trendelenburg position. Robotic surgery, obesity, and increased tracheal secretions could displace and obstruct the Tritube® easily (Figs. 4, 5, and 6).

Other important clinical pearls:

- Change in abdominal pressure, thoracic and lung compliance during Trendelenburg position, insufflation/de-sufflation of abdominal gas, and surgical manipulation can lead to abrupt and excessively high or immediately reduced tidal volumes.
- Leakage due to repositioning or leakage of the cuff (high PEEP levels/ Trendelenburg position, pressures on the cuff etc.) can result in reduced tidal volumes, and absence of cycling to expiratory phase (only pressure checks). The warning during leakage handling is dependent on leakage and peak pressure/flow.
- Anaesthesia for FCV has been advised to be administered using total intravenous anaesthesia (TIVA) or Target Controlled Infusion (TCI) as it is not possible to administer anaesthesia gases through the same system.

6.1 Recovery from Anaesthesia and Extubation of Tritube®

For emergence, potential techniques have been well described and published in a previous review [33]. The authors of the review advise to either (1) Continue with FCV until extubation (or) (2) Switch to jet ventilation mode in flow controlled ventilator after deflating the cuff (or) (3) Use the Tritube® as subglottic insufflation catheter with FiO_2 of 1.0 and with cuff deflated for apnoeic oxygenation (or) (4) Establish spontaneous breathing and, if needed, provide ventilatory support with a standard airway device such as a facemask or laryngeal mask airway (LMA), either after removing the Tritube® or with cuff deflated and the Tritube® left in place.

However, in laparoscopic surgeries, where the patient may have an increased risk for regurgitation and pulmonary aspiration, it is essential to, if possible, deflate the stomach with a gastric tube under anaesthesia and not to deflate the cuff until the patient is fully awake. Thus, it is advisable to continue FCV with cuff inflated until the patient is fully awake and spontaneously breathing.

6.2 Recovery from Anaesthesia and Extubation of CTA®

Additional advantage of CTA® and conventional ETT is to connect them to the ventilator and extubate the patient conventionally (reversal of muscle relaxant, switch the ventilator to spontaneous respiration mode and extubate the patient as in regular practice).

7 Future Perspectives

Most of the previously-mentioned details have been extrapolated from existing studies which described use of FCV in different clinical settings. However, no study has yet been published that prospectively examined the effects of FCV in patients during laparoscopy surgery. Until such data becomes available, we would urge physicians to practice extreme caution while using FCV in such patients. Additionally, to generate evidence for the utility of FCV in laparoscopic surgeries, the authors of this chapter have proposed a Randomized Controlled Study, comparing the use of Tritube® and FCV mode in flow-controlled ventilator, with cuffed endotracheal tube and conventional volume-controlled ventilation, for assessing oxygenation and ventilation efficiency in ASA physical status 1 and 2 patients undergoing elective laparoscopic surgery. This is, as of the time of writing this article, still a work in progress.

8 Conclusion

In conclusion, the use of Flow Controlled Ventilation (FCV) strategy for mechanical ventilation, has been well described with multiple benefits to patients such as better and more homogenous lung aeration, improved CO_2 clearance and ventilator efficiency, reduced lung injury and stable haemodynamics. However, till date no study has compared FCV with other conventional ventilator modes for use in patients during laparoscopic surgery or robotic abdominal surgery. Until such data becomes available, we would urge physicians to practice extreme caution while using FCV in such patients.

Disclaimer In this chapter we introduced the flow-controlled manual ventilator (FCmV), exemplified frequently by the Ventrain®, merely because there is no alternative of its kind available commercially and thus, the readers may find a particular focus on the only commercially available FCV ventilator: the "Evone®" ventilator. Moreover the use of 'Tritube®' instead of ultra-thin or straw sized ETT nomenclature may be found due to the lack of other examples and is not intended as commercial endorsement of the products.

References

1. Hayden P, Cowman S. Anaesthesia for laparoscopic surgery. Contin Educ Anaesth Crit Care Pain. 2011;11(5):177–80.
2. Loring SH, Behazin N, Novero A, Novack V, Jones SB, O'Donnell CR, Talmor DS. Respiratory mechanical effects of surgical pneumoperitoneum in humans. J Appl Physiol. 2014;117(9):1074–9.
3. Atkinson TM, Giraud GD, Togioka BM, Jones DB, Cigarroa JE. Cardiovascular and ventilatory consequences of laparoscopic surgery. Circulation. 2017;135(7):700–10.
4. Carey BM, Jones CN, Fawcett WJ. Anaesthesia for minimally invasive abdominal and pelvic surgery. BJA Educ. 2019;19(8):254–60.
5. Jo YY, Kwak HJ. What is the proper ventilation strategy during laparoscopic surgery? Korean J Anesthesiol. 2017;70(6):596–600.
6. Park HP, Hwang JW, Kim YB, Jeon YT, Park SH, Yun MJ, Do SH. Effect of pre-emptive alveolar recruitment strategy before pneumoperitoneum on arterial oxygenation during laparoscopic hysterectomy. Anaesth Intensive Care. 2009;37(4):593–7.
7. Futier E, Constantin J-M, Pelosi P, Chanques G, Kwiatkoskwi F, Jaber S, Bazin J-E. Intraoperative recruitment maneuver reverses detrimental pneumoperitoneum-induced respiratory effects in healthy weight and obese patients undergoing laparoscopy. Anesthesiology. 2010;113(6):1310–9.
8. Reinius H, Jonsson L, Gustafsson S, Sundbom M, Duvernoy O, Pelosi P, et al. Prevention of atelectasis in morbidly obese patients during general anesthesia and paralysis: a computerized tomography study. Anesthesiology. 2009;111(5):979–87.
9. Maltby JR, Beriault MT, Watson NC. Use of the laryngeal mask is not contraindicated for laparoscopic cholecystectomy. Anaesthesia. 2001;56(8):799–820.
10. Asai T. Editorial II: who is at increased risk of pulmonary aspiration? Br J Anaesth. 2004;93(4):497–500.
11. Viira D, Myles PS. The use of the laryngeal mask in gynaecological laparoscopy. Anaesth Intensive Care. 2004;32(4):560–3.
12. Beleña JM, Ochoa EJ, Núñez M, Gilsanz C, Vidal A. Role of laryngeal mask airway in laparoscopic cholecystectomy. World J Gastrointest Surg. 2015;7(11):319–25.
13. Eschertzhuber S, Brimacombe J, Hohlrieder M, Keller C. The Laryngeal Mask Airway Supreme™–a single use laryngeal mask airway with an oesophageal vent. A randomised, cross-over study with the Laryngeal Mask Airway ProSeal™ in paralysed, anaesthetised patients. Anaesthesia. 2009;64(1):79–83.
14. Keller C, Brimacombe J, Bittersohl J, Lirk P, von Goedecke A. Aspiration and the laryngeal mask airway: three cases and a review of the literature. Br J Anaesth. 2004;93(4):579–82.
15. Lim Y, Goel S, Brimacombe JR. The ProSeal laryngeal mask airway is an effective alternative to laryngoscope-guided tracheal intubation for gynaecological laparoscopy. Anaesth Intensive Care. 2007;35(1):52–6.
16. Tyagi A, Kumar R, Sethi AK, Mohta M. A comparison of pressure-controlled and volume-controlled ventilation for laparoscopic cholecystectomy. Anaesthesia. 2011;66(6):503–8.
17. Oğurlu M, Küçük M, Bilgin F, Sizlan A, Yanarateş O, Eksert S, et al. Pressure-controlled vs volume-controlled ventilation during laparoscopic gynecologic surgery. J Minim Invasive Gynecol. 2010;17(3):295–300.
18. Veerasamy S, Kumar L, Kartha A, Rajan S, Kumar N, Purushottaman SS. Comparison of arterial to end-tidal carbon dioxide gradient P (a-ET)CO(2) in volume versus pressure controlled ventilation in patients undergoing robotic abdominal surgery in the Trendelenburg position. A randomised controlled study. Indian J Anaesth. 2022;66(Suppl 5):S243–s9.
19. Singer BD, Corbridge TC. Pressure modes of invasive mechanical ventilation. South Med J. 2011;104(10):701–9.

20. Wang P, Zhao S, Gao Z, Hu J, Lu Y, Chen J. Use of volume controlled vs. pressure controlled volume guaranteed ventilation in elderly patients undergoing laparoscopic surgery with laryngeal mask airway. BMC Anesthesiol. 2021;21(1):69.
21. Weber J, Straka L, Borgmann S, Schmidt J, Wirth S, Schumann S. Flow-controlled ventilation (FCV) improves regional ventilation in obese patients - a randomized controlled crossover trial. BMC Anesthesiol. 2020;20(1):24.
22. Grassetto A, Pettenuzzo T, Badii F, Barzaghi F, Carlon R, Dellarole S, et al. A new perspective during laryngo-tracheal surgery: the use of an ultra-thin endotracheal tube (Tritube®) and flow-controlled ventilation—a retrospective case series and a review of the literature. J Anesth Analg Crit Care. 2022;2(1):39.
23. Goebel U, Haberstroh J, Foerster K, Dassow C, Priebe HJ, Guttmann J, Schumann S. Flow-controlled expiration: a novel ventilation mode to attenuate experimental porcine lung injury. Br J Anaesth. 2014;113(3):474–83.
24. Abram J, Spraider P, Mathis S, Wagner J, Ranalter M, Putzer G, et al. Improved ventilation efficiency due to continuous gas flow compared to decelerating gas flow in mechanical ventilation: results of a porcine trial. Am J Physiol. 2023;324(6):L879–L85.
25. Schmidt J, Wenzel C, Mahn M, Spassov S, Cristina Schmitz H, Borgmann S, et al. Improved lung recruitment and oxygenation during mandatory ventilation with a new expiratory ventilation assistance device: a controlled interventional trial in healthy pigs. Eur J Anaesthesiol. 2018;35(10):736–44.
26. Weber J, Schmidt J, Straka L, Wirth S, Schumann S. Flow-controlled ventilation improves gas exchange in lung-healthy patients—a randomized interventional cross-over study. Acta Anaesthesiol Scand. 2020;64(4):481–8.
27. Spraider P, Martini J, Abram J, Putzer G, Glodny B, Hell T, et al. Individualized flow-controlled ventilation compared to best clinical practice pressure-controlled ventilation: a prospective randomized porcine study. Crit Care. 2020;24(1):662.
28. Bialka S, Palaczynski P, Szuldrzynski K, Wichary P, Kowalski D, Van Der Hoorn JW, et al. Flow-controlled ventilation – a new and promising method of ventilation presented with a review of the literature. Anaesthesiol Intensive Ther. 2022;54(1):62–70.
29. Wittenstein J, Scharffenberg M, Ran X, Keller D, Michler P, Tauer S, et al. Comparative effects of flow vs. volume-controlled one-lung ventilation on gas exchange and respiratory system mechanics in pigs. Intensive Care Med Exp. 2020;8(S1):24.
30. Sebrechts T, Morrison SG, Schepens T, Saldien V. Flow-controlled ventilation with the evone ventilator and tritube versus volume-controlled ventilation: a clinical cross-over pilot study describing oxygenation, ventilation and haemodynamic variables. Eur J Anaesthesiol. 2021;38(2):209–11.
31. Nucci G, Suki B, Lutchen K. Modeling airflow-related shear stress during heterogeneous constriction and mechanical ventilation. J Appl Physiol. 2003;95(1):348–56.
32. Barnes T, Enk D. Ventilation for low dissipated energy achieved using flow control during both inspiration and expiration. Trends Anaesth Crit Care. 2019;24:5–12.
33. Schmidt J, Günther F, Weber J, Wirth S, Brandes I, Barnes T, et al. Flow-controlled ventilation during ear, nose and throat surgery: a prospective observational study. Eur J Anaesthesiol. 2019;36(5):327–34.
34. Van Dessel ED, De Meyer GR, Morrison SG, Jorens PG, Schepens T. Flow-controlled ventilation in moderate acute respiratory distress syndrome due to COVID-19: an open-label repeated-measures controlled trial. Intensive Care Med Exp. 2022;10(1):19.
35. Berlin DA, Manoach S, Oromendia C, Heerdt PM. Automated expiratory ventilation assistance through a small endotracheal tube can improve venous return and cardiac output. Intensive Care Med Exp. 2019;7(1):6.
36. Shallik N, Elarref M, Khamash O, Abdelaal A, Radi Alkhafaji M, Makki H, Menon A. Management of critical tracheal stenosis with a straw sized tube (Tritube): case report. Qatar Med J. 2020;2020(3):48.
37. Shallik N, Labib A, Ganaw A, Shaikh N, Moustafa A, Hammad Y. Virtual bronchoscopy and 3D reconstruction in the critical care setting. Qatar Med J. 2019;2:81. https://doi.org/10.5339/qmj.2019.qccc.81.

Flow Controlled Ventilation in ICU Settings

Ans Alamami, Ahmed Labib Shehatta, and Nadir Kharma

1 Introduction

Conventional invasive mechanical ventilation (IMV) and extracorporeal life support (ECLS) are established making for the management of severe acute respiratory distress syndrome (ARDS) albeit with potential for significant complications. Flow controlled ventilation (FCV), a novel approach to IMV, offers several physiological advantages over conventional IMV and may negate the need for ECLS and hence may pose a potential role in the management of such conditions. In this chapter we will go over the principles, application and current evidence for FCV utilization in the critically ill patient.

A flow-controlled ventilator mediates its effect by controlling specific ventilator preset variables, specifically the flow rate, peak airway pressure (PIP), end-expiratory pressure, oxygen concentration, and inspiratory to expiratory (I:E) ratio of the respiratory cycle [1, 2]. On the other hand, the tidal volume and respiratory rate (RR) are reflections of the respiratory mechanics. Such a reflection of the primary effect has been evaluated in multiple studies, and it has been postulated that the flow-controlled ventilator and its active control of inspiratory and expiratory arm of the respiratory cycle's flow can help in more homogenous gas exchange in the lungs via a constant linear change. Controlling the expiratory flow linearly is achievable by regulating the tracheal pressure. Such a flow pattern will lead to more evenly distributed mechanical power through the lungs, and to some extent, the stored power at the elastance component of the respiratory system will be able to release the energy in a controlled fashion. Additionally, the heterogeneous distributed energy force through different lung components within a normal pressure limit

A. Alamami · A. L. Shehatta · N. Kharma (✉)
Department of Critical Care, Hamad Medical Corporation, Doha, Qatar
e-mail: nkharma@hamad.qa

N. A. Shallik (ed.), *Flow Controlled Ventilation Mode Through a Straw Size Tube*, https://doi.org/10.1007/978-3-031-77477-5_14

will be less significant, and this mechanism could explain the flow-controlled ventilation key role in patients with ARDS [3].

The hemodynamic effect of the positive pressure ventilation is determined by the level of PEEP and mean airway pressure provided. The major difference between the FCV and the other modes of mechanical positive pressure ventilation is the mean airway pressure, as the FCV would have a relatively higher mean airway pressure as a reflection of the high tracheal pressure. This effect has been evaluated by Weber et al. [4], and there was no significant difference in the hemodynamic parameters in terms of systolic, diastolic, and mean arterial pressures.

2 Technical Aspect

The application of FCV starts by identification of the patient in whom FCV would be beneficial and safe, that depend on several factor from the underlying insult to the patient respiratory mechanics, and the patient effort and work of breathing, the readiness of the patient to specific interventions requirement of the initiation and maintenance of the FCV, one the main challenges is the patient selection as FCV effectiveness would depend on the airway restiveness force and the presence of patient active effort, as that will result in alteration of the main idea of evenly distributed flow during the respiratory cycle. The application of FCV can be achieved by the utilization of small type of endotracheal tube or ultrathin tube such as the Ventinova ETT (Tritube®) (Ventinova Medical B.V., Eindhoven, The Netherlands) or with the help of conventional tube adapter (CTA®) (Ventinova Medical B.V., Eindhoven, the Netherlands) (Figs. 1, 2, 3, and 4). This manoeuvre would help maintain a constant flow at a rate of 1:1 during both phase of the respiratory cycle.

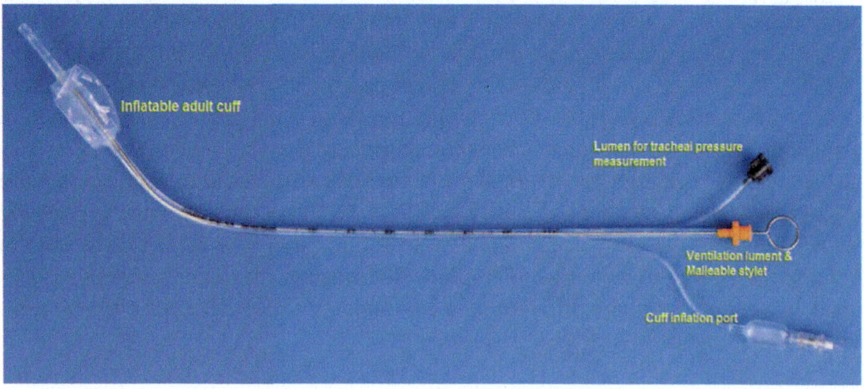

Fig. 1 Ultra-thin or Straw-size cuffed endotracheal tube. The ID of the tube is less than 3 mm, and the outer diameter (OD) is 4.4 mm, its length is 50 cm and it has three independent ports: a ventilatory lumen that opens at the tip of the tube and has a Murphy eye, a pressure-monitoring lumen that continuously measures the intra-tracheal pressure, and a cuff-inflation channel to inflate/deflate the cuff (Tritube® Ventinova Medical, Eindhoven, The Netherlands)

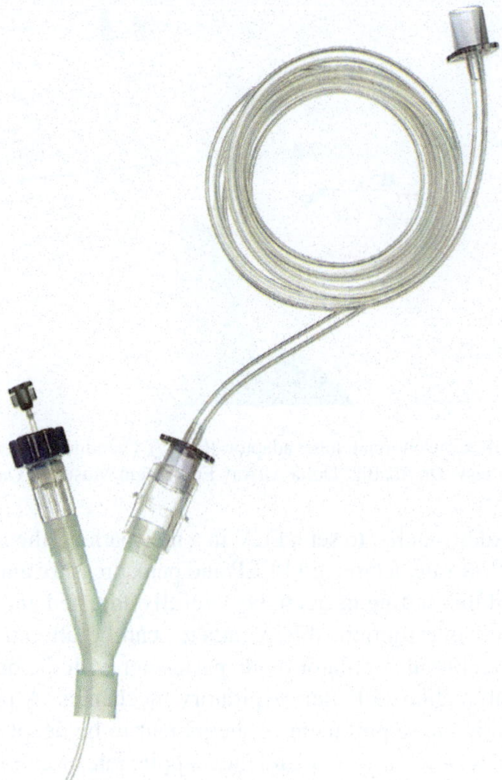

Fig. 2 Conventional tube adaptor (CTA®) for conventional adult endotracheal tube with an ID of at least 5 mm, can be used with flow-controlled ventilator (FCV) (Evone®) (Ventinova Medical, Eindhoven, The Netherlands)

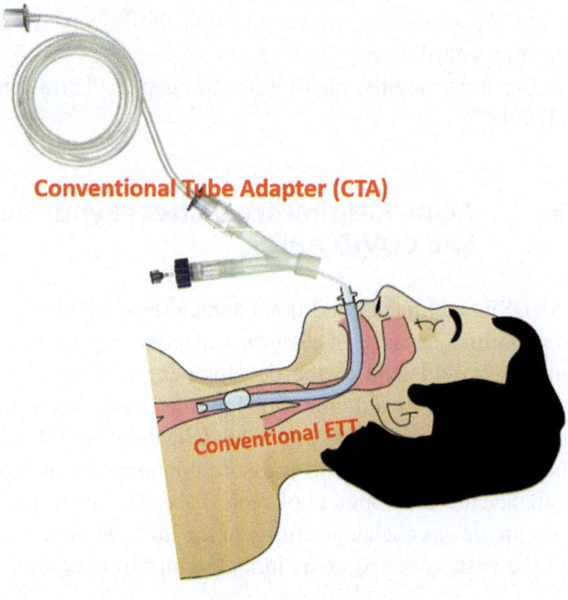

Fig. 3 Conventional tube adaptor (CTA®) for conventional adult endotracheal tube with an ID of at least 5 mm, can be used with flow-controlled ventilator (FCV) (Evone®) (Ventinova Medical, Eindhoven, The Netherlands)

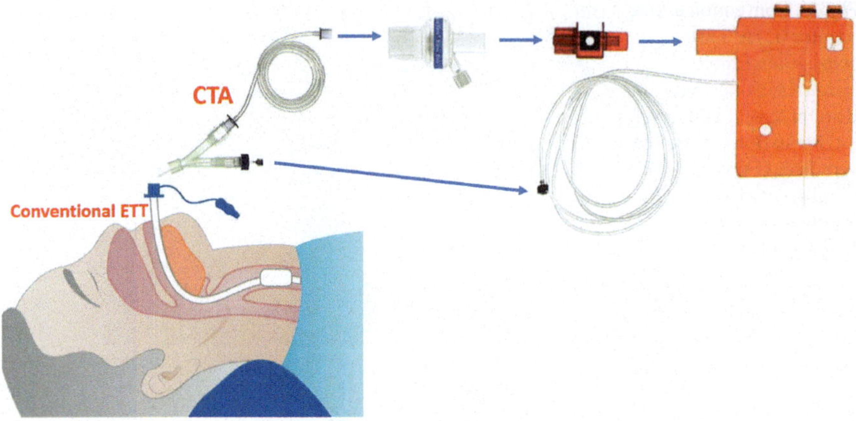

Fig. 4 Conventional tube adaptor (CTA®) (Ventinova Medical, Eindhoven, the Netherlands) (Courtesy, Dr. Shallik, Doha Airway Equipment Museum, Qatar)

Additionally, to set a FCV in a new patient, the main parameter to be tackled is the flow rate, a targeted PEEP and peak pressure and a targeted minute ventilation, all of this setting needs to be carefully adjusted and in specific intervals after each circuit interruption, this parameter can be altered in a similar way to the other conventional ventilator mode parameter with the best values corresponding to the highly achieved better respiratory mechanics. A potentially negative side of the FCV is the requirement of the patient to be deeply sedated in order not to intervene with the flow rate and the inapplicable circuit break in term of neutralization, bronchoscopy or suctioning as all of this can result in a significant change in the underlying ventilatory parameter and would require close monitoring over short intervals in order to make sure that the FCV setting would not result in a suboptimal ventilation.

For more details, please refer to chapter "Ultra-thin Cuffed Endotracheal Tube (Tritube®)".

3 Acute Respiratory Distress Syndrome (ARDS) and COVID ARDS

ARDS is a clinical condition characterized by lung inflammation-induced respiratory failure because of disturbed alveolar-capillary integrity. Such diffuse inflammation would lead to the development of heterogenous non-aerated lung areas, which in turn would affect the lung mechanics in terms of increased elastance and decreased compliance, and that delicately would affect the conditional relation between the volume and pressure containment in the alveolar space, as it would enhance the development of dead space. The dead space areas, which do not participate in the gas exchange ability of the lung, would result in shifting the blood supply to the better aerated areas in an attempt to overcome the ventilation limitation of such a space, and hence the pulmonary shunt mechanism ensues. The clinical criteria to diagnose ARDS are based on the Berlin definition [5] of acute onset presentation within less than 1-week, diffuse opacities on chest imaging not explained by pleural effusion or lung collapse, and a PO_2/FIO_2 ratio of less than 300 mmHg with a PEEP greater than 5 cmH_2O. The management of ARDS has to be simultaneously orchestrated toward ceasing the injuries underlying pathology and minimizing further lung insult, which can be achieved by treating the main cause of the presentation, providing a form of non-injurious controlled respiratory support to deliver a low tidal volume ventilation, prone positioning as both have been recommended for proven mortality benefit [6, 7]. Other suggested interventions such as utilization of non-depolarizing muscle relaxants and avoiding volume overload and balanced intravascular volume status have demonstrated a reduction of IMV duration and improvement in survival [8–10]. Contrarily, an inhaled pulmonary vasodilator such as nitric oxide has not been shown to improve outcome in ARDS [11, 12]. Mechanical ventilation remains the cornerstone for ARDS management specifically for a patient with an extensive and more severe form of lung injury despite perceived risks of ventilator-induced lung injury.

The clinical choice of using FCV for ARDS management is based on several physiological concepts and to what extent the injurious process has affected lung compliance along with the requirement of neuromuscular block and deep sedation. FCV generates the ability to have a continuous constant flow during the inspiratory and the expiratory phase of the respiratory cycle which leads to a more linear decrease in the peak and driving pressure [13, 14]. In a feasibility study, 11 patients with moderate ARDS due to severe acute respiratory syndrome-covirus 2 SARS-Cov2 were assigned to receive FCV through the Ventinova® ventilator with tube compensation mode after the initial application of pressure-controlled ventilation (PCV). Through the application of FCV, the gas flow was adjusted to achieve a RR and PIP similar to the initial PCV settings the total duration of the FCV was 30 min then the ventilation mode was shifted to the volume-controlled ventilation (VCV). The study revealed the feasibility of applying an FCV in patient with moderate ARDS though the result showed no difference in $PaO_2{:}FiO_2$ ratio and the average mean airway pressure were higher in the FCV. This can be attributed to the I:E ratio of 1:1 during the FCV and 1:1.5 during the VCV. Another finding was a lower minute ventilation and tidal volume during the FCV but with similar PCO_2 levels at the end of the 30-min trial [15]. In another application trial a case report by Spraider et al., on evaluating the feasibility of utilization of an FCV in COVID-19 induced moderate ARDS patients, the FCV initiation with a preset value mimicking the already used parameters on a PCV resulted in a linear and more stable airway pressure drop across the respiratory cycle evidenced by improved the peak and driving pressure and along with improvement in compliance and mechanical power, though this improvement was witnessed in the few hours after the institution of FCV which was intended for 30 min but nevertheless was extended to 2 and 4 h before reverting the mode to PCV due to drop in the PO_2/FiO_2 ratio readings [16]. Additionally, porcine studies have shown the improvement in oxygenation, lung recruitment and the reduction of the process of further lung injury with the utilization of FCV (Evone®,

Ventinova Medical, Eindhoven, The Netherlands) in terms of a significant increase in the PO_2 and the significant reduction in the alveolar wall and cellular infiltrate when compared to VCV [17]. In the same context, the use of expiratory flow-assisted ventilation (Ventrain®, Ventinova Medical, Eindhoven, The Netherlands) in the porcine model yielded a significant improvement in lung aeration (recruitment and in turn lung oxygenation capabilities in comparison to VCV [18].

4 Obesity

Obesity is global health issue in terms of cost, social and psychological impact, mortality and morbidity. In the critically ill; obesity poses significant risks, and these risks are related to the multiorgan impact of obesity, patient comorbidity and the practical and technical challenges in this category of patients. One of the difficulties that carries a significant risk is the airway and respiratory management [19].

Hypoxia is considered among the most frequently encountered disorder in morbidly obesity patient in the intensive care unit. Oxygenation decreases because of the higher work of breathing and increased oxygen consumption in addition to atelectasis which would reduce the functional residual capacity and further deteriorate the gas exchange. Taking that into consideration, the application of FCV has shown an improvement in the regional ventilation in obese patients. In a study by Weber et al., 23 obese patients were randomly allocated to a cross-over VCV vs FCV with comparable ventilator setting except the I: E ratio of 1:2 in VCV and passive expiratory flow, on the other hand in FCV group, the I: E ratio was set at 1:1 with active expiration. The study was powered to evaluate the difference in end-expiratory lung volume as a primary outcome. The study results were significant in terms of decreased loss of end-expiratory and mean lung volume with the application of FCV with a higher mean tracheal pressure which suggests improved recruitment and probably more homogenous aeration in FCV and that effect is likely related to the higher mean tracheal pressure and the linear expiratory flow in the FCV [20], this findings were supported by another trial involving 18 diabetic and obese patient with the similar finding of the loss of end-expiratory and mean lung volumes being less in FCV with higher tracheal mean pressure which plays a key role in maintaining the aeration through reservations the lung volumes and homogeneity [21].

The findings, despite study limitations, support the rule of FCV in obese patients and how it can overcome the major issue of preserving lung volume and overcoming decreased chest wall compliance in obese patients.

5 Laryngotracheal Stenosis

The management of patients with upper airway obstruction/ stenosis depends on the magnitude to which it compromises the air flow and whether the patient can generate inspiratory flow enough to maintain normal gas exchange or not. There is a remarkable difference between the acute life-threatening obstruction which is more likely to require an invasive intervention and the chronic limitation in term of the tumour, or infection-related tracheal stenosis.

FCV through standard endotracheal tube (ETT) and CTA® can be utilized in upper airway narrowing such as that caused by tracheal stenosis. FCV can also be applied in critical upper airway compromise where a specially designed ultra-thin endotracheal tube (Tritube®) can bypass the very narrow airway, achieve adequate oxygenation and decarboxylation and facilitate surgery.

The FCV in such a case can be utilized using a propriety ETT-the Tritube®-with an external diameter of only 4.4 mm and inner diameter of 2.4 mm. This ETT can pass through a significant narrow upper airway with the addition of sufficient ventilation with less risk of barotrauma [22].

In a systematic review of 17 studies by Mangahas et al., evaluating the different modalities for upper airway stenosis, 17 studies were included and the outcome determinant were technique failure, intra-operative hypoxia with the FCV (Evon®, Ventinova Medical, Eindhoven, The Netherlands) through Tritube® showed a low rate of technique failure similar to nonocclusive balloon dilator and superior to total intravenous anaesthesia (TIVA) with high flow nasal cannula (HFNC), laryngeal mask airway (LMA) and jet ventilation. Regarding intra operative hypoxia, the Tritube® was similar to HFNC with TIVA having a lower rate of hypoxia and superior to occlusive balloon dilator, LMA, and jet ventilator [23].

5.1 Minimize Aerosol Exposure During Percutaneous Tracheostomy in Highly Infectious Situations

SARS-CoV-2 ARDS patients has a more prolonged course of mechanical ventilation. This has led to challenges related to timing and performance of tracheostomy [24]. As tracheostomy is a high-risk aerosol generating procedure, infectious risk to the health care staff was leading to delays in performance of the procedure until the patient is negative for SARS-CoV-2. Many patients continued to be positive beyond 2–3 weeks of their hospital stay [25]. There is a significant need to find innovative approaches to decrease aerosolization while performing tracheostomy. Magasich-Airola described a new technique that utilizes FCV and Tritube® to achieve a more protective environment while performing tracheostomy in a COVID patient who is endotracheally intubated and on invasive mechanical ventilation [26]. The technique is briefly described in Fig. 5.

The intubated and sedated patient will receive a muscle relaxant and subsequently the endotracheal tube (ETT) is severed at its proximal end. This facilitates the simpler insertion of the Tritube® through the standard endotracheal tube (ETT) at the desired depth. Upon verifying the length marks of both tubes, the Tritube® is inserted into the ETT and pushed distally as far as feasible into the trachea. The Tritube® cuff has been inflated. Patient will be ventilated using the Evone® FCV system and the Tritube®. The ETT cuff can be safely deflated and the ETT can be pulled above the vocal cords. This will create a convenient and safe working area for the operator without the possibility of aerosolization by inflating the Tritube® cuff, which isolates the lower airways being

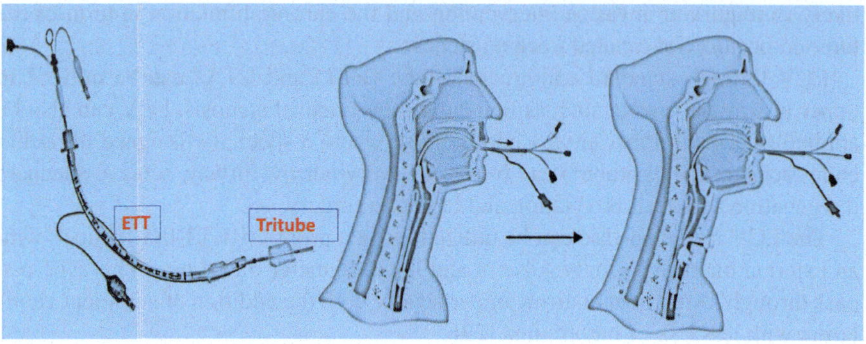

Fig. 5 Tritube® (Ventinova Medical B.V., Eindhoven, The Netherlands) in a tube for tracheostomy in COVID-19 patients to reduce the risk of aerosol exposure

ventilated. The narrow diameter of the Tritube® enables the tracheal cannula to be inserted without removing the Tritube®. The cuff of the cannula can be expanded, allowing the patient to be ventilated using a standard ventilator. Once the tracheostomy procedure is concluded and the tracheostomy cannula is in place, the cuff of Tritube® can be deflated, and along with the ETT withdrawn. Tritube® will easily pass alongside the inflated cuff of a tracheostomy cannula. In addition to significantly reducing the aerosolization of virus particles, the duration of apnoea is reduced when the patient is ventilated continuously on FCV, even during the insertion of the cannula. This enables the safe performance of tracheostomy in patients with severe hypoxia. This method can also be utilized for both surgical and percutaneous tracheostomy, providing a secure means of fiberoscopic visualization. Additional research should be undertaken to investigate the efficacy of using FCV with Tritube® as a protective measure in ENT surgery and at the ICU bedside for health care personnel.

5.2 Tritube® for Difficult Extubation in ICU

A study published in 2017, demonstrated that Tritube® (Ventinova Medical B.V., Eindhoven, The Netherlands) could be left in situ, after deflating the cuff, while performing face-mask ventilation. This use is rendered practical by virtue of an ultra-thin tube that does not interfere with the mask seal with the face. In this study, the vast majority of the patients tolerated the presence of the tube intratracheally and were able to talk and transferred to the recovery unit (PACU) until deemed fit for extubation [27].

5.3 Ultra-Thin Tube in "Cannot Intubate, Cannot Oxygenate" (CICO) Scenario in ICU

CICO is one of the most feared and better avoided airway emergencies. There are several ways to evaluate and secure the airway in a CICO situation. The most recognized technique for front of neck access (FONA) is the Scalpel cricothyroidotomy. Another way is the Surgical tracheostomy. The Tritube® cannula used with FCV can be used to facilitate Cannula cricothyroidotomy.

Cannula cricothyroidotomy involves creating an airway by inserting a small tube, typically as a 2 mm or 4 mm cannula, into the cricothyroid membrane. The cricothyroid membrane (CTM) is located by palpation and punctured to create a route for either a narrow bore (with an internal diameter of about 2 mm) or wide bore (with an internal diameter of approximately 4 mm) cannula. This allows for easier oxygenation [28]. Each technique has its unique advantages and drawbacks.

Performing a narrow bore cricothyroidotomy necessitates the use of a specialized high-pressure ventilation device, to provide low frequency, transtracheal jet ventilation (TTJV). This technique however is plagued with several problems. According to the data from the Fourth National Audit Project (NAP4) of the Royal College of Anaesthetists (RCoA) and the Difficult Airway Society (DAS), 63% of the narrow bore cannula cricothyroidotomies done were unsuccessful due to problems like incorrect placement of the device, bending of the cannula, and detachment of the cannula from the source of ventilation [29]. Furthermore, a comprehensive analysis of TTJV in CICO revealed a significant occurrence of procedure failure, barotrauma when TTJV is used and other complications [30]. If this technique is used in FONA during CICO, it should utilize a kink resistant cannula.

6 Weaning in FCV and Tritube®

The FCV mode necessitates profound sedation and precludes the patient's autonomous respiration, so ICU weaning regimens necessitate the utilization of alternative ventilation modalities. Following a brief period of breathing in FVC mode using a specialized Tritube® and considering other criteria, such as the possibility of aspiration, it may be feasible to cautiously awaken the patient with an inflated cuff. Upon regaining consciousness, deflate the cuff and remove the endotracheal tube from the patient, taking into consideration that the patient is unable to breathe while the cuff is inflated. To awaken the patient while utilizing the Tritube® with a deflated cuff, a breathing mode other than Forced Vital Capacity (FVC) is necessary.

All in all, the weaning process for the FCV does not differ from the weaning of the conventional modes of ventilation, starting by checking the reversal of the underlying reason of ventilation, maintain a near normal physiological parameter of respiration and hydrodynamics, then to proceed with shifting the patient to another conventional mode of ventilation in order to titrate the sedation and the NMB doses down aiming to stop them. The last step cannot be applied during the FCV phase of ventilation.

7 Weaning in FCV and CTA®

Evone® cannot be directly connected to traditional Endotracheal Tubes (ETT). However, this issue can be resolved by connecting a standard tube adapter (CTA®) with the classic ETT (Figs. 3 and 4). Therefore, FCV can be employed in intubated patients using a conventional tube adapter (CTA®) and Evone® with an endotracheal tube (ETT) that has an internal diameter (ID) greater than 5 mm. One of the added benefits of CTA® is its ability to link a traditional ETT to a Flow Controlled Ventilator (Evone®). Therefore, you can gradually reduce the patient's dependence on the ventilator and free them from it, just as you would in any other typical circumstances, by transitioning to a standard ventilator and removing the breathing tube as part of the usual procedure.

For more details, please refer to chapter "Liberation from Mechanical Ventilator: Art and Science of Weaning and Winning".

8 Conclusion

FCV aligns with the theoretical concepts of lung protective ventilation and can mitigate the difficulties associated with mechanical ventilation. It has been explored in different clinical settings including ARDS, obesity and in tracheal stenosis with favourable outcomes on oxygenation and mean airway pressure optimization while offering lung protective ventilation. An added benefit of FCV is the option to utilize a specialized ultra-thin tube with a compact outer diameter or traditional endotracheal tube with CTA® adaptor. This tube enables the ventilation of patients with abnormal airway structure, for whom conventional methods are impractical or notably challenging.

However, FCV method does have several drawbacks, including an increased workload for ICU staff, a larger chance of circuit obstruction due to secretions, limited access to ventilation data, and difficulty of weaning NMB and sedation. Future clinical trials are needed to further demonstrate the utility and impact of FCV on clinical endpoints like mortality, successful weaning, length of ICU stay and reductions in utilization of ECLS. As this will take time to be conducted, FCV use in academic institutions should be encouraged while local protocols are developed and improved based on gathered safety and use data.

References

1. Wittenstein J, Scharffenberg M, Ran X, et al. Comparative effects of flow vs. volume-controlled one-lung ventilation on gas exchange and respiratory system mechanics in pigs. Intensive Care Med Exp. 2020;8(1):24. https://doi.org/10.1186/s40635-020-00308-0.
2. Enk D, Abram J, Spraider P, Barnes T. Dynamic compliance in flow-controlled ventilation. Intensive Care Med Exp. 2021;9(1):26. https://doi.org/10.1186/s40635-021-00392-w.
3. Barnes T, van Asseldonk D, Enk D. Minimisation of dissipated energy in the airways during mechanical ventilation by using constant inspiratory and expiratory flows – flow-controlled ventilation (FCV). Med Hypotheses. 2018;121:167–76. https://doi.org/10.1016/j.mehy.2018.09.038.
4. Weber J, Schmidt J, Straka L, Wirth S, Schumann S. Flow-controlled ventilation improves gas exchange in lung-healthy patients— a randomized interventional cross-over study. Acta Anaesthesiol Scand. 2020;64(4):481–8. https://doi.org/10.1111/aas.13526.

5. The ARDS Definition Task Force. Acute respiratory distress syndrome: the berlin definition. JAMA. 2012;307(23):2526–33. https://doi.org/10.1001/jama.2012.5669.
6. Brower RG, Matthay MA, Morris A, Schoenfeld D, Thompson BT, Wheeler A, Acute Respiratory Distress Syndrome Network. Ventilation with lower tidal volumes as compared with traditional tidal volumes for acute lung injury and the acute respiratory distress syndrome. N Engl J Med. 2000;342(18):1301–8. https://doi.org/10.1056/NEJM200005043421801.
7. Guérin C, Reignier J, Richard JC, Beuret P, Gacouin A, Boulain T, Mercier E, Badet M, Mercat A, Baudin O, Clavel M, Chatellier D, Jaber S, Rosselli S, Mancebo J, Sirodot M, Hilbert G, Bengler C, Richecoeur J, Gainnier M, Bayle F, Bourdin G, Leray V, Girard R, Baboi L, Ayzac L, PROSEVA Study Group. Prone positioning in severe acute respiratory distress syndrome. N Engl J Med. 2013;368(23):2159–68. https://doi.org/10.1056/NEJMoa1214103. Epub 2013 May 20.
8. Papazian L, Forel JM, Gacouin A, Penot-Ragon C, Perrin G, Loundou A, Jaber S, Arnal JM, Perez D, Seghboyan JM, Constantin JM, Courant P, Lefrant JY, Guérin C, Prat G, Morange S, Roch A, ACURASYS Study Investigators. Neuromuscular blockers in early acute respiratory distress syndrome. N Engl J Med. 2010;363(12):1107–16. https://doi.org/10.1056/NEJMoa1005372.
9. Silversides JA, Fitzgerald E, Manickavasagam US, et al. Deresuscitation of patients with iatrogenic fluid overload is associated with reduced mortality in critical illness. Crit Care Med. 2018;46:1600.
10. Liu X, Jiang Y, Jia X, et al. Identification of distinct clinical phenotypes of acute respiratory distress syndrome with differential responses to treatment. Crit Care. 2021;25:320.
11. Adhikari NK, Burns KE, Friedrich JO, et al. Effect of nitric oxide on oxygenation and mortality in acute lung injury: systematic review and meta-analysis. BMJ. 2007;334:779.
12. Afshari A, Brok J, Møller AM, Wetterslev J. Inhaled nitric oxide for acute respiratory distress syndrome and acute lung injury in adults and children: a systematic review with meta-analysis and trial sequential analysis. Anesth Analg. 2011;112:1411.
13. Grasselli G, Calfee CS, Camporota L, et al. ESICM guidelines on acute respiratory distress syndrome: definition, phenotyping and respiratory support strategies. Intensive Care Med. 2023;49(7):727–59. https://doi.org/10.1007/s00134-023-07050-7.
14. Roehrig S, Ait Hssain A, Shallik NAH, et al. Flow controlled ventilation in acute respiratory distress syndrome associated with COVID-19: a structured summary of a study protocol for a randomised controlled trial. Trials. 2020;21:781. https://doi.org/10.1186/s13063-020-04708-1.
15. Van Dessel ED, De Meyer GR, Morrison SG, Jorens PG, Schepens T. Flow-controlled ventilation in moderate acute respiratory distress syndrome due to COVID-19: an open-label repeated-measures controlled trial. ICMx. 2022;10(1):19. https://doi.org/10.1186/s40635-022-00449-4.
16. Spraider P, Putzer G, Breitkopf R, et al. A case report of individualized ventilation in a COVID-19 patient – new possibilities and caveats to consider with flow-controlled ventilation. BMC Anesthesiol. 2021;21(1):145. https://doi.org/10.1186/s12871-021-01365-y.
17. Schmidt J, Wenzel C, Mahn M, et al. Improved lung recruitment and oxygenation during mandatory ventilation with a new expiratory ventilation assistance device: a controlled interventional trial in healthy pigs. Eur J Anaesthesiol. 2018;35(10):736–44. https://doi.org/10.1097/EJA.0000000000000819.
18. Schmidt J, Wenzel C, Spassov S, et al. Flow-controlled ventilation attenuates lung injury in a porcine model of acute respiratory distress syndrome: a preclinical randomized controlled study. Crit Care Med. 2020;48(3):e241–8. https://doi.org/10.1097/CCM.0000000000004209.
19. De Jong A, Chanques G, Jaber S. Mechanical ventilation in obese ICU patients: from intubation to extubation. Crit Care. 2017;21(1):63. https://doi.org/10.1186/s13054-017-1641-1.
20. Weber J, Straka L, Borgmann S, Schmidt J, Wirth S, Schumann S. Flow-controlled ventilation (FCV) improves regional ventilation in obese patients – a randomized controlled crossover trial. BMC Anesthesiol. 2020;20(1):24. https://doi.org/10.1186/s12871-020-0944-y.
21. Dmytriiev D, Dmytriiev K, Dmytriieva K. Flow-controlled ventilation (FCV) improves regional ventilation in obese patients with diabetis type 1 and 2. Eur Respir J. 2020;56(64):339. https://doi.org/10.1183/13993003.congress-2020.339.

22. Schmidt J, Günther F, Weber J, et al. Flow-controlled ventilation during ear, nose and throat surgery: a prospective observational study. Eur J Anaesthesiol. 2019;36(5):327. https://doi.org/10.1097/EJA.0000000000000967.
23. Mangahas AM, Talugula S, Husain IA. Anesthesia considerations during management of airway stenosis: a systematic review. Am J Otolaryngol. 2023;44(2):103767. https://doi.org/10.1016/j.amjoto.2022.103767.
24. Lamb CR, Desai NR, Angel L, et al. Use of tracheostomy during the COVID-19 pandemic: American College of Chest Physicians/American Association for Bronchology and Interventional Pulmonology/Association of Interventional Pulmonology Program Directors Expert Panel Report. Chest. 2020;158:1499–514.
25. Pichi B, Mazzola F, Bonsembiante A, et al. CORONA-steps for tracheotomy in COVID-19 patients: a staff-safe method for airway management. Oral Oncol. 2020;105:104682.
26. Magasich-Airola NP, Rosal Martins M, Desuter GR, Van Boven MJ. Novel technique for safe tracheostomy during COVID-19 pandemic using Evone® flow-controlled ventilation system. Int J Clin Pract. 2021;75(6):e13863.
27. Kristensen MS, de Wolf MWP, Rasmussen LS. Ventilation via the 2.4 mm internal diameter Tritube with cuff – new possibilities in airway management. Acta Anaesthesiol Scand. 2017;61(6):580–9.
28. Price TM, McCoy EP. Emergency front of neck access in airway management. BJA Educ. 2019;19(8):246–53.
29. Cook TM, Woodall N, Frerk C. Fourth National Audit Project of the Royal College of Anaesthetists and Difficult Airway Society. In: Cook TM, Woodall N, Frerk C, editors. Major complications of airway management in the United Kingdom. Report and findings. London: Royal College of Anaesthetists; 2011.
30. Duggan LV, Ballantyne Scott B, Law JA, Morris IR, Murphy MF, Griesdale DE. Transtracheal jet ventilation in the 'can't intubate can't oxygenate' emergency: a systematic review. Br J Anaesth. 2016;117(1):28–38.

Flow Control Ventilation in Intensive Care Unit: ARDS, COVID, and Alternative Uses

Piotr Palaczynski, Denis Kowalski, and Szymon Bialka

1 Introduction

As modern mechanical ventilation base on applying positive pressure to the lungs of the patient it is vastly different from physiological respiration [1]. Throughout the years, many efforts were undertaken to identify and limit modalities influencing lung injury during artificial ventilation [2]. One of the theories see energy dissipated in the lung tissue and originating from the mechanical power applied via respirators as a key factor. Barnes et al. calculated that ventilation with constant, controlled inspiratory and expiratory flow, inspiration to expiration ratio 1:1 and without ventilation pauses is most favourable in terms of utilized energy [3]. The development of technology led to creation of dedicated ventilator (Evone®, Ventinova Medical, Eindhoven, Netherlands), narrow bore breathing circuit and thin endotracheal tube (Tritube®, Ventinova Medical, Eindhoven, Netherlands) or alternatively tube adapter (Conventional Tube Adapter (CTA), Ventinova Medical, Eindhoven, Netherlands). These devices operate in flow control ventilation (FCV) mode with intratracheal pressures measured via separate pressure line. The conducted trials on short-term FCV in Operative Theatre indicated potentially lung protective characteristics of this method [4, 5].

Acute respiratory distress syndrome (ARDS) is a significantly heterogeneous disease with persistently high mortality despite the efforts undertaking to mitigate its effects of respiratory system [6]. A lot of attention is brought to ventilation practices in ARDS as the risk of secondary lung injury is high [7, 8]. Experimental studies have shown that some characteristics of FCV may be especially beneficial in ARDS [9].

P. Palaczynski · D. Kowalski · S. Bialka (✉)
Faculty of Medical Sciences in Zabrze, Department of Anaesthesiology and Intensive Care, Medical University of Silesia, Zabrze, Poland

N. A. Shallik (ed.), *Flow Controlled Ventilation Mode Through a Straw Size Tube*, https://doi.org/10.1007/978-3-031-77477-5_15

2 Feasibility

The starting point of discussion over the feasibility of FCV in ARDS are preclinical studies that use porcine model of respiratory system. Schmidt et al. have presented a study where conventional volume-controlled ventilation (VCV) was compared with FCV in terms of attenuation of lung injury in a model of induced ARDS. The results are favourable towards FCV as tissue markers of lung injury were significantly lower and lung aeration, gas exchange significantly higher in this group [10]. In addition, another study by Abram et al. examined the influence of individualized FCV and best clinical practice pressure-controlled ventilation (PCV) over the porcine respiratory system damaged by oleic acid infusion. The oxygenation, CO_2 removal, and haemodynamic stability were improved when FCV was performed [11]. These studies are valid foundation of continued efforts to translate and showcase the possible benefits of FCV in clinical studies.

However, there is extremely scarce evidence regarding the use of FCV in ARDS in humans. Up to date, only two case reports and two clinical trials were presented regarding this subject [12–15]. Chronologically, first report described the course of critical illness of a young 22-year-old patient admitted to the ICU after traumatic brain injury and blunt chest trauma [12]. The patient subsequently suffered from severe ARDS not responding to conventional mechanical ventilation and proning. As extracorporeal membrane oxygenation (ECMO) was contradicted due to administered anticoagulation the clinical team of Bergold et al. decided for alternative approach. Flow control ventilation was used with meticulous personalization of ventilator settings every 60–90 min. Throughout next 77 h patient's respiratory efficiency gradually improved leading to successful weaning from conventional ventilation in consecutive days. In the following years global pandemic of SARS-Co-2 virus hit and clinicians around the world were faced with new challenges regarding critically ill patients in need of protective ventilation.

The first case report of FCV application in ARDS due to severe acute respiratory syndrome coronavirus 2 (SARS-CoV-2) is presented by Spraider et al. [13]. A 50-year-old patient with a known SARS-CoV-2 infection 3 weeks prior to deterioration of respiratory function required mechanical ventilation and was moved to university hospital. Diagnostic imaging revealed vast ground glass opacities, however, at this point with protective ventilation strategy and proning ECMO therapy was not indicated. Due to further deterioration ventilator settings had to be readjusted and concerns were raised about the invasiveness of ventilation. To prevent secondary lung injury, FCV was initiated firstly with corresponding settings as in conventional PCV, and then personalized. At first improvement of PaO_2/FiO_2 ratio was observed with ventilator settings enabling reduction of mechanical power to 7.7 J/min (compared to 16.9 J/min in conventional mode). However, over the course of hours lung compliance decreased, the patient was proned and switched to pressure control ventilation. Hospitalization led to ECMO therapy and ultimately death due to secondary complications. Although unsuccessful in terms of patient outcome this case report brilliantly demonstrates the potential protective effect of FCV on lungs in terms of dissipated mechanical energy.

Moving on to recent clinical trials the study group of Van Dessel et al. [14] presented the feasibility and safety of FCV in moderate ARDS due to SARS-CoV-2 infection. Altogether 11 patients that presented symptoms of moderate ARDS according to the Berlin definition (100–200 mmHg PaO_2/FiO_2 ratio) with mechanical ventilation applied for no more than 10 days were included in the study. Issues that could influence respiratory function such as ECMO therapy, prone position or obesity were set as exclusion criteria. The patients were ventilated in PCV mode with settings determined by attending physician. The intervention consisted of ventilating the patients in FCV mode and VCV mode in turn for 30 min with corresponding settings as in PCV. Data around oxygenation, ventilation and haemodynamics was obtained and compared. No differences were found in terms of oxygenation and CO_2 removal with significantly lower tidal and minute volume in FCV group. What draws attention is the fact that no optimalization of ventilator settings were performed and secondly that no adverse events were noted throughout the investigation.

Finally, the most recent clinical trial by Grassetto et al. explores the feasibility of FCV even further in a group of ten COVID-19 ARDS patients with refractory hypoxemia ($PaO_2/FiO_2 < 150$ mmHg) placed in a prone position [15]. The study design was comparable to the previously described with several differences: intervention time was longer and lasted 4 h of each ventilation period and data was obtained during volume-controlled ventilation before and after switching to FCV. Ventilator settings were set with same PEEP/EEP values and equivalent driving pressure. The results demonstrated safety of FCV in a critical coronavirus disease of 2019 (COVID-19) ARDS and proned patient as well as significantly lower mechanical power and minute ventilation in FCV mode thus upholding improved ventilation efficiency claim.

To summarize existing evidence, the patients undergoing FCV in ICU setting were usually suffering from critical illness and moderate to severe ARDS, in most cases due to SARS-CoV-2 infection. In some instances, the decision to start FCV was an alternative for ECMO therapy. The overall period of ventilation was usually short, ranging from 30 min up to 72 h. No adverse events or complications regarding use of ventilator device or airway management were reported, constituting the safety and feasibility of FCV in these scenarios [12–15]. Some authors emphasize the need of optimalization of ventilation settings as the mechanics of FCV somewhat differs from conventional ventilation modes [13]. As this method of ventilation is novel, it does not yet have strong representation in literature. The benefit of FCV in terms of strong clinical endpoints such as long-lasting improvement of oxygenation or mitigation of lung injury is yet to be shown in future trials.

3 Perspectives for the Future

We still await results of a biggest clinical trial that planned to analyse and compare 20 patients with moderate to severe COVID-19 ARDS ventilated in FCV versus conventional ventilation mode for 48 h (NCT04399317 in ClinicalTrials.gov registry) [16]. The trial's main focus is a possible improvement of oxygenation throughout the analysed period. More recent trial that begun the recruitment of patients in September 2023 plans to enrol 28 participants suffering from moderate to severe ARDS of any aetiology and intubated for no more than 72 h (ClinicalTrials.gov Identifier: NCT06051188). The special emphasis of this study is given to the effects of FCV on respiratory physiology as the intervention includes Electrical Impedance Tomography imaging and transpulmonary pressure measurements. Also, as was shown in preclinical study by Schranc et al., use of FCV may be possible in paediatric populations in the near future both for ventilation of healthy and injured lungs [17].

Aside from studies strictly regarding ventilation in ARDS a number of ongoing trials concerning short-term ventilation during one lung ventilation (ClinicalTrials.gov Identifier: NCT04534933) or energy dissipation to respiratory system during abdomen surgeries (ClinicalTrials.gov Identifier: NCT06222463) may improve our understanding of this innovative technique. The true position of FCV in ARDS ventilation remains to be seen as more reliable data will be presented in literature.

4 Possible Shortcomings

One of the possible setbacks in the usage of FCV in ICU is that this mode does not allow and incorporate spontaneous respiratory drive of the patient. The clinical consequence of this fact is that deep sedation and in some instances muscle paralysis may be needed to achieve appropriate conditions. So with commencement of weaning protocols that may improve the patient outcomes the sedation has to be reduced and ventilation switched to conventional modes [18]. As the weaning from the ventilation is an important process in recovery from critical illness the existing technology of FCV does not offer any solution.

Previous studies have shown the enhanced benefits of FCV when precise optimalization of ventilation settings is being done [11–13]. Some reports advice on adjusting the parameters every 60–90 min [12]. As the process of optimizing ventilation may be laborious and time-consuming, the workload of tending to patient increases. What is more every disconnection of the breathing circuit, bronchofiberoscopy or nebulisation trigger the temporary need of conventional ventilation and when switching back to FCV optimalization may be needed.

Although the design of breathing circuit may seem simple the current cost of the disposable equipment for ventilating the patient is considerable. What is more, the equipment is usable up to 72 h. The noise generated by the FCV work is significantly higher compared to standard ventilators according to our experiences. As noise pollution may influence several physiological factors another source of sound in close proximity to the patient may be disadvantageous [19].

Several aspects of FCV need special attention as this method is novel and slightly differ from the conventional existing modes. The intratracheal pressure measurement allow insight into respiratory mechanics, however not all data regarding ventilation are available to users, example being pressure-volume loops [13]. We hope that future generation of ventilators compatible with FCV will provide more in-depth information.

One of the issues faced when using FCV is associated with precision of the intra-tracheal measurements and narrowness of the breathing circuit. The excessive amounts of secretion in the airways may prove the ventilation highly inconvenient, as it can partially obstruct the narrow endotracheal tube, the pressure line of CTA or even the circuit. Every time the secretions are suctioned the circuit has to be disconnected or ventilation switched to conventional. In case of ARDS caused by lung inflammation or other respiratory diseases the issue of secretion may prove problematic.

5 How Do We Do It?

Based on the data reported in the literature regarding the use of FCV and our own experiences, we would like to present our approach to clinical management of this novel method. Decision-making while treating the patient in critical condition is often difficult and requires tailored and individualized approach [8]. Therefore, the presented information is more of a guiding principle rather than a step-by-step recipe.

First is the decision to initiate the FCV. Usually, the trigger to debate the viability of this method is newly recognized ARDS, regardless of aetiology, with PaO_2/FiO_2 ratio less than 150 mmHg. Additional reason would be the invasiveness of the current conventional ventilation that can cause secondary lung injury.

Currently, it is possible to apply FCV through a Conventional Tube Adapter (CTA) or a "tube in tube" technique, where a thin endotracheal tube Tritube® (Tritube®, Ventinova Medical, Eindhoven, Netherlands) is inserted into a standard tube. As a method of choice, we use CTA as we perceive this method as easier and more convenient. What we see as crucial is to minimize the moments of apnoea and loss of PEEP as it may contribute to generate atelectasis and de-recruitment of alveoli. As a standard before switching to FCV from conventional ventilation we clamp the endotracheal tube with surgical instrument, only when the seal over the airways is secured, we introduce pressure measurement line into the tube and open the instrument. If the airways are managed with tracheostomy tube our procedure is analogous to the described above without clamping the tube.

As a general rule while ventilating in FCV mode, we maintain deep sedation. The choice of sedatives depends on patient's characteristics, however, usually multimodal sedation with additional opioid is chosen. We monitor the level of sedation maintaining the Richmond Agitation-Sedation score between −4 and −5 [20]. If it is indicated, we introduce neuromuscular blocking agents [21]. What is important, the respiratory drive of the patient should be non-existent or significantly decreased as the FCV mode do not incorporate patient's spontaneous breathing.

The proper management of ventilator's settings is one of the main concerns. The conventional mechanical ventilation is being set according to the principles of lung protective ventilation and optimal PEEP decided as standard of care. When switching to FCV we start the ventilation with the same PEEP value, corresponding driving pressure, inhalation to exhalation ratio 1:1 and flow rate of 12 l/min. Thus, we begin the adjustment of the ventilator settings, first determining the optimal PEEP with incremental or decremental PEEP trial while maintaining same driving pressure. The highest tidal volume or best dynamic compliance defines optimal PEEP. Then we identify optimal P_{peak} by increasing its value and observing the tidal volume up to the point where no over-proportional increase regarding measured dynamic compliance is seen. This strategy is also used by several authors and may help determine lower and upper inflection point of pressure/volume loop [13, 22, 23]. Next, we adjust flow rate, starting from 12 l/min we check arterial blood gases around 30 min from the onset of ventilation targeting pH at no less than 7.2 if no other modalities influence this decision. Finally, we check overall ventilation parameters and if no extremes are present, we continue the FCV up to another optimalization. The interval between interventions is usually set at 2 h, however, if alarming trends are present, it is shortened. Also, every suction of excessive secretions or disconnection of the tubes causes the need to reassess the ventilation parameters. Additional interventions such as prone positioning may be performed according to our standard of care; however, no nebulized medications can be administered. If there is need for fibre-optic bronchoscopy the patient is temporarily switched to conventional ventilation.

If the benefits of FCV use are observed the ventilation is carried out for 72 h on a single set of equipment. The decision to reduce the sedation or beginning to wean the patient from the respirator that outweighs the benefits of FCV usually results in switching to conventional ventilation. Just as initiation, the termination of FCV is a choice based on numerous modalities and has to be "tailored" to suit the patient needs.

6 Alternative Uses of FCV in Intensive Care Unit

6.1 FCV for Stenosed Airway in ICU

There are several alternative uses for FCV and armamentarium of thin endotracheal tubes. Among others, the thin endotracheal tube with outer diameter of 4.4 mm enables airway management of high-risk patients with distorted anatomy of upper airways. In literature, there are a number of case reports and observational studies describing handling of the patients with tracheal stenosis and difficult airways [24–27]. Such procedures may be easily implemented to suit the needs of Intensive Care Therapy, especially if the postoperative thoracic and laryngo-surgery patients are treated. What is more, the thin endotracheal tube can be left in the trachea with deflated cuff after emergence from anaesthesia or sedation securing the airways as tube exchanger [28].

6.2 FCV for COVID-19

During COVID-19 pandemic, several issues influenced procedures performed in ICU. One of them was possible contamination of hospital environment with aerosols containing highly contagious particles of respiratory viruses [29]. Exposure to

SARS-CoV-2 could influence both patients and healthcare workers, thus steps were undertaken to minimize the risk [30]. One of the frequent interventions in critically ill with prolonged respiratory insufficiency is percutaneous tracheostomy, however, in COVID-19 patients, a higher prevalence of complications is observed [31]. Combing this with a risk of aerosol generation, a safe bedside percutaneous tracheostomy may be challenging even for experienced operators. A new technique of this procedure was proposed by Magasich-Airola et al. that utilize thin endotracheal tube (Tritube®, Ventinova Medical, Eindhoven, Netherlands) and FCV [32]. This technique was being adapted and practiced in our hospital.

6.3 FCV for Percutaneous Tracheostomy

Before the onset of percutaneous tracheostomy, we clamp the endotracheal tube with surgical instrument and decrease its length by cutting at proximal end. We continue conventional mechanical ventilation and introduce the thin endotracheal tube with outer diameter of 4.4 mm into the endotracheal tube, ideally with the cuff over bifurcation of trachea. The cuff is inflated and FCV initiated. A thin fibre-optic bronchoscope is used to ensure the correct position of the cuff and to identify the optimal location of the tracheostomy. If needed, the endotracheal tube is being retracted; however, we prefer that it remains in the trachea. While the FCV continues under the guidance of fibre-optic bronchoscopy, the stoma is created. Afterwards, the correct position of the tracheostomy tube is visualized by bronchoscope. We evacuate the Tritube® with deflated cuff and as it passes tracheostomy tube its cuff is inflated and conventional ventilation is initiated. The distinctiveness of this method is based on continuous ventilation throughout the operation that may limit the apnoea time and loss of PEEP. Also, the constant seal over the airways possibly reduces the environment contamination with aerosols. However, as the rationale for these effects is strong, they are yet to be proven in clinical trials.

7 FCV Weaning

The FVC mode requires deep sedation and does not allow the patient's own breathing, so ICU weaning protocols require the use of other ventilation methods. If ventilation was provided using Evone CTA and a conventional tube during weaning, the adapter should be disconnected from the tube and another method of oxygenating the patient should be used.

After short-term ventilation in FVC mode while using a dedicated Tritube and the presence of additional factors, such as the risk of aspiration, it is possible to gently awaken the patient with a filled cuff. After awakening, empty the cuff and extubate the patient, keeping in mind that the patient is not capable of breathing while the cuff is inflated. From our own experience, we know that a Tritube with an deflated cuff can remain in place in the event of expected complications as an airway safety device and is usually well tolerated by the patient in such a case.

Awakening the patient while using the Tritube with deflated cuff requires a ventilation mode other than FVC.

In difficult cases, especially after cardiac surgery, it may be useful to use a withdrawal protocol prior to extubation with a half-hour spontaneous breathing trial (SBT) along with an analysis of accepted weaning criteria/patient status and the performance and evaluation of an arterial blood gas test. This is only an applied and proposed protocol and should be adapted to local conditions.

8 Conclusion

FCV is consistent with the theoretical principles of lung protective ventilation and can reduce the complications secondary to the use of mechanical ventilation, and in some cases be an alternative to the introduction of ECMO therapy. An additional advantage is the possibility of using a dedicated tube with a small external diameter that allows not only the ventilation of patients with abnormal airway anatomy, for which the use of conventional methods is impossible or significantly difficult, but can also be used for the new method of percutaneous tracheostomy. This method is not without disadvantages, such as increased workload for staff, more noise, greater risk of obstruction of the circuit with secretions, limited availability of ventilation data and inability to take into account the patient's spontaneous respiratory drive. Popularizing the use of this method, increasing the amount of available data, creating appropriate standards, and developing the used devices can reduce their impact when using this method.

References

1. Pham T, Brochard LJ, Slutsky AS. Mechanical ventilation: state of the art. Mayo Clin Proc. 2017;92(9):1382–400. https://doi.org/10.1016/j.mayocp.2017.05.004.
2. Tonetti T, Vasques F, Rapetti F, Maiolo G, Collino F, Romitti F, Camporota L, Cressoni M, Cadringher P, Quintel M, Gattinoni L. Driving pressure and mechanical power: new targets for VILI prevention. Ann Transl Med. 2017;5(14):286. https://doi.org/10.21037/atm.2017.07.08. PMID: 28828361; PMCID: PMC5537108.
3. Barnes T, van Asseldonk D, Enk D. Minimisation of dissipated energy in the airways during mechanical ventilation by using constant inspiratory and expiratory flows - flow-controlled ventilation (FCV). Med Hypotheses. 2018;121:167–76. https://doi.org/10.1016/j.mehy.2018.09.038. Epub 2018 Sep 24.
4. Weber J, Schmidt J, Straka L, Wirth S, Schumann S. Flow-controlled ventilation improves gas exchange in lung-healthy patients- a randomized interventional cross-over study. Acta Anaesthesiol Scand. 2020;64(4):481–8. https://doi.org/10.1111/aas.13526. Epub 2019 Dec 30.
5. Weber J, Straka L, Borgmann S, Schmidt J, Wirth S, Schumann S. Flow-controlled ventilation (FCV) improves regional ventilation in obese patients - a randomized controlled crossover trial. BMC Anesthesiol. 2020;20(1):24. https://doi.org/10.1186/s12871-020-0944-y. PMID: 31992213; PMCID: PMC6986135.
6. Bellani G, Laffey JG, Pham T, Fan E, Brochard L, Esteban A, Gattinoni L, van Haren F, Larsson A, McAuley DF, Ranieri M, Rubenfeld G, Thompson BT, Wrigge H, Slutsky AS,

Pesenti A, LUNG SAFE Investigators; ESICM Trials Group. Epidemiology, patterns of care, and mortality for patients with acute respiratory distress syndrome in intensive care units in 50 countries. JAMA. 2016;315(8):788–800. https://doi.org/10.1001/jama.2016.0291.

7. Banavasi H, Nguyen P, Osman H, Soubani AO. Management of ARDS - what works and what does not. Am J Med Sci. 2021;362(1):13–23. https://doi.org/10.1016/j.amjms.2020.12.019. Epub 2020 Dec 26. PMID: 34090669; PMCID: PMC7997862.
8. Pelosi P, Ball L, Barbas CSV, Bellomo R, Burns KEA, Einav S, Gattinoni L, Laffey JG, Marini JJ, Myatra SN, Schultz MJ, Teboul JL, Rocco PR. Personalized mechanical ventilation in acute respiratory distress syndrome. Crit Care. 2021;25(1):250. https://doi.org/10.1186/s13054-021-03686-3. PMID: 34271958; PMCID: PMC8284184.
9. Wenzel C, Frey C, Schmidt J, Lozano-Zahonero S, Urban G, Schumann S. A linearized expiration flow homogenizes the compartmental pressure distribution in a physical model of the inhomogeneous respiratory system. Physiol Meas. 2020;41(4):045005. https://doi.org/10.1088/1361-6579/ab83e6.
10. Schmidt J, Wenzel C, Spassov S, Borgmann S, Lin Z, Wollborn J, Weber J, Haberstroh J, Meckel S, Eiden S, Wirth S, Schumann S. Flow-controlled ventilation attenuates lung injury in a porcine model of acute respiratory distress syndrome: a preclinical randomized controlled study. Crit Care Med. 2020;48(3):e241–8. https://doi.org/10.1097/CCM.0000000000004209. PMID: 31856000; PMCID: PMC7017946.
11. Abram J, Martini J, Spraider P, Putzer G, Ranalter M, Wagner J, Glodny B, Hell T, Barnes T, Enk D. Individualised flow-controlled versus pressure-controlled ventilation in a porcine oleic acid-induced acute respiratory distress syndrome model. Eur J Anaesthesiol. 2023;40(7):511–20. https://doi.org/10.1097/EJA.0000000000001807. Epub 2023 Feb 7. PMID: 36749046; PMCID: PMC10256303.
12. Bergold M, Otterburg T, Woitzik J, Byhahn C. Flow-controlled ventilation – a novel approach to treating acute respiratory distress syndrome. Trends Anaesth Crit Care. 2020;30:e93. https://doi.org/10.1016/j.tacc.2019.12.231. Epub 2020 Feb 25. PMCID: PMC10044019.
13. Spraider P, Putzer G, Breitkopf R, Abram J, Mathis S, Glodny B, Martini J. A case report of individualized ventilation in a COVID-19 patient - new possibilities and caveats to consider with flow-controlled ventilation. BMC Anesthesiol. 2021;21(1):145. https://doi.org/10.1186/s12871-021-01365-y. PMID: 33980178; PMCID: PMC8113787.
14. Van Dessel ED, De Meyer GR, Morrison SG, Jorens PG, Schepens T. Flow-controlled ventilation in moderate acute respiratory distress syndrome due to COVID-19: an open-label repeated-measures controlled trial. Intensive Care Med Exp. 2022;10(1):19. https://doi.org/10.1186/s40635-022-00449-4. PMID: 35608696; PMCID: PMC9127816.
15. Grassetto A, Pettenuzzo T, Badii F, Carlon R, Sella N, Navalesi P. Flow-controlled ventilation may reduce mechanical power and increase ventilatory efficiency in severe coronavirus disease-19 acute respiratory distress syndrome. Pulmonology. 2023;29(2):154–6. https://doi.org/10.1016/j.pulmoe.2022.05.006. Epub 2022 Jun 10. PMID: 35864057; PMCID: PMC9186429.
16. Roehrig S, Ait Hssain A, Shallik NAH, Elsaid IMA, Mustafa SF, Smain OAM, Molokhia AA, Lance MD. Flow controlled ventilation in acute respiratory distress syndrome associated with COVID-19: a structured summary of a study protocol for a randomised controlled trial. Trials. 2020;21(1):781. https://doi.org/10.1186/s13063-020-04708-1. PMID: 32917259; PMCID: PMC7483072.
17. Schranc Á, Balogh ÁL, Diaper J, Südy R, Peták F, Habre W, Albu G. Flow-controlled ventilation maintains gas exchange and lung aeration in a pediatric model of healthy and injured lungs: a randomized cross-over experimental study. Front Pediatr. 2022;10:1005135. https://doi.org/10.3389/fped.2022.1005135.
18. Moraes FDS, Marengo LL, Moura MDG, Bergamaschi CC, de Sá Del Fiol F, Lopes LC, Silva MT, Barberato-Filho S. ABCDE and ABCDEF care bundles: a systematic review of the implementation process in intensive care units. Medicine. 2022;101(25):e29499. https://doi.org/10.1097/MD.0000000000029499. PMID: 35758388; PMCID: PMC9276239.

19. Pal J, Taywade M, Pal R, Sethi D. Noise pollution in intensive care unit: a hidden enemy affecting the physical and mental health of patients and caregivers. Noise Health. 2022;24(114):130–6. https://doi.org/10.4103/nah.nah_79_21. PMID: 36124521; PMCID: PMC9743307.
20. Ely EW, Truman B, Shintani A, Thomason JW, Wheeler AP, Gordon S, Francis J, Speroff T, Gautam S, Margolin R, Sessler CN, Dittus RS, Bernard GR. Monitoring sedation status over time in ICU patients: reliability and validity of the Richmond Agitation-Sedation Scale (RASS). JAMA. 2003;289(22):2983–91. https://doi.org/10.1001/jama.289.22.2983.
21. Torbic H, Krishnan S, Harnegie MP, Duggal A. Neuromuscular blocking agents for ARDS: a systematic review and meta-analysis. Respir Care. 2021;66(1):120–8. https://doi.org/10.4187/respcare.07849. Epub 2020 Aug 25
22. Spraider P, Abram J, Martini J, Putzer G, Glodny B, Hell T, Barnes T, Enk D. Flow-controlled versus pressure-controlled ventilation in cardiac surgery with cardiopulmonary bypass - a single-center, prospective, randomized, controlled trial. J Clin Anesth. 2023;91:111279. https://doi.org/10.1016/j.jclinane.2023.111279. Epub 2023 Oct 3.
23. Spraider P, Martini J, Abram J, Putzer G, Glodny B, Hell T, Barnes T, Enk D. Individualized flow-controlled ventilation compared to best clinical practice pressure-controlled ventilation: a prospective randomized porcine study. Crit Care. 2020;24(1):662. https://doi.org/10.1186/s13054-020-03325-3. PMID: 33239039; PMCID: PMC7686826.
24. Bailey JR, Lee C, Nouraei R, Chapman J, Edmond M, Girgis M, De Zoysa N. Laryngectomy with a Tritube® and flow-controlled ventilation. Anaesth Rep. 2021;9(1):86–9. https://doi.org/10.1002/anr3.12114. PMID: 33982000; PMCID: PMC8103228.
25. Grassetto A, Pettenuzzo T, Badii F, Barzaghi F, Carlon R, Dellarole S, Pipitone M, Versaci A, Sella N, Lionello M, Bertolin A. A new perspective during laryngo-tracheal surgery: the use of an ultra-thin endotracheal tube (Tritube®) and flow-controlled ventilation-a retrospective case series and a review of the literature. J Anesth Analg Crit Care. 2022;2(1):39. https://doi.org/10.1186/s44158-022-00066-3. PMID: 37386531; PMCID: PMC9411832.
26. Shallik N, Elarref M, Khamash O, Abdelaal A, Radi Alkhafaji M, Makki H, Abusabeib A, Moustafa A, Menon A. Management of critical tracheal stenosis with a straw sized tube (Tritube): case report. Qatar Med J. 2021;2020(3):48. https://doi.org/10.5339/qmj.2020.48. PMID: 33598418; PMCID: PMC7842837.
27. Nouraei SAR, Girgis M, Shorthouse J, El-Boghdadly K, Ahmad I. A multidisciplinary approach for managing the infraglottic difficult airway in the setting of the coronavirus pandemic. Oper Tech Otolayngol Head Neck Surg. 2020;31(2):128–37. https://doi.org/10.1016/j.otot.2020.04.009. Epub 2020 May 30. PMID: 32572325; PMCID: PMC7260599.
28. Kristensen MS, Abildstrøm HH. Endotracheal video-laryngoscope guided intubation with a 2.4 mm cuff'ed tube and active expiration by a dedicated ventilator versus a standard tube/ventilator. A randomized single blinded study in patients with a predicted difficult airway. A paradigm shift in airway management? Euroanaesthesia. 2019;2019:3755.
29. Wang CC, Prather KA, Sznitman J, Jimenez JL, Lakdawala SS, Tufekci Z, Marr LC. Airborne transmission of respiratory viruses. Science. 2021;373(6558):9149. https://doi.org/10.1126/science.abd9149. PMID: 34446582; PMCID: PMC8721651.
30. Thiruvenkatarajan V, Wong DT, Kothandan H, Sekhar V, Adhikary SD, Currie J, Van Wijk RM. Airway management in the operating room and interventional suites in known or suspected COVID-19 adult patients: a practical review. Anesth Analg. 2020;131(3):677–89. https://doi.org/10.1213/ANE.0000000000005043. PMID: 32502132; PMCID: PMC7288783.
31. Bertini P, Forfori F, Bruschini L, Corradi F, Ribechini A, Brogi E, Guarracino F. Percutaneous tracheostomy in COVID-19 critically ill patients: experience from 30 consecutive procedures. Int Arch Otorhinolaryngol. 2021;25(1):e135–40. https://doi.org/10.1055/s-0040-1718528. Epub 2021 Feb 1. PMID: 33552294; PMCID: PMC7851370.
32. Magasich-Airola NP, Rosal Martins M, Desuter GR, Van Boven MJ. Novel technique for safe tracheostomy during COVID-19 pandemic using Evone® flow-controlled ventilation system. Int J Clin Pract. 2021;75(6):e13863. https://doi.org/10.1111/ijcp.13863. PMID: 33245817; PMCID: PMC7744873.

Liberation from Mechanical Ventilator: Art and Science of Weaning and Winning

Nissar Shaikh, Abdelrahman Balal, Umme Nashrah, M. A. Rahman, Seema Nahid, and Nabil A. Shallik

1 Introduction

Invasive and non-invasive mechanical ventilation were first used during the polio epidemic and have saved millions of lives by supporting patients with respiratory insufficiency and failure. However, invasive ventilation is not free from complications, and the significant clinical issue is dependency. Delays in weaning increase the length of stay in the hospital and intensive care unit, morbidity, and mortality [1].

In clinical practice, 70% of patients can be easily weaned from the ventilator. The remaining patients are challenging to wean and extubate due to underlying comorbidities, acute due to muscular changes due to critical illness, such as neuromuscular abnormalities (CINMA) [2]. Clinical issues: The weaning takes approximately 42% of the total duration of mechanical ventilation (MV) [3].

N. Shaikh (✉)
Surgical Intensive Care, Hamad Medical Corporation, Doha, Qatar

Clinical Anaesthesiology Department, Weill Cornell Medical College in Qatar, Doha, Qatar
e-mail: smaheboob@hamad.qa

A. Balal · M. A. Rahman · S. Nahid
Surgical Intensive Care, Hamad Medical Corporation, Doha, Qatar

U. Nashrah
The Deccan College of Medical Sciences, Hyderabad, India

N. A. Shallik
Anaesthesia, ICU and Perioperative Medicine Department, Hamad Medical Corporation, Doha, Qatar

Clinical Anaesthesiology Department, Weill Cornell Medical College in Qatar, Doha, Qatar

Clinical Anaesthesiology Department, College of Medicine Qatar University, Doha, Qatar

Anaesthesia and SICU Department, Tanta University, Tanta, Egypt
e-mail: nshallik@hamad.qa

N. A. Shallik (ed.), *Flow Controlled Ventilation Mode Through a Straw Size Tube*, https://doi.org/10.1007/978-3-031-77477-5_16

The term weaning is milder and does not define all stages of removing the patients from the mechanical ventilator; hence, the appropriate terminology is "Liberation from mechanical ventilation," and ventilator liberation is a three-stage procedure first of checking the readiness to wean from MV, weaning strategies and a third one is final extubation of the trachea. The stages will be described in the following paragraphs:

2 Testing Readiness to Wean

It is essential to know which patient is ready to wean. The patient's readiness to wean is frequently underestimated, resulting in unnecessary ventilation.

Secondly, fear from reintubation and self-extubation are also frequent causes of prolonged MV. The preparedness to wean testing is the objective clinical criteria, and physiological tests are used to determine the readiness of MV patients. Testing the MV patient's readiness to liberate is essential as it identifies these patients who can be weaned and thus avoid prolonged ventilation, preventing the complications of prolonged MV, avoid complications of premature weaning, reintubation, and self-extubation. Lastly, testing readiness to wean is applicable to the patients intubated and ventilated for more than 24 h [4].

3 Liberation Vs. Weaning

In the late 80s, it was realized that traditional weaning takes a long time and is unnecessary as gradual weaning or withdrawal from the mechanical ventilator and, at the same time, resumption of spontaneous presenting [5]. The daily assessment of mechanically ventilated patients for readiness to withdraw the support, followed by successfully removing the endotracheal tube, is more rapid successful weaning and withdrawal from the ventilatory support as the primary etiology requiring mechanical ventilation is reversed. Therefore, it is called liberation from mechanical ventilation.

4 Stages of Liberation from Mechanical Ventilation

As mentioned earlier, liberation from mechanical ventilation comprises three stages: Readiness testing, weaning, and extubation.

4.1 Testing Readiness to Liberate

The readiness testing uses clinical and physiological tests to identify that the patient is ready to be weaned from the mechanical ventilator. These readiness tests aim to identify patients who are prepared to wean and patients who are not ready to be weaned from MV to avoid premature weaning and its complications.

4.2 The Clinical Criteria

The following clinical criteria are used to identify those patients ready to wean from MV:

1. Improvement in the underlying cause requires ventilatory support.
2. Adequate oxygenation.
3. Arterial pH >7.25.
4. Hemodynamically stable or requiring a minimal dose of vasopressor.
5. Able to initiate spontaneous breathing.
6. Hemoglobin >7.0 g/dl.
7. Core body temperature of <38.5.
8. Awake or Glasgow Coma Scale (GCS) >8 or can protect the airway.

It is essential that there should be a significant improvement in the disease or clinical condition requiring invasive mechanical ventilation, such as sepsis, septic shock, acute respiratory distress syndrome, fluid overload, or pneumonia. Adequate oxygenation and the patient's ability to maintain oxygenation are essential to prevent hypoxia and reintubation in the post-liberation period. When the patient can maintain the SPO_2 (oxygen saturation) >90% on 40% FiO_2 (fraction of inspired oxygen) or PF ratio >150 on PEEP of 5 or less (positive end-expiratory pressure), a higher PEEP of 8 and FiO_2 0.5 may be acceptable in patients intubated with a narrow tube, obese patients, and patients with abdominal distention or in patients with lung disease.

Arterial pH >7.25: Severe acute acid-base imbalance should be corrected to the baseline for the patient. An arbitrary value of 7.25 is based on the observation that PH 7.25 is reasonably tolerated well without extra burden on the respiratory system.

Stable hemodynamics: Once the patient is hemodynamically stable or on minimal dosage of vasopressors or inotropes without myocardial ischemia or injury, they are ready to wean from MV. The mean arterial pressure is >60 mmHg, systolic blood pressure is >90 mmHg and <180 mmHg, or maintaining the patient's borderline hemodynamics with or without minimal vasopressors.

Spontaneous breathing attempts: Patients should be able to breathe spontaneously, with minimal support, to compensate for the tube resistance and decrease the work of breathing with minimal anxiolytic or sedation, which is a primary requirement to initiate weaning in MV patients.

4.3 Additional or Optional Requirements

Apart from the above criteria, there are other clinical entities in which, when fulfilled, there will be a greater chance of initiation of weaning and successful liberation from mechanical ventilation.

4.3.1 Hemoglobin Levels

In the past, anemia was considered one of the contraindications for weaning as it adversely affects the weaning and liberation from MV. As Hébert et al. demonstrated, there were no differences in the weaning success of patients with restrictive or liberative transfusions. Hence, hemoglobin >7.0 g/dl is considered sufficient for weaning patients from MV [6].

4.3.2 Core Body Temperature

Although the temperature threshold for weaning from MV is not proposed, the raised temperature or fever has adverse effects on initiation and weaning as it increases the work of breathing, diminishes respiratory muscle function, and increases minute ventilation. Hence, it is advisable to have a core body temperature of less than 38.5 °C to initiate the weaning from mechanical ventilation [7].

4.3.3 Mental Status

Due to sedation or delirium, it may not be possible for the patient to be fully awake or easily arousable. It has been shown that the Glasgow Coma Scale (GCS) of 8–15 or Richmond agitation sedation scale (RAAS) of −2 to +1 is not associated with a high extubation failure rate. Therefore, it is advisable that if the patient can protect the airway, their impaired mental status does not preclude the initiation of weaning from MV [8, 9].

4.4 Predictors of Weaning/Weaning Trial

Clinicians use a predicting physiological test combined with the clinical criteria to assess readiness to wean from MV. Few clinicians use these predictors in cases of doubts about patients' readiness to wean from MV.

4.4.1 Rapid Shallow Breathing Index (RSBI)

RSBI is the most widely used and extensively studied predictor for readiness to wean from MV. It is the ratio of respiratory rate to tidal volume in liters (F/Vt). It can be measured by a handheld spirometer attached to the endotracheal tube while the patient breathes on room air for one minute without any ventilatory assistance [10]. The newer ventilators can calculate it when the patient spontaneously breathes without or with support. A negative RSBI is a ratio of more than 10^5, indicating that the patient may fail or is likely to fail the weaning. In contrast, a positive RSBI test is a ratio of less than 10^5 breaths/min, likely indicative of weaning success. Several factors affect RSBI, such as a narrow endotracheal tube, sepsis, fever, anxiety, supine posture, female gender, and chronic restrictive lung disease [11, 12].

A review of RSBI in predicting the extubation found it to be 83% sensitive and 58% specific, with a corresponding likelihood ratio of LR + 2.0 and LR of 0.3, respectively [13]. A rule of 60 is a good predictor of successful weaning in patients above 60 years of age with an RSBI of <60.

4.4.2 Respiratory Parameters and Predictors

Several predictors have poor predictive value, poorly defined thresholds, need special instruments, and are complex to calculate; therefore, they are not valuable for routine use.

1. **Gas exchange and oxygenation parameters**:

    Although adequate oxygenation is essential to determining readiness to wean, it is a poor predictor of weaning when used alone.

    PaO_2/FiO_2: Arterial oxygen, jugular oxygen tension

    PaO_2/PaO_2: Arterial oxygen jugular oxygen tension

    A-a gradient: Alveolar-arterial gradient and dead space
2. **Respiratory load and capacity measurement**

    They require special instruments, and none has consistently predicted failure or successful weaning. Minute ventilation 14, respiratory system compliance 15, work of breathing 16, and Breathing oxygen costs [14].
3. **Maximum inspiratory pressure**:

    Although a poor predictor of weaning, it may be useful as supplementary information in patients with neuromuscular weakness.
4. **Respiratory system compliance:** inconsistent predictive value
5. **Gastric pH:** Not useful
6. **Multicomponent integrative indices:**

    Inspiratory Effect quotient (IEQ)

    The CROP index (compliance, rate, oxygenation, and pressure)

    The CORE index (compromise, oxygenation, respiration, and effort)
7. **Minute ventilation:**

    Older studies have shown that minute ventilation of less than 10 L/min indicates weaning success, but the higher tidal volume has negative predictions and weaning failure. The time of recovery of minute ventilation after 2 h of spontaneous breathing trial to return to baseline is 3–4 min, a good indicator of respiratory reserve and predictor of weaning success [15].
8. **Maximum inspiratory pressure Pimax (negative inspiratory force):**

    Pimax of <−20 to −30 cm of H_2O is highly sensitive (up to 100%) but not specific (up to 69%) for the prediction of liberation from MV. Due to its low specificity, it is not enough alone to predict the weaning [16].
9. **Tidal volume:**

    Vt of >5 mL/kg is a good indicator of the weaning process. Moreover, the approximate entropy of tidal volume, breathing pattern, frequency, and regularity is a valuable indicator of reversibility of respiratory failure and weaning success [16].
10. **Respiratory rate:**

    Tachypnea (respiratory rate >30 breaths/min) is a sensitivity factor and marker of respiratory distress and weaning failure. Moreover, the absolute number or value is unimportant; the breathing pattern is essential, and the irregular breathing pattern is a more accurate predictor of failure to wean [16].

11. **Airway pressure:**

    The airway occlusion pressure is a good indicator of central respiratory drive. The ratio of $P_{0.1}/Pi_{max}$ <0.3 is found to be an excellent early indicator of liberation from MV.
12. **CROP index:**

    The CROP index includes dynamic respiratory compliance, respiratory rate, arterial to alveolar oxygenation, and Pi_{max}. The CROP Index assesses the relationship between the respiratory system's demand and the ability of the respiratory muscles to handle it. CROP values of more than 13–16 ml/breath/min were a good predictor of weaning. The CROP index disadvantage is a complex and cumbersome calculation with the potential risk of measurement errors [16].
13. **Weaning index and integrative index**

    All these indexes are complex, and none of them has confirmed higher accuracy levels in the literature.
14. **Use of ultrasonography (USG) and point-of-care ultrasound (POCUS):**

    Diaphragmatic thickness:

    POCUS or USG of the diaphragm, showing atrophy and dysfunction, is correlated with weaning and extubation, liberation failure, and the need for a more extended study. More recently, the intercostal muscle thickness has been found to be associated with weaning [17].

5 Weaning Strategies

Weaning is the process of decreasing the ventilatory support and, at the same time, increasing the patient's spontaneous breathing efforts. Weaning from the ventilator is classified into three groups [18]:

1. Simple weaning: It is considered that the patient underwent simple weaning when the patient passed their first weaning trial.
2. Difficult to wean: Patients are considered challenging to wean when they fail the first weaning trial and then need up to three SBTs or seven days to pass SBT.
3. Prolonged weaning: Patient fails three SBTs or requires more than a week pass SBT.

The patient intubated for more than 24 h and cleared the readiness to wean should undergo a weaning trial. There are various methods used to wean patients from mechanical ventilators. The following are the methods used to wean from MV:

1. Daily spontaneous breathing trial is the preferred method.
2. T-tube use.
3. Progressively reducing the ventilatory rate and pressure support.
4. Newer compliance-assisted alternative automatic weaning of pressure support and applying an intermittent non-invasive ventilator (NIV) or high-flow nasal cannula (HFNC)

5.1 Daily Spontaneous Breathing Trial (SBT)

Daily spontaneous breathing trial (SBT) with mild analgo-sedation is the preferred method to wean; compared to other methods, it is safe, effective, and efficient [19]. In daily SBT, patients connected to spontaneous breathing (Fig. 1) or pressure support ventilation for 30 min to 2 h. In up to 75% of patients, SBT is successful in the first attempt and extubated [20]. This SBT with PSV has the advantage of overcoming the work of breathing; although the exact pressure support to optimize the workload and assist in alleviating the work of breathing is unknown, it is considered around 8 cmH_2O. The higher-pressure support may over-assist the patient and lead to extubation failure. In contrast, the lower PS will not help overcome the systemic resistance and, thus, the exhaustion and failure of SBT [21]. Esteban et al., while comparing the methods of weaning from MV, found that the daily SBT was helpful in sooner extubation compared to the gradual decrease of PS or IMV [22]. Patients who failed the SBT trial should be rested, and another SBT should be performed the next day to avoid exhaustion and recovery of respiratory muscles.

5.2 T-Piece Weaning Trial

It is a weaning process where the patient breaths spontaneously through T-shaped corrugated tubing with an oxygen supply connected with an adaptor to the endotracheal tube (Fig. 2). Although it is suggested to have a better outcome and successful extubation in patients with prolonged weaning [23], the main issue of T-piece weaning from MV is no work of breathing compensation; hence, these T-piece weaning patients during a trial of 30–120 min may get exhausted and sink or fail or swim or victorious in weaning.

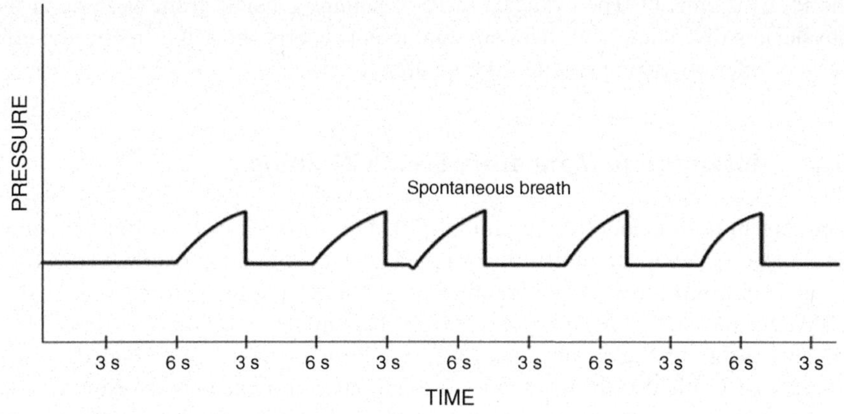

Fig. 1 Spontaneous breathing

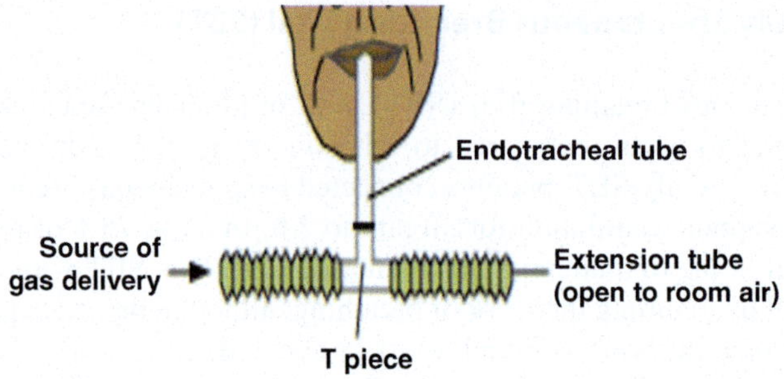

Fig. 2 T-piece

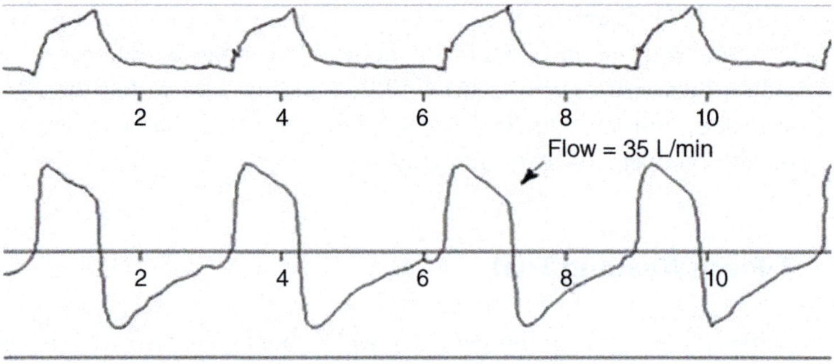

Fig. 3 Typical pressure support curve

5.3 Pressure Support Ventilation (Fig. 3)

In this method of weaning, initially, the patient will be allowed to breathe spontaneously with PS of 12–18 cmH_2O, then gradually, every 2 h or more (per day), reduce the PS by 2 cmH_2O. The evidence of PS weaning is mainly from weaning at the physician's discretion, and there are conflicting reports about its superiority, efficacy, or inferiority compared to SBT weaning.

5.4 Intermittent Mandatory Breath Weaning

The intermittent mandatory breath (IMV) (Fig. 4) is set to 12–14 breaths/min. Gradually, either twice daily or every 24 h, 1 or 2 breaths decrease the IMV breath rate until the IMV is six breaths/min, and then the patient is shifted to PSV ventilation, followed by extubation. This mode of weaning is reported to be successful in the usual care [24]. Therefore, it is recommended by the Society of Critical Care Medicine to combine a spontaneous awakening trial (by decreasing or changing to an analog-sedative agent) with a spontaneous breathing trial [25].

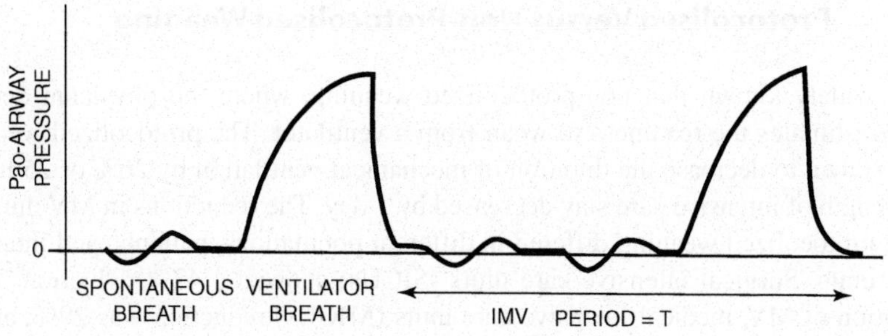

Fig. 4 Intermittent mandatory breath

5.5 Spontaneous Awakening Test (SAT)

The wean-safe study shows that higher sedation scores delay weaning from the ventilator and are associated with weaning failure. Delayed weaning is associated with longer ICU stays and increased morbidity and mortality [26]. Hence, it is a famous quote in the ICU to tell the patient in the weaning trial to "wake up and breathe" and decrease the sedation level. By checking the readiness to liberate from mechanical ventilation and weaning trial, patients can be on lighter sedation; as we practice, starting Dexmedetomidine significantly decreasing opioid analgesia to a minimal level, and stopping other sedatives would help [24].

5.6 Newer Automated Modes of Weaning

Now, various automated weaning machines are available. Hence, once the patient is confirmed to be ready for weaning, the physician or respiratory therapist adjusts the level of IMV, rate, exhaled carbon dioxide, and tidal volume. The ventilator uses proprietary, computerized, closed-loop weaning and weans the PS level, indicating that the patient is ready for extubation. These types of weaning are unsuitable for surgical patients as they would be extubated after a shorter ventilation period. As most of these automatic weaning modes take PCO_2 of 60 mmHg as an upper limit, those patients with baseline PCO_2 >60 mmHg may not be suitable for automatic weaning. The automatic weaning modes vary from adoptive supportive ventilation (ASV), Smart Care/PS, Proportional assist ventilation (PAV), and neurally adjusted ventilation assist (NAVA) [17].

The manually adjusted pressure support during the weaning process provides a constant pressure support level, which may undercompensate or overcompensate for breathing and endotracheal tube compensation. In contrast, the automatic tube compensation (ATC) compensates for endotracheal tube resistance according to the gas flow [27]. ATC compensates continuously for the tube resistance; hence, it is called electronic extubation [26]. The smaller studies about ASV and Smart Care show that they have slightly earlier extubation but need further research [28].

6 Protocolised Versus Non-Protocolised Weaning

It is widely known that non-protocolized weaning, where the physician decides underestimates the readiness to wean from a ventilator. The protocolized weaning was shown to decrease the duration of mechanical ventilation by 26% or 25 h, and the length of intensive care stay decreased by 1 day. The reductions in MV duration with protocolized weaning differed in different populations, patients, and intensive care units. Surgical intensive care units (SICUs) showed a 47% reduction in the duration of MV, medical intensive care units (MICUs) reduction was 29%, and in mixed ICUs, the duration of MV reductions was 21%. In contrast, there was limited or no effect introduction of MV (1%) [29].

7 Weaning Failure

Patients should not be extubated during weaning as it has a negative impact. When SBT fails, give at least 24 h before the second SBT. SBT may be repeated in patients who are drowsy and wake up from the sedative effects.

7.1 Clinical Findings (Table 1)

7.2 Causes of Failed Weaning

Following are the common etiologies of failure of SBT and inability to wean critically ill patients from mechanical ventilation.

7.2.1 Nutritional Factors

Always calculate the nutritional needs of critically ill patients, and adequate administration of either parenteral or enteral nutrition is essential for successful weaning from mechanical ventilation. Protein catabolism and underfeeding cause respiratory

Table 1 The weaning trial failure

Clinical manifestations [30–33]	Body system
Drowsy/delirium/agitated	Neurological
Uses accessory muscles of respiration or paradoxical breathing pattern	Respiratory
Tachypnea >35 breaths/min	Hemodynamics
Tachycardia >140 beats/min	Gas exchange
Bradycardia <50 beats/min	Others
Hypertensive >180 mmHg hypotension <90 mmHg	
Lower oxygenation (sPO_2 90%) or PO_2 less than 50 mmHg	
Inadequate ventilation (raised PCO_2 by 10%, or pH by 0.1)	
Sweating/anxious	

muscle wasting. The overfeeding causes increased PCO_2 production and increases the respiratory load [30].

7.2.2 Cardiac Factors

Continuous ICU monitoring is essential during weaning with the optimization of cardiac medications. The weaning process can cause myocardial ischemia and pulmonary edema. Even fluid balance or negative fluid balance will be better in these patients [31].

7.2.3 Respiratory Factors

Monitoring of respiratory rate, chest examination, chest radiography, and arterial blood gas with optimization of different pathologies causing the need for mechanical ventilation is essential. The increased ventilatory demand due to basal collapse of the lung, abdominal distention, increased dead space (due to dehydration or hyperventilation), and metabolic factors are the main reasons for increased ventilatory demand and causing weaning failure. Bronchospasm, airway edema, increased secretions, and respiratory tract can cause an increase in resistive load, leading to weaning failure. Lung hyperinflation, pulmonary edema, pleural effusions, decreased chest wall compliance, and abdominal distention cause increased elastic load, leading to weaning failure. The electrolyte imbalance, steroids, muscle relaxants, neuropathies, and myopathies decrease neuromuscular capacities and can cause weaning failure. Excess sedation, metabolic alkalosis, encephalopathy, shock, and obstructive sleep apnea cause decreased respiratory drive and can cause weaning failure [31].

7.2.4 Psychological Factors

Patient education, control and prevention of delirium, optimizing lighter sedation, and appropriate analgesia are essential for weaning success [32].

7.2.5 Ventilatory Circuit Factors

The examination of breathing patterns, ventilatory waveform if needed, and change of tubing, ventilator, or pulmonary toilet should be considered in the preweaning period. Exhalation valve dysfunction, circuit compliance, water, and increased endotracheal tube resistance due to inspissated secretions can cause weaning failure [32].

8 Extubation

The final step in liberation from mechanical ventilation is safely removing the endotracheal tube. The steps for successful extubation and, finally, liberation from ventilation are assessing the safety to extubate, selecting a method of extubation, and managing post-extubation.

8.1 Stability of the Clinical Conditions

The patient should not be extubated unless the clinical or medical conditions requiring intubation improve and the patient has passed the readiness tests and weaning criteria.

8.2 Passed Weaning Trial or SBT

Except for postoperative patients with ventilation for a maximum of 24 h, all patients in intensive care setup should not be extubated unless they successfully pass the SBT. Moreover, Fernandez et al. showed that after successful SBT, these patients can be reconnected to mechanical ventilation and given rest for 1 h, significantly decreasing the reintubation rate [33].

8.3 Airway Protection Assessment

To guard or prevent aspiration during spontaneous breathing is airway protection. To prevent this (aspiration during spontaneous breathing), it is essential that the patient is awake and has adequate or strong cough reflexes; hence, for safe and successful extubation, the two things should be assessed separately. There is no universally accepted level of consciousness. Cough strength and endotracheal suctioning frequency that recommend extubation are not established. It is generally accepted not to extubate patients with weaker cough or whose Glasgow Coma Scale (GCS) is lower than eight and require ETT suctioning more frequently than 2 h. A note of caution is that all of the above factors should be evaluated on a case-by-case basis to avoid the complication of delayed extubation. The combination of factors such as impaired neurological function (inability to obey commands), increased amount of endotracheal secretions >2.5 ml/h, and decreased expiratory peak flow of <60 l/min in combination had extubation failure rates of 100% [34].

8.4 Testing of this Strength and Clearance of Secretions

Level of consciousness is quickly evaluated using GCS, following a description of assessing strength and secretions clearance before extubation.

8.4.1 Mental Status

If the patient is awake and obeying commands, it is ideal for extubation, but nowadays, Dexmedetomidine or Remifentanil in small doses are used during weaning; hence, the patient should be arousable. Salam et al. demonstrated that the ability to follow eye-opening, follow objects with eye movements, and grasp hand stick tongue increases successful extubation chances [34]. Namen et al. reported a significant failed extubation rate in patients with GCS of less than 8 [35].

8.4.2 Cough Strength

Routine suctioning of the endotracheal tube gives an idea about the strength of the cough. More precisely, cough strength in patients with weaker coughs is evaluated by spirometry or index card. A spirometer is attached to the ventilator, and the patient is asked to cough, and peak expiratory flow during coughing is measured. If it is <60 l/min, there is a five times more chance of extubation failure [36]. Card method: A card, held around 2 cm from the detached ETT, should be moist and in 3–4 cough. If not, the patient had three times more risk of extubation failure [37].

8.4.3 Amount of Endotracheal Secretions

The suction canister can measure the amount of secretions from the endotracheal tube. If the patient requires suctioning from the ETT for less than 2 h, then extubation should be held. If they are thicker in combination with a weaker cough strength, then nature of secretions will result in extubation failure [37].

9 Post-extubation Stridor Risk Assessment

Post-extubation stridor occurs in 10% of the intubated patients. Hence, all intubated patients with invasive ventilations should be assessed for post-extubation stridor. The post-extubation stridor can cause extubation failure, longer ventilation, and intensive care therapy. Risk factors for post-extubation stridor are described in the following table:

1. Elderly patients (>80 years).
2. Prolonged intubation (>36 h).
3. Larger size of endotracheal tube.
4. Elevated severity scores.
5. Lower GCS.
6. Female gender.
7. Difficult and traumatic intubations.
8. Excessive endotracheal tube mobility.

9.1 Cuff Leak Test

Patients at risk of having post-extubation stridor should be assessed by cuff leak test; otherwise, if there is no risk for post-extubation stridor, this test may not be needed.

The cuff leak test is the normal airflow around the ETT. After deflation, if reduced, it indicates a decrease in the space between the ETT and laryngeal wall, which means the presence of secretions, edema, injury, or stenosis. Quantitative assessment of cuff leak is done by deflating the cuff of ETT and measuring the difference between inspired and expired volume during the volume cycle mechanical ventilation. The cuff leak volume of less than 110 ml or less than 12–24% of the delivered tidal volume proposed failed extubation [38]. The combination of cough and cuff leak improves the ability to predict post-extubation failure due to stridor. The absence of audible cough and cuff leak indicates patient has a ten times more chance of developing post-extubation stridor [39]. Laryngeal ultrasonography is another simple, rapid, non-invasive method for evaluating the air column around the larynx during cuff deflation. It is subjective and needs a more controlled trial before it is recommended [40].

9.2 Use of Steroids

Shaikh et al. demonstrated that patients with lower or negative cuff leaks had more significant post-extubation stridor than those with sufficient cuff leaks [41].

They also compared and concluded that the most effective steroid is methylprednisolone in preventing and treating post-extubation stridor and failure [41]. As multiple dosages of steroids are required to treat and prevent post-intubation laryngeal oedema, the last dose of steroid therapy should be post-extubation. The recommended dose of methylprednisolone is 20 mg every 4 h, starting in the evening of the day before extubation, and the last dose will land in the postoperative period [42]. Alternatives in unplanned admissions include a single 40 mg dose of methylprednisolone and extubation after 4 h in unplanned extubation with lesser or no cuff leak [41, 43].

9.3 Day or Nighttime Extubation

The impact of day/night time in all steps of weaning is unknown, and the patient should be ready for extubation. Generally, extubation is done in the morning hours. If the chance of re-reintubation is low and the patient is prepared, he can be extubated at night hours [44].

Meanwhile, Gershengorn et al., in their retrospective study, concluded that extubation during the night increases reintubation and mortality [45].

9.4 Assessment of Difficult Intubation and Reintubation

Suppose the patient is difficult to intubate or may not protect the airway in post-extubation operator fatigue. In that case, a skilled person's availability should be considered in extubation, and appropriate arrangements should be made.

9.5 Post-Extubation Issues and Treatment

Extubated patients should be closely monitored. There'll be varying in post-extubation support. The protocolized approach for all patients with either non-invasive ventilation (NIV) or high-flow nasal cannula (HFNC) has not been shown to impact the outcome [46].

Most patients do well with low-flow oxygen by nasal cannula or mask. Still, a few high-risk patients (up to 20%) need aggressive medical therapy, oxygenation, and airway patency maneuvers to prevent reintubation. For up to 40% of patients who develop post-extubation respiratory failure, treatment should be directed to correct the cause of respiratory failure, such as excessive secretions, heart failure, or increased in work of breathing. This includes nasopharyngeal airway and frequent suctioning of secretions, diuresis, bronchodilators, and non-invasive ventilation or high-flow nasal cannula therapy.

9.6 Euobalance and Extubation

As dry lungs are happy, it is always preferred to have a negative or at least equal balance in patients for planned extubation. More recently, Dos Santos et al. reported that the post-extubation positive fluid balance is associated with extubation failure [47].

9.7 Nil Per Oral (NPO) Status and Extubation

We hold enteral feeding for 1–4 h (NPO) before extubation in critically ill patients. Still, again, the most recent study did not show any benefits of holding enteral feeding for a few hours or feeding just before extubation [48].

9.8 Post-extubation Respiratory Failure

Extubation failure occurs in around 14% of patients, commonly in the first 12–24 h of extubation. Prompted reintubation and therapy to correct the cause should be started immediately.

9.9 Unplanned or Self-Extubation

Unplanned or self-extubation occurs most during weaning and is reported to be around 3–12%. More frequent in oral than nasal intubations, on lower sedation levels, and if ETT is not appropriately fixed and during restlessness. One should have a low threshold for reintubation. Delays are associated with an increase in mortality, longer duration of mechanical ventilation, and longer ICU stay. Unplanned/self-extubation requires lower oxygen and a patent airway; the ability to protect the airway should be monitored carefully [49].

9.10 Stridor and Post-extubation Failure

In these patients with post-extubation stridor and respiratory failure, immediate intubation should be done frequently with a smaller size tube. The upper airway

Table 2 Doha protocol for extubation

1. SAT and SBT, RSBI < 110 or < in age >60
2. Awake or arousable, GCS >8, and patent airway
3. Hand grip/head lift
4. Able to clear secretions/suction requirements >2 hourly
5. Good cough reflex

should be examined for edema, lesions, trauma, and secretions. A short course of methylprednisolone in four doses should be administered [38, 39]. If an appropriate leak is present, the patient can safely be extubated in the ICU. If a cuff leak is absent, extubation in a controlled atmosphere or operation theater and extubation over an airway exchange catheter is advised [50].

9.11 Resumption of the Feeding

There is no protocol for predicting swallowing dysfunction following extubation. The physician must balance the risks and benefits of oral intake in the post-extubation period.

The restarting of feed or oral intake following extubation depends upon mental status, duration of intubation, associated comorbidities, and admission diagnosis.

Generally, the patient intubated for a short period (less than 7 days) can take oral fluids initially if swallowing is satisfactory, then quickly progress to an oral diet. Those patients intubated for 2 weeks or more are delayed in oral intake. In these groups of patients, a swallowing test or fiber-optic endoscopic evaluation of the swallowing (FEES) is recommended before the patient is put on an oral diet. All of the above maneuvers delay receiving adequate nutrition under the pretext of prevention of aspiration, and only 25% of patients receive adequate nutrition in the first week post-extubation [51]. We follow the Doha protocol for extubation (Table 2).

10 Flow Control Ventilation in ICU Settings

Flow control ventilation (FCV) is a novel ventilatory mode used in the ventilation of acute respiratory distress syndrome (ARDS) and found to be equally effective [52].

The use of FCV in intensive care patients is limited to case reports or small case series, mainly in COVID-19 patients and few clinical trials, like our institutional-controlled clinical trial in COVID-19 patients [53]. When it is individualized to ventilator compliance, FCV has been shown to increase ventilator efficiency with decreased mechanical support.

Ventilation can easily be individualized initially by the end-expiratory pressure (EEP) optimization by changing both EEP and peak pressure increments of 1–2 mbar or cmH_2O (keeping driving pressure constant). The lowest EEP, resulting in the highest tidal volume, has been chosen and is compliant. Then, the peak pressure (and hence the driving pressure) is increased stepwise. If the measured dynamic compliance is 50 ml/mbar, then an increase in driving pressure of 1 mbar would lead to an increase in tidal volume of 50 ml. However, lung mechanics are improved if the tidal volume increases significantly more than 50 ml. This step is repeated until tidal volume rises proportionally. Peak pressure should then be set at the previous setting. The FCV should be optimized within the limits of alveolar derecruitment and over-distention. Flow should be adjusted according to CO_2 measurements. The I: E (inspiratory: expiratory) ratio in FCV should always be set at 1:1. The minute volume will be half of the set flow, so while adjusting the flow, the respiratory frequency will change accordingly. The minute volumes will be lower with FCV compared to volume control ventilation (VCV) or pressure-controlled ventilation (PCV) [54].

FCV with Evone® can be used when the intratracheal pressures are continuously monitored, and the ventilating lumen has a Luer lock connection. Endotracheal tubes (ET) cannot be directly connected to Evone®. This can be overcome by connecting a conventional tube adapter (CTA®) with a conventional endotracheal tube. So, FCV can be used in conventionally intubated patients with a conventional tube adapter (CTA®) and Evone® with ETT of more than 5 mm internal diameter (ID) [55] (Figs. 5 and 6).

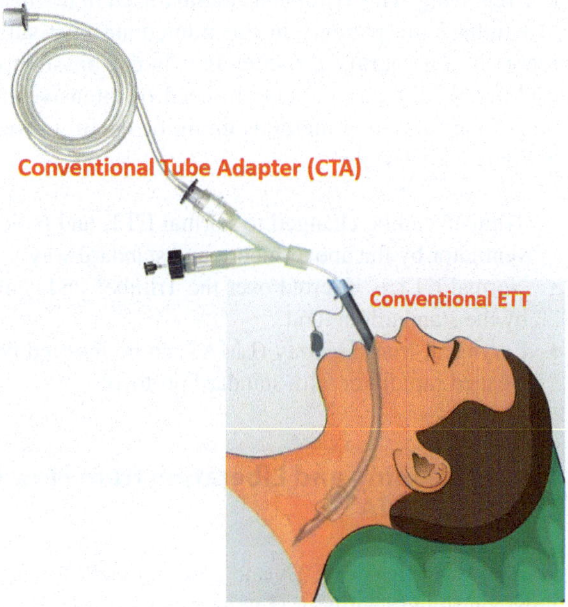

Fig. 5 Conventional tube adaptor (CTA®) (Ventinova Medical, Eindhoven, the Netherlands) (Courtesy, Dr. Shallik, Doha Airway Equipment Museum, Qatar)

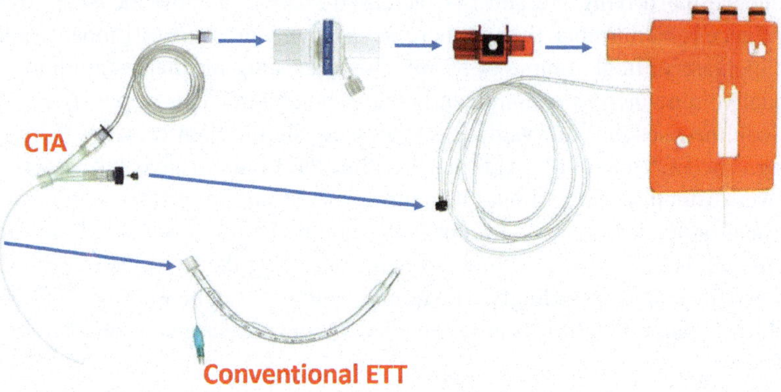

Fig. 6 Schematic diagram showing CTA® connection with conventional ETT & Evone® ventilation (Courtesy, Dr. Shallik, Doha Airway Equipment Museum, Qatar)

11 Weaning from Flow Control Ventilation and Tritube®

Scanty literature about weaning patients with FCV and Tribute® weaning or weaning difficulties exists. Hence, it is a potential area for research and prospective reporting. The Tritube® is mainly used in tracheal and upper airway surgeries to extubate the patients in the immediate post-surgical period, as in this case report in our facility [56–59]. If it is not possible to ventilate the patient with traditional ETT and patients in need of intensive care therapy, in this scenario, one of the following methods might be useful in weaning and liberation of FCV patients with Tritube®.

- Tritube® can be changed to normal ETT, and patients can be liberated from the ventilator by the above-mentioned standard way
- Normal ETT is inserted over the Tritube® and can be liberated from ventilation by the standard method
- Laryngeal Mask Airway (LMA) can be inserted beside the Tritube® and can be weaned rapidly or with standard protocols

12 Weaning and Liberation from Flow Control Ventilation and CTA®

Another advantage of CTA and conventional ETT is that they can be connected to flow-controlled ventilator (Evone®). So, you can wean and liberate the patient like any other traditional case after switching to a conventional ventilator to extubate the patient as a routine practice (Please refer to the section "Protocols and Techniques" for more details).

13 Conclusion

Invasive ventilation helps to improve patients with respiratory failure due to various etiological reasons. The appropriate weaning and extubation will prevent the complications of prolonged intubation and ventilation. Meanwhile, premature weaning is a risk for complications. The term liberation from mechanical ventilator seems more appropriate than "weaning." The liberation from the mechanical ventilator is a three-stage process. First, it is essential to check the readiness for weaning. The second step is the weaning trial, and the third is tracheal extubation and liberation from mechanical ventilation. A combination of clinical criteria and various respiratory parameters does the readiness to wean. As far as the weaning strategies are concerned, SBT is the best option. Newer modes of weaning need more validation. Weaning from ~~the~~ flow-controlled ventilation requires further research. Protocolized weaning is a better option. There are several factors associated with weaning failure. Before extubation, see that the patient does not have many secretions and a good cough reflex. Apart from liberation from mechanical ventilation, preventing post-extubation stridor and resumption of feeding is essential for better patient outcomes.

Disclaimer Here, we introduce the flow-controlled manual ventilator (FCmV), exemplified frequently by the Ventrain®, merely because there is no alternative of its kind on the market. Also, you may find a particular focus on the only commercially available FCV ventilator, the "Evone®" ventilator, moreover using (Tritube®) instead of ultra-thin or straw sized ETT nomenclature due to the lack of other examples and not as commercial endorsement of the products.

References

1. Wawrzeniak IC, Regina Rios Vieira S, Almeida Victorino J. Weaning from mechanical ventilation in ARDS: aspects to think about for better understanding, evaluation, and management. Biomed Res Int. 2018;2018:5423639.
2. Shaikh N, Ummunnisa F, Safak MG. HELLP needs aggressive help. Qat Med J. 2011;20(2):47–52.
3. Augustus Oglesby HJ, Cataldo SH, Pedro MJ. Automated near real-time ventilator data feedback reduces incidence of ventilator-associated events: a retrospective observational study. Crit Care Explor. 2021;3:e0379.
4. Epstein SK, Ciubotaru RL, Wong JB. Effect of failed extubation on the outcome of mechanical ventilation. Chest. 1997;112:186–92.
5. Hall JB. Liberation of the patient from mechanical ventilation. JAMA J Am Med Assoc. 1987;257:1621.
6. Hébert PC, et al. Do blood transfusions improve outcomes related to mechanical ventilation? Chest. 2001;119:1850–7.
7. Netzer G, et al. Fever is associated with delayed ventilator liberation in acute lung injury. Ann Am Thorac Soc. 2013;10:608–15.
8. Beuret P, et al. Interest of an objective evaluation of cough during weaning from mechanical ventilation. Intensive Care Med. 2009;35:1090–3.
9. Coplin WM, Pierson DJ, Cooley KD, Newell DW, Rubenfeld GD. Implications of extubation delay in brain-injured patients meeting standard weaning criteria. Am J Respir Crit Care Med. 2000;161:1530–6.

10. Yang KL, Tobin MJ. A prospective study of indexes predicting the outcome of trials of weaning from mechanical ventilation. N Engl J Med. 1991;324:1445–50.
11. Epstein SK, Ciubotaru RL. Influence of gender and endotracheal tube size on preextubation breathing pattern. Am J Respir Crit Care Med. 1996;154:1647–52.
12. Seymour CW, Cross BJ, Cooke CR, Gallop RL, Fuchs BD. Physiologic impact of closed-system endotracheal suctioning in spontaneously breathing patients receiving mechanical ventilation. Respir Care. 2009;54:367–74.
13. Trivedi V, et al. The usefulness of the rapid shallow breathing index in predicting successful extubation: a systematic review and meta-analysis. Chest. 2022;161:97–111.
14. Hubmayr RD, Loosbrock LM, Gillespie DJ, Rodarte JR. Oxygen uptake during weaning from mechanical ventilation. Chest. 1988;94:1148–55.
15. Martinez A, Seymour C, Nam M. Minute ventilation recovery time: a predictor of extubation outcome. Chest. 2003;123:1214–21.
16. El-Khatib MF, Bou-Khalil P. Clinical review: liberation from mechanical ventilation. Crit Care. 2008;12:221.
17. Nakanishi N, et al. Change in diaphragm and intercostal muscle thickness in mechanically ventilated patients: a prospective observational ultrasonography study. J Intensive Care. 2019;7:56.
18. Boles J-M, et al. Weaning from mechanical ventilation. Eur Respir J. 2007;29:1033–56.
19. Esteban A, et al. Evolution of mechanical ventilation in response to clinical research. Am J Respir Crit Care Med. 2008;177:170–7.
20. Perkins GD, et al. Effect of protocolized weaning with early extubation to non-invasive ventilation vs invasive weaning on time to liberation from mechanical ventilation among patients with respiratory failure: the breathe randomized clinical trial. JAMA. 2018;320:1881–8.
21. Ouellette DR, et al. Liberation from mechanical ventilation in critically ill adults: an official American College of Chest Physicians/American Thoracic Society Clinical Practice Guideline: inspiratory pressure augmentation during spontaneous breathing trials, protocols minimising sedation, and non-invasive ventilation immediately after extubation. Chest. 2017;151:166–80.
22. Esteban A, et al. A comparison of four methods of weaning patients from mechanical ventilation. N Engl J Med. 1995;332:345–50.
23. Pellegrini JAS, et al. Spontaneous breathing trials with T-piece or pressure support ventilation. Respir Care. 2016;61:1693–703.
24. Sheikh N, et al. Analgesic sparing effects of dexmedetomidine in surgical intensive care patients. Qatar Med J. 2019;2019:58.
25. Girard TD, et al. Efficacy and safety of a paired sedation and ventilator weaning protocol for mechanically ventilated patients in intensive care (awakening and breathing controlled trial): a randomised controlled trial. Lancet. 2008;371:126–34.
26. Pham T, et al. Weaning from mechanical ventilation in intensive care units across 50 countries (WEAN SAFE): a multicentre, prospective, observational cohort study. Lancet Respir Med. 2023;11:465–76.
27. Kuhlen R, et al. Breathing pattern and workload during automatic tube compensation, pressure support and T-piece trials in weaning patients. Eur J Anaesthesiol. 2003;20:10–6.
28. Rose L, et al. Automated versus non-automated weaning for reducing the duration of mechanical ventilation for critically ill adults and children: a cochrane systematic review and meta-analysis. Crit Care. 2015;19:48.
29. Blackwood B, Burns KE, Cardwell CR, O'Halloran P. Protocolized versus non-protocolised weaning for reducing the duration of mechanical ventilation in critically ill adult patients. Cochrane Database Syst Rev. 2014;11:CD006904. https://doi.org/10.1002/14651858.CD006904.pub3.
30. Heunks LM, van der Hoeven JG. Clinical review: the ABC of weaning failure–a structured approach. Crit Care. 2010;14(6):245.
31. Routsi C, Stanopoulos I, Kokkoris S, et al. Weaning failure of cardiovascular origin: how to suspect, detect and treat—a literature review. Ann Intensive Care. 2019;9:6.

32. Carlucci A, Navalesi P. Weaning failure in critical illness. In: Webb A, et al., editors. Oxford textbook of critical care. 2nd ed. Oxford: Oxford Academic; 2016.
33. Fernandez MM, et al. Reconnection to mechanical ventilation for 1 h after a successful spontaneous breathing trial reduces reintubation in critically ill patients: a multicenter randomised controlled trial. Intensive Care Med. 2017;43:1660–7.
34. Salam A, Tilluckdharry L, Amoateng-Adjepong Y, Manthous CA. Neurologic status, cough, secretions and extubation outcomes. Intensive Care Med. 2004;30:1334–9.
35. Namen AM, et al. Predictors of successful extubation in neurosurgical patients. Am J Respir Crit Care Med. 2001;163:658–64.
36. Smina M, et al. Cough peak flows and extubation outcomes. Chest. 2003;124:262–8.
37. Khamiees M, Raju P, DeGirolamo A, Amoateng-Adjepong Y, Manthous CA. Predictors of extubation outcome in patients who have successfully completed a spontaneous breathing trial. Chest. 2001;120:1262–70.
38. Schnell D, et al. Cuff leak test for the diagnosis of post-extubation stridor: a multicenter evaluation study. J Intensive Care Med. 2017; https://doi.org/10.1177/0885066617700095.
39. Maury E, et al. How to identify patients with no risk for postextubation stridor? J Crit Care. 2004;19:23–8.
40. Sutherasan Y, Theerawit P, Hongphanut T, Kiatboonsri C, Kiatboonsri S. Predicting laryngeal edema in intubated patients by portable intensive care unit ultrasound. J Crit Care. 2013;28:675–80.
41. Shaikh N. Use of steroid for extubation failure due to stridor in surgical intensive care patients. Int J Crit Care Emerg Med. 2016;2:13.
42. François B, et al. 12-h pretreatment with methylprednisolone versus placebo for prevention of postextubation laryngeal oedema: a randomised double-blind trial. Lancet. 2007;369:1083–9.
43. Cheng K-C, Hou C-C, Huang H-C, Lin S-C, Zhang H. Intravenous injection of methylprednisolone reduces the incidence of postextubation stridor in intensive care unit patients. Crit Care Med. 2006;34:1345–50.
44. Krebs ED, et al. Is routine extubation overnight safe in cardiac surgery patients? J Thorac Cardiovasc Surg. 2019;157:1533–42.
45. Gershengorn HB, Scales DC, Kramer A, Wunsch H. Association between overnight extubations and outcomes in the intensive care unit. JAMA Intern Med. 2016;176:1651.
46. Casey JD, et al. Protocolised postextubation respiratory support to prevent reintubation: a randomised clinical trial. Am J Respir Crit Care Med. 2021;204:294–302.
47. Santos PAD, Ribas A, Quadros TCC, Blattner CN, Boniatti MM. Postextubation fluid balance is associated with extubation failure: a cohort study. Rev Bras Ter Intensiva. 2021;33(3):422–7.
48. Landais M, et al. Continued enteral nutrition until extubation compared with fasting before extubation in patients in the intensive care unit: an open-label, cluster-randomised, parallel-group, non-inferiority trial. Lancet Respir Med. 2023;11:319–28.
49. Krinsley JS, Barone JE. The drive to survive. Chest. 2005;128:560–6.
50. Mort TC. Continuous airway access for the difficult extubation: the efficacy of the airway exchange catheter. Anesth Analg. 2007;105:1357–62.
51. Peterson SJ, et al. Adequacy of oral intake in critically ill patients 1 week after extubation. J Am Diet Assoc. 2010;110:427–33.
52. Van Dessel ED, De Meyer GR, Morrison SG, Jorens PG, Schepens T. Flow-controlled ventilation in moderate acute respiratory distress syndrome due to COVID-19: an open-label repeated-measures controlled trial. Intensive Care Med Exp. 2022;10(1):19.
53. Roehrig S, Ait Hssain A, Shallik NAH, et al. Flow controlled ventilation in acute respiratory distress syndrome associated with COVID-19: a structured summary of a study protocol for a randomised controlled trial. Trials. 2020;21:781. https://doi.org/10.1186/s13063-020-04708-1.
54. Abram J, Martini J, Spraider P, Putzer G, Ranalter M, Wagner J, Glodny B, Hell T, Barnes T, Enk D. Individualised flow-controlled versus pressure-controlled ventilation in a porcine oleic acid-induced acute respiratory distress syndrome model. Eur J Anaesthesiol. 2023;40(7):511–20.

55. Bialka S, Palaczynski P, Szuldrzynski K, Wichary P, Kowalski D, van der Hoorn J, et al. Flow-controlled ventilation – a new and promising method of ventilation presented with a review of the literature. Anaesthesiol Intensive Ther. 2022;54(1):62–70. https://doi.org/10.5114/ait.2022.112889.
56. Shallik N, Elarref M, Khamash O, Abdelaal A, Radi Alkhafaji M, Makki H, Abusabeib A, Moustafa A, Menon A. Management of critical tracheal stenosis with a straw sized tube (Tritube): case report. Qatar Med J. 2021;3:48.
57. Meade M, et al. Predicting success in weaning from mechanical ventilation. Chest. 2001;120:400S–24S.
58. Nemer SN, et al. A new integrative weaning index of discontinuation from mechanical ventilation. Crit Care. 2009;13:R152.
59. Levy MM, Miyasaki A, Langston D. Work of breathing as a weaning parameter in mechanically ventilated patients. Chest. 1995;108:1018–20.

Index

N. A. Shallik (ed.), *Flow Controlled Ventilation Mode Through a Straw Size Tube*, https://doi.org/10.1007/978-3-031-77477-5

The manufacturer's authorised representative in the EU is Springer Nature Customer Service Centre GmbH, Europaplatz 3, 69115 Heidelberg, Germany. If you have any concerns regarding our products, please contact ProductSafety@springernature.com

Printed and bound by CPI Group (UK) Ltd, Croydon, CR0 4YY
30/09/2026
02225594-0001